PCCN Certification Review

Ann J. Brorsen, RN, MSN, CCRN, CEN
Menifee, California

Keri R. Rogelet, RN, MSN, MBA/HCM, CCRN
Menifee, California

JONES AND BARTLETT PUBLISHERS
Sudbury, Massachusetts
BOSTON   TORONTO   LONDON   SINGAPORE

World Headquarters
Jones and Bartlett Publishers
40 Tall Pine Drive
Sudbury, MA 01776
978-443-5000
info@jbpub.com
www.jbpub.com

Jones and Bartlett Publishers Canada
6339 Ormindale Way
Mississauga, Ontario L5V 1J2
Canada

Jones and Bartlett Publishers International
Barb House, Barb Mews
London W6 7PA
United Kingdom

Jones and Bartlett's books and products are available through most bookstores and online booksellers. To contact Jones and Bartlett Publishers directly, call 800-832-0034, fax 978-443-8000, or visit our website www.jbpub.com.

Substantial discounts on bulk quantities of Jones and Bartlett's publications are available to corporations, professional associations, and other qualified organizations. For details and specific discount information, contact the special sales department at Jones and Bartlett via the above contact information or send an email to specialsales@jbpub.com.

The authors, editor, and publisher have made every effort to provide accurate information. However, they are not responsible for errors, omissions, or for any outcomes related to the use of the contents of this book and take no responsibility for the use of the products and procedures described. Treatments and side effects described in this book may not be applicable to all people; likewise, some people may require a dose or experience a side effect that is not described herein. Drugs and medical devices are discussed that may have limited availability controlled by the Food and Drug Administration (FDA) for use only in a research study or clinical trial. Research, clinical practice, and government regulations often change the accepted standard in this field. When consideration is being given to use of any drug in the clinical setting, the health care provider or reader is responsible for determining FDA status of the drug, reading the package insert, and reviewing prescribing information for the most up-to-date recommendations on dose, precautions, and contraindications, and determining the appropriate usage for the product. This is especially important in the case of drugs that are new or seldom used.

Production Credits

Publisher: Kevin Sullivan
Acquisitions Editor: Emily Ekle
Acquisitions Editor: Amy Sibley
Associate Editor: Patricia Donnelly
Editorial Assistant: Rachel Shuster
Supervising Production Editor: Carolyn F. Rogers
Associate Production Editor: Katie Spiegel
Production Assistant: Lisa Cerrone
Senior Marketing Manager: Barb Bartoszek
Manufacturing and Inventory Control Supervisor: Amy Bacus
Composition: Arlene Apone
Cover Design: Brian Moore
Printing and Binding: Courier Stoughton
Cover Printing: Courier Stoughton

Library of Congress Cataloging-in-Publication Data
Brorsen, Ann J.
  PCCN certification review / Ann J. Brorsen & Keri R. Rogelet.
      p. ; cm.
  Includes bibliographical references.
  ISBN 978-0-7637-5935-3 (pbk.)
   1. Critical care nursing—Examinations—Study guides. I. Rogelet, Keri R. II. Title.
   [DNLM: 1. Critical Care—Examination Questions. 2. Critical Illness—nursing—Examination Questions. 3. Nursing Assessment—Examination Questions. WY 18.2 B873p 2009]
  RT120.I5B75 2009
  616.07'5076—dc22
                                                        2008029519
6048

Printed in the United States of America
13 12 11 10 09 10 9 8 7 6 5 4 3

Contents

About the Authors

Ann J. Brorsen, RN, MSN, CCRN, CEN

Ann is a nationally known speaker and has presented certification review courses for the Adult and Pediatric CCRN, PCCN, and CEN. Ann has worked as a staff nurse, manager, nurse executive, consultant, and entrepreneur. Ann's clinical practice includes trauma ED and ICU. Ann holds memberships in Sigma Theta Tau, the American Association of Critical-Care Nurses, the Emergency Nurses Association, the Society of Critical Care Medicine, and the National Nurses in Business Association. Ann is co-author of the *Adult CCRN Certification Review*. She is also the Chief Operating Officer and Director of Clinical Applications for Pro Ed in Menifee, California.

Keri R. Rogelet, RN, MSN, MBA/HCM, CCRN

Keri has presented national programs on adult health issues, the Neonatal CCRN, the Pediatric CCRN, and neonatal developmental care. Keri has worked in an adult cardiothoracic ICU and currently works as a team leader in a Level III NICU. Keri holds memberships in Sigma Theta Tau, the American Association of Critical-Care Nurses, the National Association of Neonatal Nurses, and the Academy of Neonatal Nursing. In addition, she works as a consultant for adult, pediatric, and neonatal product applications. Keri recently co-authored the *Adult CCRN Certification Review*, also published by Jones and Bartlett. She is currently the Chief Financial Officer and Director of Clinical Development for Pro Ed in Menifee, California.

Contact Information

Web site: www.forproed.com
Email: proedcertify@yahoo.com

Contributor

Melissa R. Christiansen, RN, MSN, NP-C, CCRN, CNRN

Melissa has more than 23 years of experience as a critical care nurse in neurological, cardiac, and trauma ICUs. She is currently working as a family nurse practitioner in Southern California. Melissa has presented programs on neurological-neuroscience topics, adult critical care certification reviews, and courses on post-anesthesia nursing. Melissa is a member of Sigma Theta Tau, the American Association of Critical-Care Nurses, the American Association of Neuroscience Nurses, and the American Academy of Nurse Practitioners. Melissa served as the regional Vice President of the California Association for Nurse Practitioners. Melissa is also on the faculty for the BSN and MSN programs at the University of Phoenix.

Acknowledgments

Mary Margaret Forsythe, RN, and Nancy O. Roberts, RN
Two instructors who were ultimate professionals
and passed before their time

⁌ • ⁍

This book is for all progressive care nurses. Thank you for caring,
working against seemingly insurmountable odds, long hours
and missed breaks, and your courage and professionalism
in being willing to get up every day and do it again.

Preface

Congratulations! Preparing for certification as a PCCN is a great step to take. Even if you plan to use this book simply as a study guide for progressive or critical care nursing, it will be an invaluable resource. This book introduces the PCCN credential, guides you through the process of registering for the PCCN exam, and offers some valuable test-taking strategies. We will even provide you with the resources and paperwork you need to complete the process.

This book contains test questions with answers and their rationales that cover a broad range of topics and are representative of the type of questions you will find on the actual PCCN examination. In addition, two written 125-question practice exams with answers and rationales appear at the end of the book. These exams are also available on the enclosed CD. The questions on the CD will be randomly selected and will enable you to time yourself and practice as if you were taking the actual examination.

We are dedicated to helping you successfully pass this exam and achieve certification as a PCCN. Please feel free to contact us if you have any questions or you would like to schedule a PCCN Review for your facility or group.

Ann and Keri

Introduction to the PCCN Credential

Traditionally, nurses have worked in a variety of roles and environments. When nurses graduated from their programs, they had spent many hours in multiple clinical situations and were prepared to practice in any area. Nursing eventually had to adjust from the general practitioner to a nurse who would concentrate practice in one area. Nurses worked in emergency rooms, operating rooms, recovery rooms, obstetrics, and medical surgical units. Those nurses who worked in operating rooms or who administered anesthesia, were considered specialized. With the advent of emerging technology, a post-war population boom, and increasingly more acute patients, nursing and hospitals adjusted by placing patients in more subspecialized areas.

In the early twentieth century, patients with poliomyelitis were increasing in numbers and special needs. The "iron lung" had been around for years. In the 1930s, the machine cost $1,500, which was also the median cost for a home at that time. Patients who could afford such treatment began to recover and developed sequelae that required specialized care. Tilt beds and hot pack treatments were initiated. At one time, even curare was used to combat the severe muscle spasms suffered by polio victims. All these treatments required time and resources, including larger numbers of nurses.

In 1931, the American Association of Nurse Anesthetist (no "s" on the end) was formed. On June 4, 1945, the organization held the first-ever certification examination for a nursing specialty. In 1952, the first accredited program for nurse anesthetists was started.

In 1955, Jonas Salk announced the discovery of a vaccine for polio. The vaccine would help prevent spread of the disease, but thousands of victims still required care. Technology in general was also improving and becoming more widely available. Although the first EKG machines were available in the United States as early as 1909, they were not widely used until the late 1950s.

In the 1960s, many patients required around-the-clock specialized care that required resources and practitioners who were experts or who had a great deal of experience with the particular condition or disease process. Veterans of previous wars and the escalating Vietnam War required increasingly more medical resources. Hospitals began placing cardiac, trauma, burn, and acute medical patients in areas of the hospital designated as providing more "intensive" care. As patient survival rates improved, the numbers of specialized areas increased.

In 1967, nurses from the Nashville Baptist Hospital became frustrated at the lack of educational opportunities for continuing education for intensive care nurses. In response, they sent inquiries to other nurses to see if interest existed in forming an association or some type of national association to provide education to other intensive care nurses. At the time, cardiac patients accounted for the majority of patients treated in intensive care units (ICUs). A year later, more than 400 nurses attended a symposium and affirmed the need for an organization. In 1969, the American Association of Cardiovascular Nurses was formed. In 1971, its name was changed to the American Association of Critical-Care Nurses (AACN) in recognition of the broad areas covered by critical care.

AACN is now the largest specialty nursing organization in the world. In 1975, the AACN Certification Corporation was established and began offering the CCRN examination. Nursing has continued to evolve and many patients who were relegated to an ICU or CCU are now being cared for in areas recognized as progressive care. To recognize the contributions and skills required in the progressive care setting, the PCCN certification was developed.

We invite you to visit the AACN Web site at (www.aacn.org) and learn more about the PCCN credential. We are here to help you become successful. The next section will explain the registration procedure for the PCCN examination. You have taken the first step, so keep going!

REFERENCES

http://www.aacn.org
(accessed February 19, 2008).

http://www.aacn.org/AACN/mrkt.nsf/vwdoc/HistoryofAACN?opendocument
(accessed February 19, 2008).

http://americanhistory.si.edu/polio/howpolio/index.htm
(accessed February 20, 2008).

http://www.anesthesia-nursing.com/wina.html
(accessed February 20, 2008).

The Synergy Model

The Synergy Model was originally developed to match clinical competency with patient needs and outcomes. The nurse and the care provided are driven by the needs of the patients and their families. Nurses begin practice as novices and, as they gain experience, may reach the expert level. The expert nurse is able to synthesize information, integrate that information, and then formulate a plan of care based on the patient's needs. A patient may have simple needs or very complex needs. Each patient also has characteristics that reflect their physical, emotional, cultural, family, financial, and social resources. The nurse must take all of the patient's characteristics into consideration.

The patient must be the focus of the care, and the patient's needs must come first. When the needs and characteristics of the patient are matched with the competencies of the nurse, synergy is the result. For example, it would not be in the best interest of a critically ill patient who requires multiple medications and hemodynamic monitoring to assign them to a new graduate who lacks the experience and knowledge to care for such a complex patient.

Synergy is applicable to education, the corporate world, small business, and anywhere the characteristics of the individual must be matched by the competencies of another entity. In nursing, we are looking for optimal outcomes for the patient and the nurse.

Until 1999, certification exams were based on clinical judgment. If you could memorize a lot of facts, you would probably be successful on the exam. Now, the PCCN certification examination consists of 80% of questions relying on clinical judgment; the other 20% focuses on "professional caring and ethical practice."

Without question, the Synergy Model can be confusing and intimidating. There are excellent resources available that can help you understand the model and its underlying concepts. At the end of this section is a list of those resources and we hope you will take the time to investigate each of them. There are two excellent books about the Synergy Model: *Critical Care Nursing: Synergy for Optimal Outcomes* by Roberta Kaplow, RN, PhD, CCRN, CCNS, and Sonya R. Hardin, RN, PhD, CCRN, and *Synergy for Clinical Excellence: The AACN Synergy Model for Patient Care* by Sonya R. Hardin, RN, PhD, CCRN and Roberta Kaplow, RN, PhD, CCRN, CCNS.

AACN has posted on its Web site the information about nurse and patient characteristics that follows. Recently, AACN expanded the information about the Synergy Model patient and nurse characteristics. We thank them for the information that appears in the tables on pages 2–7.

Remember, the PCCN exam does not test you on your knowledge of terminology, but rather on your ability to integrate these concepts into the care of patients.

PATIENT CHARACTERISTICS

Resiliency

The capacity to return to a restorative level of functioning using compensatory/coping mechanisms; the ability to bounce back quickly after an insult.

Level 1—Minimally resilient

Unable to mount a response; failure of compensatory/coping mechanisms; minimal reserves; brittle

Level 3—Moderately resilient

Able to mount a moderate response; able to initiate some degree of compensation; moderate reserves

Level 5—Highly resilient

Able to mount and maintain a response; intact compensatory/coping mechanisms; strong reserves; endurance

Vulnerability

Susceptibility to actual or potential stressors that may adversely affect patient outcomes.

Level 1—Highly vulnerable

Susceptible; unprotected, fragile

Level 3—Moderately vulnerable

Somewhat susceptible; somewhat protected

Level 5—Minimally vulnerable

Safe; out of the woods; protected, not fragile

Stability

The ability to maintain steady-state equilibrium.

Level 1—Minimally stable

Labile; unstable; unresponsive to therapies; high risk of death

Level 3—Moderately stable

Able to maintain steady state for limited period of time; some responsiveness to therapies

Level 5—Highly stable

Constant; responsive to therapies; low risk of death

Complexity

The intricate entanglement of two or more systems (e.g., body, family, therapies).

Level 1—Highly complex

Intricate; complex patient/family dynamics; ambiguous/vague; atypical presentation

Level 3—Moderately complex

Moderately involved patient/family dynamics

Level 5—Minimally complex

Straightforward; routine patient/family dynamics; simple/clear cut; typical presentation

Resource availability

Extent of resources (e.g., technical, fiscal, personal, psychological, and social) the patient/family/community bring to the situation.

Level 1—Few resources

Necessary knowledge and skills not available; necessary financial support not available; minimal personal/psychological supportive resources; few social systems resources

Level 3—Moderate resources

Limited knowledge and skills available; limited financial support available; limited personal/psychological supportive resources; limited social systems resources

Level 5—Many resources

Extensive knowledge and skills available and accessible; financial resources readily available; strong personal/psychological supportive resources; strong social systems resources

PATIENT CHARACTERISTICS (CONTINUED)

Participation in care	**Extent to which patient/family engages in aspects of care.**
Level 1—No participation	Patient and family unable or unwilling to participate in care
Level 3—Moderate level of participation	Patient and family need assistance in care
Level 5—Full participation	Patient and family fully able to participate in care
Participation in decision-making	**Extent to which patient/family engages in decision-making.**
Level 1—No participation	Patient and family have no capacity for decision-making; requires surrogacy
Level 3—Moderate level of participation	Patient and family have limited capacity; seeks input/advice from others in decision-making
Level 5—Full participation	Patient and family have capacity, and makes decision for self
Predictability	**A characteristic that allows one to expect a certain course of events or course of illness.**
Level 1—Not predictable	Uncertain; uncommon patient population/illness; unusual or unexpected course; does not follow critical pathway, or no critical pathway developed
Level 3—Moderately predictable	Wavering; occasionally-noted patient population/illness
Level 5—Highly predictable	Certain; common patient population/illness; usual and expected course; follows critical pathway

Source: American Association of Critical-Care Nurses. (n.d.) *The AACN Synergy Model for patient care.* Available at: http://www.aacn.org/WD/Certifications/content/synmodel.content. Used with permission.

NURSE COMPETENCIES

Clinical judgment	**Clinical reasoning, which includes clinical decision-making, critical thinking, and a global grasp of the situation, coupled with nursing skills acquired through a process of integrating formal and informal experiential knowledge and evidence-based guidelines.**
Level 1	Collects basic-level data; follows algorithms, decision trees, and protocols with all populations and is uncomfortable deviating from them; matches formal knowledge with clinical events to make decisions; questions the limits of one's ability to make clinical decisions and delegates the decision-making to other clinicians; includes extraneous detail

NURSE COMPETENCIES (CONTINUED)

Level 3	Collects and interprets complex patient data; makes clinical judgments based on an immediate grasp of the whole picture for common or routine patient populations; recognizes patterns and trends that may predict the direction of illness; recognizes limits and seeks appropriate help; focuses on key elements of case, while shorting out extraneous details
Level 5	Synthesizes and interprets multiple, sometimes conflicting, sources of data; makes judgment based on an immediate grasp of the whole picture, unless working with new patient populations; uses past experiences to anticipate problems; helps patient and family see the "big picture"; recognizes the limits of clinical judgment and seeks multidisciplinary collaboration and consultation with comfort; recognizes and responds to the dynamic situation
Advocacy and moral agency	**Working on another's behalf and representing the concerns of the patient/family and nursing staff; serving as a moral agent in identifying and helping to resolve ethical and clinical concerns within and outside the clinical setting.**
Level 1	Works on behalf of patient; self assesses personal values; aware of ethical conflicts/issues that may surface in clinical setting; makes ethical/moral decisions based on rules; represents patient when patient cannot represent self; aware of patients' rights
Level 3	Works on behalf of patient and family; considers patient values and incorporates in care, even when differing from personal values; supports colleagues in ethical and clinical issues; moral decision-making can deviate from rules; demonstrates give and take with patient's family, allowing them to speak/represent themselves when possible; aware of patient and family rights
Level 5	Works on behalf of patient, family, and community; advocates from patient/family perspective, whether similar to or different from personal values; advocates ethical conflict and issues from patient/family perspective; suspends rules—patient and family drive moral decision-making; empowers the patient and family to speak for/represent themselves; achieves mutuality within patient/professional relationships
Caring practices	**Nursing activities that create a compassionate, supportive, and therapeutic environment for patients and staff, with the aim of promoting comfort and healing and preventing unnecessary suffering. Includes, but is not limited to, vigilance, engagement, and responsiveness of caregivers, including family and healthcare personnel.**

NURSE COMPETENCIES (CONTINUED)

Level 1	Focuses on the usual and customary needs of the patient; no anticipation of future needs; bases care on standards and protocols; maintains a safe physical environment; acknowledges death as a potential outcome
Level 3	Responds to subtle patient and family changes; engages with the patient as a unique patient in a compassionate manner; recognizes and tailors caring practices to the individuality of patient and family; domesticates the patient's and family's environment; recognizes that death may be an acceptable outcome
Level 5	Has astute awareness and anticipates patient and family changes and needs; fully engaged with and sensing how to stand alongside the patient, family, and community; caring practices follow the patient and family lead; anticipates hazards and avoids them, and promotes safety throughout patient's and family's transitions along the healthcare continuum; orchestrates the process that ensures patient's/family's comfort and concerns surrounding issues of death and dying are met
Collaboration	**Working with others (e.g., patients, families, healthcare providers) in a way that promotes/encourages each person's contributions toward achieving optimal/realistic patient/family goals. Involves intra- and interdisciplinary work with colleagues and community.**
Level 1	Willing to be taught, coached and/or mentored; participates in team meetings and discussions regarding patient care and/or practice issues; open to various team members' contributions
Level 3	Seeks opportunities to be taught, coached, and/or mentored; elicits others' advice and perspectives; initiates and participates in team meetings and discussions regarding patient care and/or practice issues; recognizes and suggests various team members' participation
Level 5	Seeks opportunities to teach, coach, and mentor and to be taught, coached, and mentored; facilitates active involvement and complementary contributions of others in team meetings and discussions regarding patient care and/or practice issues; involves/recruits diverse resources when appropriate to optimize patient outcomes
Systems thinking	**Body of knowledge and tools that allow the nurse to manage whatever environmental and system resources exist for the patient/family and staff, within or across healthcare and non-healthcare systems.**
Level 1	Uses a limited array of strategies; limited outlook—sees the pieces or components; does not recognize negotiation as an alternative; sees patient and family within the isolated environment of the unit; sees self as key resource

NURSE COMPETENCIES (CONTINUED)

Level 3	Develops strategies based on needs and strengths of patient/family; able to make connections within components; sees opportunity to negotiate but may not have strategies; developing a view of the patient/family transition process; recognizes how to obtain resources beyond self
Level 5	Develops, integrates, and applies a variety of strategies that are driven by the needs and strengths of the patient/family; global or holistic outlook—sees the whole rather than the pieces; knows when and how to negotiate and navigate through the system on behalf of patients and families; anticipates needs of patients and families as they move through the healthcare system; utilizes untapped and alternative resources as necessary
Response to diversity	**The sensitivity to recognize, appreciate, and incorporate differences into the provision of care. Differences may include, but are not limited to, cultural differences, spiritual beliefs, gender, race, ethnicity, lifestyle, socioeconomic status, age, and values.**
Level 1	Assesses cultural diversity; provides care based on own belief system; learns the culture of the healthcare environment
Level 3	Inquires about cultural differences and considers their impact on care; accommodates personal and professional differences in the plan of care; helps patient/family understand the culture of the healthcare system
Level 5	Responds to, anticipates, and integrates cultural differences into patient/family care; appreciates and incorporates differences, including alternative therapies, into care; tailors healthcare culture, to the extent possible, to meet the diverse needs and strengths of the patient/family
Facilitation of learning	**The ability to facilitate learning for patients/families, nursing staff, other members of the healthcare team, and community. Includes both formal and informal facilitation of learning.**
Level 1	Follows planned educational programs; sees patient/family education as a separate task from delivery of care; provides data without seeking to assess patient's readiness or understanding; has limited knowledge of the totality of the educational needs; focuses on a nurse's perspective; sees the patient as a passive recipient
Level 3	Adapts planned educational programs; begins to recognize and integrate different ways of teaching into delivery of care; incorporates patient's understanding into practice; sees the overlapping of educational plans from different healthcare providers' perspectives; begins to see the patient as having input into goals; begins to see individualism

NURSE COMPETENCIES (CONTINUED)

Level 5	Creatively modifies or develops patient/family education programs; integrates patient/family education throughout delivery of care; evaluates patient's understanding by observing behavior changes related to learning; is able to collaborate and incorporate all healthcare providers' and educational plans into the patient/family educational program; sets patient-driven goals for education; sees patient/family as having choices and consequences that are negotiated in relation to education
Clinical inquiry (innovator/evaluator)	**The ongoing process of questioning and evaluating practice and providing informed practice. Creating practice changes through research utilization and experiential learning.**
Level 1	Follows standards and guidelines; implements clinical changes and research-based practices developed by others; recognizes the need for further learning to improve patient care; recognizes obvious changing patient situation (e.g., deterioration, crisis); needs and seeks help to identify patient problem
Level 3	Questions appropriateness of policies and guidelines; questions current practice; seeks advice, resources, or information to improve patient care; begins to compare and contrast possible alternatives
Level 5	Improves, deviates from, or individualizes standards and guidelines for particular patient situations or populations; questions and/or evaluates current practice based on patients' responses, review of the literature, research and education/learning; acquires knowledge and skills needed to address questions arising in practice and improve patient care (The domains of clinical judgment and clinical inquiry converge at the expert level; they cannot be separated)

Source: American Association of Critical-Care Nurses. (n.d.) *The AACN Synergy Model for patient care.* Available at: http://www.aacn.org/WD/Certifications/content/synmodel.content. Used with permission.

REFERENCES

American Association of Critical-Care Nurses. (2008). *General information regarding certification.* Retrieved July 29, 2008, from http://www.aacn.org/WD/Certifications/Content/basiccertinfo.pcms

Becker, D., Kaplow, R., Muenzen, P. M., & Hartigan, C. (2006). Activities performed by acute and critical care advanced practice nurses: American Association of Critical-Care Nurses study of practice. *American Journal of Critical Care, 15*(2), 130–148.

Brewer, B. B., Wojner-Alexandrov, A. W., Triola, N., Pacini, C., Cline, M., Rust, J. E., et al. (2007). AACN Synergy Model's characteristics of patients: Psychometric analyses in a tertiary care health system. *American Journal of Critical Care, 16*(2), 158–167.

Burns, S. M. (Ed.). (2007). *American Association of Critical-Care Nurses (AACN): AACN protocols for practice: Healing environments* (2nd ed.). Sudbury, MA: Jones and Bartlett.

Cline, M., Nottingham, M., & Lockhart, J. S. (2006). Synergy for clinical excellence: The AACN Synergy Model for Patient Care. *Critical Care Nurse, 26*(2), 139–140.

Copstead, L., & Banasik, J. L. (2000). *Pathophysiology: Biological and behavioral perspectives* (2nd ed.). Philadelphia: W. B. Saunders/Elsevier.

Curley, M. A. Q. (1998). Patient–nurse synergy: Optimizing patients' outcomes. *American Journal of Critical Care, 7,* 64–72.

Dossey, B. M., Keegan, L., & Guzzetta, C. (2003). *Holistic nursing: A handbook for practice* (3rd ed.). Sudbury, MA: Jones and Bartlett.

Edwards, D. F. (1999). The Synergy Model: Linking patient needs to nurse competencies. *Critical Care Nurse, 19*(1), 88–98.

Hardin, S. R., & Kaplow, R. (Eds.). (2004). *Synergy for clinical excellence: The AACN Synergy Model for Patient Care.* Sudbury, MA: Jones and Bartlett.

Kaplow, R. (2004). Applying the Synergy Model to nursing education. *Critical Care Nurse: AACN Critical Care Careers, 20,* 22, 24–26.

Kelleher, S. (2006). Providing patient-centered care in an intensive care unit. *Nursing Standard, 21*(13), 35–40.

Lipson, J. G., Dibble, S. L., & Minarik, P. A. (Eds.). (1996). *Culture and nursing care: A pocket guide.* San Francisco, CA: UCSF Nursing Press.

McQuillan, K. A., Von Rueden, K. T., Hartsock, R. L., Flynn, M. B., & Whalen, E. (Eds.). (2002). *Trauma nursing: From resuscitation through rehabilitation* (3rd ed.). Philadelphia: W. B. Saunders/Elsevier.

Smith, A. R. (2006). Using the Synergy Model to provide spiritual nursing care in critical care settings. *Critical Care Nurse, 26*(4), 41–47.

Registering for the PCCN Examination

The first thing to do is determine if you are eligible for the exam. You must not have any encumbrances on your current registered nurse license in any state. That means that there can be no restrictions, disciplinary actions, attached conditions, or provisions of any kind that would affect your ability to practice as a nurse. You need to have completed 1,750 hours of direct bedside care for a progressive care patient population during the past two years. All your practice hours for the exam must have been spent caring for progressive care patients. In other words, you cannot split the hours between, say, a pediatric ICU and a progressive care unit.

Of the 1,750 hours of direct bedside care, 875 hours must have been completed in the past year. If you are an educator, a CNS, or a manager, you can still qualify for the PCCN exam. If you directly supervise students or nurses at the bedside, you will qualify. You must, however, participate in the care of the patient. For example, if you demonstrate a procedure or supervise a nurse or student performing the procedure, that activity would be acceptable.

You should have a certain level of experience before you take the PCCN exam. Many of the questions on the exam require integration of knowledge and critical thinking. A few questions test your familiarity with technology. Although having experience with this technology might make some questions easier to understand, not every progressive care area utilizes these therapies.

The exam is broad based, so we tried to include representative questions in all appropriate areas. The relevant concepts can be learned from reading appropriate texts or by learning from another nurse with experience in the particular area. Nursing is a mobile profession, and quite often the person you work with may have experiences and qualifications unknown to you. For example, some nurses have the opportunity to work via registries or as travelers and have a wide base of experience. Other nurses seek out new experiences within their own facility or work part-time in other facilities. We are not trying to scare you—thousands of nurses have passed this exam, and it is certainly possible for you to be equally successful.

Candidates for the PCCN come from a variety of critical care settings: ICU, telemetry, DOU, oncology units, catheterization labs, PACU, step-down units, emergency rooms, and progressive care units. Critical care patients are found in all these areas. To see what the PCCN exam covers, you can download a copy of the PCCN Test Plan from our Web site at www.forproed.com. Just click on the PCCN tab, then on the link to download the current Test Plan. The Test Plan is an outline, or blueprint, of the major areas to be tested. The Test Plan also indicates the percentage of questions tested in each particular section or system. Specific conditions and pathophysiologies are listed on the Test Plan, allowing you to focus your study time and resources. If you would like us to send you an application and current PCCN Test Plan, please email us your name and address (please do not forget your ZIP code!).

When you sign up for the PCCN exam, you can sign up as either a member or a nonmember of AACN. The cost is lower if you are a member, and you can join AACN at the time you register to receive the member discount.

After your documents are received by AACN, you must allow for several weeks for their processing. You will then be sent a postcard stating the date from which you will have 90 days to complete the exam.

You will be provided with a list of examination locations near you, based on your ZIP code. The PCCN test is administered at Applied Measurement Professional (AMP) sites around the United States. The sites provided to you by AACN are suggestions—you may take the exam at any of the AMP locations.

Your next step is to call the AMP testing center you select and make an appointment for the exam. The testing center will authorize the time and day for you. Please visit the AACN Web site or the AMP Web site for updated information, as specific rules about changing appointments apply and you must have the current information.

In addition to the computer-based testing provided at the AMP sites, you may take the PCCN exam the old-fashioned way, using pencil and paper. These written exams are given only a few times each year, and require special registrations and arrangements. Please contact AACN directly if you wish to test in this manner.

Remember, other nurses have passed this examination and you can too!

Test-Taking Strategies

When preparing for the PCCN examination, the first thing to do is be absolutely honest with yourself about how you study. If you have good study habits and plenty of time, you are very fortunate. If you are a procrastinator, studying a little at a time might help. Nurses have to juggle many roles, all of which place demands on their time: parent, child, employee, student, teacher, and on and on. One of the biggest struggles is simply finding time and a place to study. Discovering your learning style will help you find a better way to absorb information.

Three types of learners are commonly identified: visual, auditory, and kinesthetic. There is no perfect strategy for learning that applies to everyone, because we are all unique. Not everyone prefers a single style of learning—you may use a mixture of several different styles.

Visual learners learn better from reading and writing than from hearing and talking about information. Background noise, such as music and television, is distracting to these kinds of learners. Unfortunately, finding a quiet space for study is a problem for some people. You may have to stay awake after family members have gone to bed. With visual learners, flashcards often work to facilitate learning and some people use colored markers to highlight important information.

Auditory learners learn information effectively by listening and talking. Playing music, listening to audiotapes, and being part of a study group are often helpful strategies for these learners.

Kinesthetic learners prefer to learn in a "hands-on" manner. Nurses often learn this way—for example, they may listen to lectures and then demonstrate skills. This learning approach may utilize models, manikins, or patients. Kinesthetic learners are often "antsy" and cannot sit still for long periods of time, so lectures may be difficult for them to tolerate without frequent breaks. Tactics that might help these learners while studying include taking frequent breaks, walking around, or riding a stationary bicycle.

No matter what your personal learning style, you can always improve your test-taking skills. How? Practice! That is why we wrote this book in a question-and-answer format. Keep practicing the questions until you can answer at least 80% correctly. Research has shown that two-thirds of study time should be spent taking sample tests, and only one-third of the time should be spent reviewing content.

Studying, like regular exercise, is good for the brain. As nurses, we must always keep abreast of the professional literature and spend time studying. Many states require nurses to complete continuing education courses to renew a professional license. Anything worthwhile takes time, effort, and sacrifice. There is no way around studying for the PCCN certification. There are no shortcuts!

If you have been out of school for a while, don't despair! You may find the process slow going at first, so take things a little at a time. Just like going to the gym regularly, you should make a plan to study in one particular place and at the same time if possible. This is your space and your time—claim it! Keep all of your books, tapes and other study materials handy. If you need snack food, make sure it is not all sugar; include some salty food. Caffeine tends to make people jittery, but if you need it, it may be right for you.

The PCCN Test Plan is a blueprint for exam content. The major sections are broken down into subheadings and topics. If you study only a little at a time, you will be fine. One day you may feel like studying cardiomyopathy, the next day, you may focus on chest tubes. You can download the current PCCN Test Plan from our Web site (www.forproed.com). We did not include a Test Plan in this book because the exam changes frequently, so it is best that you have a copy of the current plan.

If you study with a group, you can save a lot of time and effort by breaking up the topics for that study period, with each person then presenting a different topic. Each group member can provide handouts and practice questions for the rest of the group. When you can make up a test question about a subject, you really will be prepared. Study for short periods of time, say 30 to 45 minutes, and then take a break. Set small goals and, after you have accomplished each one, reward yourself!

EXAM CONTENT

The PCCN certification exam consists of 125 multiple-choice test questions. Twenty-five of those questions do not count—they are there to be validated. In other words, the question is tried out to see if it is written well and if a certain percentage of people answer the question correctly. At this point in the process, the question can still be "tweaked" for use in future exams.

Your test results will be determined by how many answers you get correct. Some answers are a bit harder than others. The final score usually indicates a pass if you get at least 70% correct. If you do not know an answer, take your best guess, because you have at least a 25% chance of guessing correctly. You get points only for questions answered.

The Test Plan shows the breakdown of the PCCN certification examination by topic and section. AACN uses the Synergy Model as a basis for practice. A brief overview of the Synergy Model appears in Section 1 of this book. Here is the good news: The PCCN exam does not include any questions that deal specifically with the Synergy Model. Instead, the answers for questions reflect best practices that utilize and synthesize the concepts included in the Synergy Model.

STUDY TIPS

A multiple-choice test question consists of three parts: an *introductory statement,* a *stem* (question), and *options* from which you must select the correct answer.

The introductory statement provides information about a clinical issue, pathophysiology, or a nursing action or duty.

Stems are worded in different ways. Some stems are in the form of a question; others take the form of an incomplete statement. Additionally, a stem will usually request one of two types of responses: a *positive response* or a *negative response.* Good news: The PCCN exam no longer includes negative stem questions! That means questions with phrases such as "all of the following except" are not part of the exam. More good news: There are no longer any multiple-multiple-choice questions on the exam! The questions you will practice from in this book may occasionally include a negative stem question to facilitate learning.

Key words are important words or phrases that help focus your attention on what the question is specifically asking. Examples of key words include *always, most, first response, earliest, priority, first, on admission, common, best, least, not, immediately,* and *initial.*

You should always be looking for a *therapeutic response.* The nurse is *always* therapeutic. Your initial response is *always* the therapeutic response—you must acknowledge and validate the patient's feelings. Communication skills learned in Nursing 101 are important components of successful test-taking strategies. More than one option may contain a therapeutic response. When in doubt, validate, validate, validate. Always validate the individual's feelings before you present information. A medical emergency would, of course, take precedence.

Who is actually the focus of the question? You need to be able to identify the person who is the focus of the question. Sometimes questions deal with a friend, relative, or significant other instead of the patient. In fact, a lot of information in the question may be deliberately distracting. Also, you must, when applicable, validate that person's feelings first.

WHEN IN DOUBT

When considering your response, think first about Maslow's hierarchy of needs and the ABCs of airway, breathing, and circulation. When these goals are met, then safety is the priority. After safety, psychological needs are a priority. Assessment always comes before diagnosis and treatment (intervention). Learning takes place only if the patient is motivated.

Eliminate incorrect options. This step gives you a 50/50 chance of guessing the correct answer. Here are some other hints:

- Select the most general, all-encompassing option.
- Eliminate similar options or those that contain words such as "always" or "never." If two options say essentially the same thing, neither is correct. If three of the four options sound similar, choose the one that sounds unusual.
- Look for the longest option. It is usually the correct answer.
- Watch for grammatical inconsistencies between the stem and the options.

IT'S TIME FOR THE PCCN EXAM!

Well, you are finally ready!

The night before the exam, get a good night's sleep. Do not cram the night before, although that is easier said than done. Do something relaxing and enjoyable such as going to a movie or out to dinner. Try to avoid caffeine or any other stimulant.

Take the exam and pass it!

Send us an email to let us celebrate, too!

REFERENCES

Kobel Lamonte, M. (2007). Test-taking strategies for CNOR certification. *AORN Journal, 85*(2), 315–332.

Ludwig, C. (2004). Preparing for certification: Test-taking strategies. *Medsurg Nursing, 13*(2), 127–128.

Section 4

Cardiovascular

QUESTIONS

1. Calculate the cardiac output for a patient with a heart rate of 70 and a stroke volume of 65 mL.

   A. 0.85%

   B. 4.6 L/min

   C. 1.07 mL/min

   D. 3,800 cc/min

   (handwritten: CO = HR × SV   70 × 0.65)

2. What percentage of the cardiac cycle is provided by the atrial kick?

   A. 15%

   B. 20%

   C. 30%

   D. 35%

3. A normal value for an ejection fraction (EF) would be

   A. 65%.

   B. 40%.

   C. 30%.

   D. 25%.

4. Lee, a 67-year-old retiree, is being admitted to your unit for chest pain after collapsing at home. He is arguing with his wife that he should not be admitted because he just "overdid it" while working in the yard. Lee's wife states to you that his chest pain is more frequent, severe, and prolonged than before. You anticipate which diagnosis?

   A. Exertional angina

   B. Unstable angina

   C. Variant angina

   D. Stable angina

5. Stroke volume is comprised of which of the following factors?

   A. Blood volume, viscosity, and impedance

   B. Cardiac output, heart rate, and compliance

   C. Contractility, preload, and afterload

   D. Compliance, impedance, and heart rate

6. A reflex tachycardia caused by stretch of the right atrial receptors is known as the
   A. Herring–Sines law.
   B. Renin–angiotensin system.
   C. Starling's law.
   D. Bainbridge reflex.

7. Diastole comprises what percentage of the cardiac cycle?
   A. Half
   B. Two-thirds
   C. One-fourth
   D. One-third

8. What is the mean arterial pressure (MAP) for a patient with a blood pressure of 120/70 and a heart rate of 80?
   A. 87
   B. 2.4
   C. 50
   D. 85

$$\frac{2(70)+120}{3}$$

9. Your patient has the following parameters:
   HR 80
   BP 110/70
   SV 60
   BSA 2.0 m²

   Use the space provided to calculate the cardiac index (CI) for this patient.
   A. 4.8 L/min
   B. 55 L/min/m²
   C. 2.4 L/min/m²
   D. 30 mL/m²

$$CO = HR \times SV$$

$$\frac{CO}{BSA}$$

10. The resistance against which the right ventricle must work to eject its volume is known as
    A. Resting heart pressure.
    B. Systemic vascular resistance.
    C. Central venous pressure.
    D. Pulmonary vascular resistance.

11. Mr. Ironclaw lives on a nearby Indian reservation. He is retired and on a fixed income without insurance. He is being discharged today after an overnight observational stay for chest pain. In planning his discharge care, which of the following should be considered first to increase compliance with his plan of care once he is home?
    A. Arrange for home nursing visits every day for 1 week
    B. Ask the physician to consider an over-the-counter antiplatelet medication
    C. Schedule his follow-up appointment with the cardiologist in 3 months
    D. Suggest a gym membership to begin exercising

12. **William was diagnosed with unstable angina. He is scheduled for an exercise stress test. He tells you that he has a "bad hip" and an old knee injury that make it difficult for him to walk or stand for more than 20 minutes. You tell him:**
    A. "You only need to walk for 10 minutes."
    B. "You can ride a bike for 20 minutes instead."
    C. "I will call the physician and ask for the Weight-lift test."
    D. "I will call the physician and ask for a stress echocardiography test."

13. **Approximately what percentage of coronary artery blockage is needed to cause angina?**
    A. 45%
    B. 60%
    C. 75%
    D. 90%

14. **A heart murmur associated with acute valvular regurgitation would be**
    A. S_3.
    B. S_2.
    C. S_1.
    D. S_4. compliance/regurg

15. **Which of the following leads is best for monitoring for a RBBB?**
    A. Lead II
    B. Lead I
    C. Lead V_1
    D. Lead V_6

16. **Tall, peaked T waves on an EKG may be indicative of**
    A. Hypocalcemia.
    B. A non-STEMI MI.
    C. Hyperkalemia.
    D. A LBBB.

17. **Ethyl P. suffered a cardiac arrest at home. The family did not perform CPR, and the paramedics arrived six minutes after the arrest. The patient was found in pulseless V-tach. Defibrillation was performed, and continuous CPR was provided during transport to the ED. The patient was transferred to the telemetry unit because of a bed shortage in the ICU. The physician initiated hypothermic measures and administered vecuronium. This medication was used to**
    A. Control ventricular dysrhythmias.
    B. Prevent shivering.
    C. Act as a sedative.
    D. Relieve pain.

paralytic to prevent shivering

18. **Your patient was admitted for malaise, severe dyspnea and he had a syncopal episode at work. The patient states he has a midline burning sensation in his chest that worsens when he is supine. You suspect**
    A. A pleural effusion.
    B. Pericardial tamponade.
    C. GERD.
    D. Myocarditis.

19. **A definitive diagnosis of myocarditis can be made via**
    A. An endomyocardial biopsy. *The only definitive way*
    B. Transesophageal ultrasound.
    C. Transmural catheterization.
    D. Chest X-ray.

20. **The volume of fluid required to cause a pericardial tamponade is**
    A. 25–50 mL.
    B. 50–75 mL. *could = or > diastolic pressures = tamponade*
    C. 100–150 mL.
    D. 200–300 mL.

21. **Beck's triad is a combination of symptoms useful in diagnosing tamponade. These symptoms include**
    A. Pericardial friction rub, hypertension, and RV failure.
    B. Increased pulse pressure, increased JVD, and tachycardia.
    C. Tachycardia, hypertension, and LV failure.
    D. Distended neck veins, muffled heart sounds, and hypotension.

22. **Which of the following hemodynamic changes will occur with cardiac tamponade?**
    A. Increased cardiac output
    B. Stroke volume decreases
    C. Contractility increases
    D. Decreased heart rate

23. **If your patient had a cardiac tamponade, which of the following findings would you expect on a chest X-ray?**
    A. A dilated superior vena cava
    B. Increased JVD
    C. Narrowed mediastinum
    D. Delineation of the pericardium and epicardium

24. **Your patient was admitted for severe dyspnea, dysphagia, palpitations, and an intractable cough. On auscultation, you hear a loud S$_1$ and a right-sided S$_3$ and S$_4$. The patient probably has** *= fluid problem + pressure problem*
    A. Mitral insufficiency.
    B. Myocarditis.
    C. Atrial stenosis.
    D. Mitral stenosis.

25. **Quincke's sign is usually seen in which of the following conditions?**
    A. Mitral stenosis
    B. Endocarditis
    C. Aortic insufficiency *incompetent valve*   *pulsation in nail bed*
    D. Pericarditis

26. **In patients with aortic insufficiency, the popliteal BP is often higher than the brachial BP by at least 40 mm Hg. This discrepancy between the measurements is known as**
    A. DeMusset's sign.
    B. Hill's sign.
    C. Holmes' sign.
    D. Rochelle's sign.

27. **In stable angina, which of the following statements is true?**
    A. A positive treadmill test will indicate CAD.
    B. A thallium test will not diagnose LV dysfunction.
    C. The treadmill test will miss as many as 20% of cases of single-vessel disease.
    D. CK-MB isoenzymes and troponins will not increase.

28. **Actions of beta blockers include**
    A. Increased myocardial oxygen demand.
    B. Increased heart rate.
    C. Increased diastolic filling time.
    D. Increased afterload.

29. **If the inferior wall of the heart is infarcted, the leads that will most directly reflect the injury are**
    A. II, II, and aVF.
    B. I, aVL.
    C. V_1–V_2. *septal wall*
    D. V_5–V_6.

30. **An anterior wall infarction may be seen in leads**
    A. V_4, R. *–R ventricular damage*
    B. V_5–V_6. *–apical injury*
    C. V_7–V_9. *–posterior wall*
    D. V_2–V_4.

31. **Pulsus alternans is most often noted with**
    A. Mitral stenosis.
    B. Constrictive pericarditis.
    C. Aortic stenosis.
    D. LV failure.

    weak myocardium can't maintain = pressure c̄ each contraction

32. **Which of the heart valves is most commonly affected by infective endocarditis?**
    A. Aortic
    B. Pulmonic
    C. Mitral
    D. Tricuspid

33. **Alpha-adrenergic effects of norepinephrine include**
    A. Increased force of myocardial contraction.
    B. Increased SA node firing.
    C. Increased AV conduction time.
    D. Peripheral arteriolar vasoconstriction.

    [handwritten: α = C]

34. **Stimulation of the vasomotor center in the medulla occurs when the partial pressure of oxygen changes. This sequence is initiated by**
    A. Baroreceptors. *[handwritten: = pressure Δs]*
    B. Chemoreceptors.
    C. The Purkinje system.
    D. The Bainbridge reflex.

35. **When attempting to auscultate the aortic area, the location of the stethoscope should be**
    A. At the second intercostal space, left sternal border. *[handwritten: pulmonic]*
    B. Over the apical area. *[handwritten: mitral valve]*
    C. At the second intercostal space, right sternal border.
    D. At the fifth intercostal space, left sternal border. *[handwritten: tricuspid]*

36. **When preparing to teach your 30-year-old female patient about goals for weight control, the BMI should be assessed. The BMI should be between**
    A. 12.6 and 15.0.
    B. 11.2 and 15.8.
    C. 18.0 and 24.9.
    D. 28.6 and 24.7.

37. **Symptoms of right-sided heart failure include**
    A. Pulmonary edema.
    B. Elevated pulmonary pressures. *[handwritten: } (L) sided]*
    C. Hepatomegaly.
    D. Orthopnea.

38. **NSAIDs are contraindicated in the treatment of patients with heart failure because they**
    A. Decrease myocardial contractility.
    B. Cause atrial fibrillation in patients with heart failure.
    C. Promote fluid retention. *[handwritten: -can contribute to renal insuff.]*
    D. May cause hypocalcemia.

39. **Joe underwent CABG surgery 4 days ago and was transferred to your care yesterday. Today he complains of dull aching around the sternum. You note increased tenderness to touch along the sternal edge and contracted intercostal muscles. You should**
    A. Contact the physician for an order for a 12-lead EKG, cardiac enzymes, and morphine.
    B. Culture-swab the wound for bacterial infection.
    C. Do nothing; his pain is normal.
    D. Administer morphine and diazepam as ordered.

40. You are using the PQRST method of pain assessment for your patient complaining of chest pain. The S in this mnemonic stands for
    A. Sensitivity.
    B. Severity.
    C. Standard.
    D. Symptoms.

    P provokes
    Q quality
    R radiation
    S severity
    T time/duration

41. An <u>absolute</u> contraindication for use of a fibrinolytic would be
    A. Traumatic CPR.
    B. Cerebrovascular disease. *i ∈ hemorrhagic*
    C. Subacute bacterial endocarditis. *i ∈ ··*
    D. Oral anticoagulants. *i ∈ ···*

42. Which of the following statements is true about lidocaine?
    A. Lidocaine causes hypotension.
    B. Lidocaine has a moderate gastrointestinal intolerance.
    C. Lidocaine has no impairment of normal contractility.
    D. Lidocaine can cause nystagmus.

43. Which drug listed below has a high iodine content?
    A. Flecanide
    B. Lidocaine
    C. Mexilitene
    D. Amiodarone

44. The drug of choice to treat AV nodal and atrioventricular re-entrant arrhythmias is
    A. Amiodarone.
    B. Clonidine.
    C. Quinidine.
    D. Adenosine.

45. Sometimes certain medications prolong the QT interval, potentially causing polymorphic ventricular tachycardia. The drug of choice to treat this rhythm is
    A. Magnesium. — *high doses, can slow AV conduction*
    B. Calcium.
    C. Digoxin.
    D. Lidocaine.

46. Calcium-channel blockers act primarily on
    A. Reduction of cardiac output.
    B. Arteries to arterioles.
    C. Lung receptors only.
    D. Venules to veins.

47. The fourth heart sound (S$_4$) is   — *"atrial gallop"*
    A. Heard as the mitral valve opens.
    B. A low-pitched murmur.
    C. Heard during atrial contraction.
    D. Produced in congestive heart failure.

48. **An example of a systolic murmur would be**
    A. Tricuspid stenosis.
    B. Tricuspid insufficiency.
    C. Mitral stenosis.
    D. Pulmonic insufficiency.

49. **An example of a pansystolic murmur is**
    A. Pulmonic insufficiency.
    B. Tricuspid insufficiency.
    C. Atrial stenosis.
    D. Mitral stenosis.

    diastolic murmur

50. **Erica was diagnosed with pericarditis on admission yesterday to the Progressive Care Unit. She is complaining of intermittent, sharp, knifelike pain in her chest. Which position would you place her in to help alleviate some of the pain?**
    A. Lay her flat with her feet elevated
    B. Sit her up and lean her forward on a stable bedside table
    C. Position her prone in Trendelenburg
    D. Position her on her right side

51. **Brenda was admitted to your unit for observation after falling 10 feet into a ravine. She was diagnosed with systemic lupus erythematosus (SLE) two years ago. Brenda suffered a concussion, three fractured ribs, a fractured radius, and a sprained ankle. She is on a Holter monitor and is receiving IV fluids and anti-biotics. Which of the following conditions would be exacerbated by the SLE?**
    A. Hypotension
    B. Constipation
    C. Pericarditis
    D. Polycythemia

    effects vascular + connective tissues

52. **If the international normalized ratio (INR) is greater than 5.0, the patient is at significant risk of bleeding. A drug that can cause a significant rise in the INR is**
    A. Ethacrinic acid.
    B. Penicillin.
    C. Amiodarone.
    D. A statin.

53. **A drug that will significantly decrease the INR would be**
    A. Naficillin.
    B. Vitamin K.
    C. High-dose vitamin C.
    D. Cyclosporine.

54. **Your patient has a temporary pacemaker and has been requiring adjustments to raise the energy output (milliamps). This is probably due to**
    A. Hyperkalemia.
    B. Necrotic tissue.
    C. Lidocaine toxicity.
    D. An atrioventricular block.

55. Kenneth is a 54-year-old dockworker who was admitted with a non-STEMI inferior wall MI. He is complaining of dyspnea, weakness, bilateral crackles, and demonstrates orthopnea. He has developed an S_3 heart sound. You suspect he has also developed
    A. A pulmonary embolus.
    B. Pulmonary hypertension.
    C. A fat embolism.
    D. Cardiogenic shock.

56. Your patient suddenly complains of chest pain. You auscultate a new holosystolic murmur at the lower left sternal border. Your patient has probably experienced a
    A. Dissecting thoracic aneurysm.
    B. Pulmonary embolus.
    C. Ventricular septal rupture.
    D. Lateral wall MI.

57. Francine was admitted three days ago for management of a deep vein thrombosis. During your initial assessment this morning, you found her sitting on the side of the bed leaning forward. Francine states that this position relieved her newly developed chest pain. She also states that the pain is worse on inspiration. You notify the physician and she orders a CXR and lab work. The lab results show that the patient's sed rate and WBCs are elevated. Francine most likely has
    A. Pericarditis.
    B. A thoracic aneurysm.
    C. A pulmonary embolus.
    D. Pulmonary edema.

58. A probable candidate for a coronary artery bypass graft might have
    A. An ejection fraction of 55% and diabetes.
    B. Right main artery disease.
    C. An ejection fraction of 35% and coronary artery disease.
    D. A previous history of cardiac surgery.

59. You are performing cardiopulmonary resuscitation on a patient with an endotracheal tube in place. The placement of the tube has been confirmed. The patient should be ventilated every
    A. 6 to 8 seconds.
    B. 5 compressions.
    C. 15 compressions.
    D. 3 to 5 seconds.

60. If you are using a biphasic defibrillator on an adult, the energy setting should be
    A. 360 joules.
    B. 50–100 joules.
    C. 300 joules.
    D. 200 joules.

61. Maria has been diagnosed with pericarditis secondary to blunt chest trauma and cardiac contusion after a motor vehicle accident. She asks you how long the pericarditis may last. Your answer will be formulated based on the fact that
    A. Acute pericarditis will self-resolve in 1 week.
    B. Acute pericarditis should self-resolve in 2–6 weeks.
    C. Acute pericarditis will always result in chronic pericarditis.
    D. Chronic pericarditis is reoccurring and not associated with any other cardiac symptoms.

62. Wellen's syndrome
    A. Is the same as Prinzmetal's angina.
    B. Occurs with proximal stenosis of the LAD.
    C. Is also called crescendo angina.
    D. Is variant angina.

63. A vasodilator used in the treatment of anginal pain is
    A. Morphine.
    B. Ticlid.
    C. Aspirin.
    D. NTG.

64. A patient is at high risk for ventricular septal defect or rupture or even a ventricular aneurysm if an infarct occurs in the
    A. Left anterior descending artery.
    B. Left main coronary artery.
    C. Left circumflex artery.
    D. Right coronary artery.

65. If a chronic fluid accumulation occurs, the pericardial sac may hold as much as _____ before the signs of cardiac tamponade will appear.
    A. 200 mL
    B. 400 mL
    C. 1,000 mL
    D. 2,000 mL

66. Which of the following statements is true about pericardial effusion?
    A. Pericardial effusion is a painless, hard-to-diagnose condition.
    B. On CXR, a "water bottle" silhouette is noted.
    C. Diastolic filling is increased.
    D. The voltage of the QRS complex is increased.

67. Increased afterload would be seen with
    A. Polycythemia.
    B. Aortic insufficiency.
    C. Hypovolemia.
    D. Sepsis.

68. Auto-regulatory control of cardiac vessels becomes impaired if the coronary perfusion pressure drops below
    A. 35 mm Hg.
    B. 40 mm Hg.
    C. 50 mm Hg.
    D. 60 mm Hg.

69. Renin is secreted by the
    A. Pancreas.
    B. Lungs.
    C. Liver.
    D. Kidneys.

70. If blood pressure is lower by at least 10–11 mm Hg on inspiration than on expiration, this is known as
    A. Pulsus alternans.
    B. Pulse pressure.
    C. Pulsus paradoxus.
    D. Pulsus parvus.

71. Your patient, Robert, suffered an MI but is now in stable condition in your progressive care unit. Seven family members arrive at the ICU, demanding to see the patient. Your best response would be to
    A. Notify social services. *HIPAA*
    B. Identify a responsible family spokesperson and contact him or her.
    C. Refuse to admit more than one person.
    D. Call security to remove the visitors.

72. Continuing with the scenario in Question 71, after you have identified Robert's significant other, his estranged wife arrives at the ICU. Robert tells you he does not want contact with his estranged wife. He even writes a note to that effect to be placed on his chart. He also states he wants no information given to the estranged wife. She became belligerent when told of Robert's wishes and threatened the staff with a lawsuit. The most appropriate nursing action would be to
    A. Request an ethics/multidisciplinary care conference to discuss communication and dissemination of the patient's medical status and to review the visitation policy.
    B. Immediately call the hospital attorney to speak with the wife.
    C. Give the wife any information she wants, but do not inform the patient that you have done so.
    D. Request that the patient's physician write a non-visitation order for the wife.

73. Rebecca, who is a Jehovah's Witness, has just undergone a cardiac surgical procedure. Her Hgb and Hct levels have been falling and are now 6.5 and 24, respectively. Her chest tubes have drained 1,750 mL in the last four hours. The anticipated treatment would be to administer
    A. One unit of type-specific whole blood.
    B. 500 cc of albumin.
    C. 250 mL of fresh frozen plasma.
    D. Continuous-circuit auto-transfusion.

74. **The major advantage of using an internal mammary artery for cardiac bypass would be**
    A. Greater ease of harvesting.
    B. Better postsurgical patency.
    C. A lowered infection rate.
    D. A lower rate of reperfusion rhythms.

75. **Your patient just underwent a percutaneous intervention for stent placement, after which he was returned to your telemetry unit. You note a rash over the patient's trunk and arms. This is probably due to**
    A. An allergic reaction to contrast dye.
    B. Petechiae from a fat emboli.
    C. A reaction to the indwelling stent.
    D. A rash secondary to a *Candida* infection.

76. **A sign of necrosis on an EKG would include**
    A. Acute ST elevation.
    B. A right BBB.
    C. A left BBB.
    D. A Q wave in Lead III.

Q wave in 6hrs = bad

77. **Holly received 4 mg of morphine IV. She is now unresponsive and her respiratory rate and depth are diminished. The antidote for morphine is**
    A. Regitine.
    B. Bicarbonate.
    C. Naloxone.
    D. Atropine.

78. **Complications associated with ventricular assist devices (VADs) include**
    A. Thromboembolism.
    B. Thrombocytopenia.
    C. Dissection of the aorta.
    D. Septicemia.

also infection + bleeding

79. **Indications for use of a VAD include**
    A. Dysrhythmias.
    B. As destination therapy.
    C. Prolonged cardiac arrest.
    D. Extensive organ damage.

all others contraindicated

80. **The most common infection in patients with a VAD is**
    A. Septicemia.
    B. Pericarditis.
    C. Pneumonia.
    D. Pericardial effusion.

d/t immobility

81. The most commonly used type of VAD is the
    A. RVAD.
    B. VAD.
    C. BIVAD.
    D. LVAD.

82. The most common major impediment to family education regarding placement of a ventricular assist device is
    A. Language.
    B. Technology.
    C. Time.
    D. Physician availability.

    usually emergent

83. The physician has just informed your patient that she needs an LVAD. The patient is crying and says, "I just know I am going to die. What's the point? It must be my time." The patient is obviously quite stressed. The priority for the nurse at this time is to
    A. Tell the patient she will not die.
    B. Explore possible suicidal ideation.
    C. Immediately place the patient in a single room.
    D. Notify the hospital's spiritual advisor.

84. Your patient has just transferred from the ICU to your unit. The patient had an abdominal aortic aneurysm repair two days ago. He is somewhat restless, and his vital signs are stable. He keeps pointing at the lumbar area of his back and saying that he has discomfort in that area. This may indicate
    A. A blister from the surgical ground pad.
    B. Need for repositioning.
    C. Irritation from the dressing.
    D. Retroperitoneal bleeding.

85. The definitive invasive diagnostic procedure to diagnose an aortic dissection is a(n)
    A. Left lateral recumbent CXR.
    B. Computerized tomography (CT) scan.
    C. Transesophageal ultrasound.
    D. Aortogram.

86. Which of the following statements about aortic aneurysms is true?
    A. The mortality increases when the patient is between 25 and 35 years old.
    B. Aortic aneurysms are more common in men than in women.
    C. There are no warning signs.
    D. Aortic aneurysms are the result of aortic stenosis.

87. An aneurysm that is dissecting upward (ascending) produces pain
    A. In the chest and midscapular area.
    B. In the back of the neck and left shoulder.
    C. From the umbilical area to the shoulder.
    D. In the left shoulder and midsternal area.

88. An aortic aneurysm that extends more than _____ will require surgical repair.
    A. 3 cm
    B. 5 cm
    C. 7 cm
    D. 9 cm

89. When an arterial aortic dissection occurs, it is usually due to weakness in which area of the artery?
    A. Tunica intima
    B. Tunica adventicia
    C. Tunica media
    D. Tunica externa

90. The area most commonly affected by aortic aneurysms is
    A. The aortic arch.
    B. The abdomen.
    C. The thoracic area.
    D. The lumbar region.

91. You are discussing EKG interpretation with your nursing orientee. She asks you why there is such a difference in the size of the waves. You tell her:
    A. "The P wave represents repolarization of the atrium and the QRS the depolarization of the ventricles; the size difference is related to lead placement."
    B. "The P wave represents repolarization of the atrium and the QRS the repolarization of the ventricles; the size difference is related to the muscle mass involved in the polarization."
    C. "The P wave represents depolarization of the atrium and the QRS the depolarization of the ventricles; the size difference is related to the muscle mass involved in the polarization."
    D. "The P wave represents depolarization of the atrium and the QRS the repolarization of the ventricles; the size difference is related to the lead placement."

92. Your patient with obstructive jaundice has no prior history of cardiac arrhythmias. He asks why he is on a cardiac monitor. Your best response is:
    A. "You may develop sinus bradycardia, which is a slower heart rate. This monitor will alert staff to any dangerous drop in your heart rate."
    B. "You may develop sinus tachycardia, and the monitor will alert staff to any increase in your heart rate."
    C. "You will develop atrial flutter, and the monitor will alert staff to changes in your heart rate."
    D. "You may develop ventricular tachycardia and the monitor will alert you to changes in your heart rate."

93. Bernard was admitted for pneumonia. He is two years post heart transplant. When you place the EKG monitoring leads, you note sinus tachycardia with PVCs and a 2-mm ST elevation. The patient denies pain. This finding is

A. Impossible.
B. Normal.
C. Indicative of an RBBB.
D. Indicative of an inferior MI.

[handwritten: ♥ transplant = denervated]

94. **The primary cause of acquired valvular heart disease is**
    A. Heredity.
    B. Smoking.
    C. Drug abuse.
    D. Rheumatic fever.

95. **A patient who is status post heart transplant may have significant bradycardia. The drug of choice in such cases is**
    A. Atropine.
    B. Isuproterenol.
    C. Apresoline.
    D. Adenosine.

96. **The most common precipitating cause of dissecting aneurysms is**
    A. Weakness of the vessel wall.
    B. Heart failure.
    C. Hypertension.
    D. Atheroembolism.

97. **Your patient is 36 hours status post right femoral bypass graft. The patient complains of pain with even slight movement of the limb. You suspect**
    A. An arterial obstruction.
    B. A DVT.
    C. A venous obstruction.
    D. A leg cramp from prolonged bed rest.

98. **You are discussing pericardial effusions with a nursing student. He asks you if fluid in the pericardial sac in normal. Your best answer is** *[handwritten: usually contains 20–25 cc]*
    A. "No; if there is any fluid in the pericardial sac, it always leads to pericarditis."
    B. "No; any fluid in the pericardial sac leads to cardiac tamponade."
    C. "Yes; there is a small amount of blood in the pericardial sac."
    D. "Yes; there is a small amount of fluid in the pericardial sac."

99. **Your patient received streptokinase about 30 minutes ago for a lateral wall STEMI. You would expect which of the following events to occur?**
    A. Lowered CPK isoenzymes
    B. Reperfusion rhythms
    C. Transient increased chest pain
    D. Mild CHF

[handwritten: Vtach, SB]

100. A quadriplegic patient has undergone a CABG and has had no complications. You are about to teach his wife how to change the chest dressings and the graft site dressings on the legs. Principles of teaching include
    A. Teaching all the information at once.
    B. Teaching the information as fast as possible.
    C. Explaining the rationale for the procedure, and then demonstrating it.
    D. Speaking slowly so that the patient can hear.

101. Your patient had a cardiac arrest. You are doing CPR near his implanted ICD generator. If the ICD defibrillates, you would feel
    A. A powerful shock.
    B. Nothing.
    C. Mild tingling.
    D. A mild shock.

102. Newer ICDs use the most efficient shock waveforms for defibrillation and cardio-version. The most efficient waveform would be
    A. Square wave technology.
    B. Monophasic.
    C. Fixed curve.
    D. Biphasic.

103. Your patient requires emergent programming of her ICD. How many joules above the defibrillation threshold should the ICD be set?
    A. 10 joules
    B. 20 joules
    C. 30 joules
    D. 40 joules

104. When you receive report on your patient, you are told his ICD was reset. You notice a large magnet on the table outside the room. What is the purpose of this magnet?
    A. It inhibits all output from the ICD.
    B. It inhibits the shocking portion only of the ICD.
    C. It inhibits the pacemaker function of the ICD.
    D. It allows timing of the ICD to be set.

105. Tachyarrhythmias that are refractive to conventional therapies may have to be treated with radio-frequency ablation. This treatment is usually successful on reentry tachyarrhythmias. The radio-frequency destroys myocardial tissue via
    A. Radiation.
    B. Heat.
    C. Cold.
    D. An overriding signal to ablate the pacemaker.

106. Your patient has atrial fibrillation and needs to be cardioverted. The patient was medicated for pain and anxiety with morphine and Versed. Which additional medication will help the process of cardioversion from atrial fibrillation to a normal sinus rhythm?
    A. Digitalis
    B. Amiodarone
    C. Pronestyl
    D. Ibutilide

107. Symptoms of chronic pericarditis most often mimic which other disease process?
    A. Chronic right-sided heart failure
    B. Pulmonary hypertension
    C. Pneumonia
    D. Cardiomyopathy

108. Helen developed infective pericarditis after renal failure and sepsis. Morning labs should show a(n):
    A. Increased WBC, decreased ESR, normal CK-MB.
    B. Normal WBC, decreased ESR, elevated CK-MB.
    C. Increased WBC, increased ESR, elevated CK-MB.
    D. Increased WBC, normal ESR, elevated CK-MB.

109. Which of the following organisms is most often the cause of myocarditis?
    A. Coxsackievirus
    B. *E. coli*
    C. *Streptococcus*
    D. *Staphylococcus*

110. During insertion of a CVP catheter, your patient has a short run of V-tach and shows unifocal PVCs. Your immediate response should be to
    A. Administer lidocaine 1 mg/kg.
    B. Hang an amiodarone drip.
    C. Notify the physician who is inserting the catheter. *needs to be pulled back*
    D. Immediately have the physician completely withdraw the catheter.

111. What percentage of acute myocardial infarctions may be considered "silent" infarcts?
    A. 5%
    B. 10%
    C. 20%
    D. 30%

112. During shift report, you are told that your patient has a 90% occlusion to the circumflex coronary artery. Which type of myocardial infarction is this patient at greatest risk of developing?
    A. Lateral wall infarction
    B. Anterior wall infarction
    C. Posterior wall infarction
    D. Septal wall infarction

113. **Laura suffered a myocardial infarction as a result of 100% occlusion of the left anterior descending and circumflex artery. Although cardiac catheterization returned some blood flow to the left side of her heart, you note a new murmur at the fifth intercostal space, midclavicular line. You suspect**
    A. Tricuspid valve stenosis.
    B. Mitral valve regurgitation.
    C. Pulmonic stenosis.
    D. Aortic regurgitation.

114. **Gina was admitted to the PCU with cough, fever, chills, anorexia, malaise, and headache. She has a pericardial friction rub. She also has a history of rheumatic fever. While examining Gina, you note fine, dark lines in her nail beds and some flat lesions on her palms. These flat lesions are known as**
    A. Janeway lesions.
    B. Roth spots.
    C. Osler's nodes.
    D. Pella's sign.

115. **Under the Fontaine classification for peripheral vascular disease, intermittent claudication occurs at**
    A. Stage I.
    B. Stage II.
    C. Stage III.
    D. Stage IV.

116. **Which of the following nursing actions would be important in the care of a patient with occlusive disease of the terminal aorta and a nonhealing wound on the left foot?**
    A. Elevate the legs
    B. Place the patient in high Fowler's position
    C. Maintain normothermia
    D. Fluid restriction

117. **In a patient with cardiogenic shock, an undesirable outcome would produce**
    A. Increased cardiac output.
    B. Increased systemic vascular resistance.
    C. Decreased ventricular preload.
    D. Decreased pulmonary artery pressures.

118. **Marvin has heard staff talking about his mitral valve regurgitation; they also mentioned that it could be mitral valve stenosis. He asks you how you can tell the difference just by listening to his heart. Your best answer is:**
    A. "Mitral stenosis produces a high-pitched murmur and mitral valve regurgitation produces a low-pitched murmur."
    B. "Mitral stenosis produces a murmur during systole and mitral valve regurgitation produces a murmur during diastole."
    C. "Mitral stenosis murmurs do not radiate their sound, whereas mitral valve regurgitation murmurs will radiate toward the left arm."
    D. "There is no difference between the presentation of mitral valve stenosis and the presentation of mitral valve regurgitation."

119. **If your patient's temporary pacemaker is not sensing, your first action should be to**
   A. Place the patient on the right side.
   B. Increase mA output.
   C. Check the sensitivity control for proper setting.
   D. Immediately turn off the pacemaker and notify the physician.

120. **A diastolic murmur will occur as a result of regurgitant blood flow over which of the following valves?**
   A. Mitral and aortic
   B. Mitral and tricuspid
   C. Pulmonic and aortic
   D. Tricuspid and pulmonic

121. **Blood flow that moves forward through stenotic valves can also cause a diastolic murmur. The valves involved are the**
   A. Mitral and aortic.
   B. Mitral and tricuspid.
   C. Pulmonic and aortic.
   D. Tricuspid and pulmonic.

122. **Sid is a 30-year-old male who lost control of his motorcycle while riding in the rain. At the time of the accident, he was wearing a helmet and protective gear. Sid suffered a fractured left femur, a fractured rib, a cervical sprain, and road rash on his face and neck. He is admitted with a blood pressure of 84/44, HR 100, RR 26 and shallow, T 98.4°F. His 12-lead EKG shows ST elevation in the anterior leads. His CXR shows a normal cardiac silhouette and no infiltrates. His Hgb is 9.0, and his Hct is 32. MB is 18%. Sid is restless and complains of pain in the chest and left leg. Which condition would you anticipate?**
   A. Systolic dysfunction
   B. Hypovolemic shock
   C. Pulmonary hypertension
   D. Pulmonary edema

123. **Four days ago, Gertrude, who is 70 years old, was admitted to your unit status post laparotomy for an unknown abdominal mass. During the surgery, Gertrude had minimal blood loss and an uneventful course. The patient's history includes smoking since she was 15 (unknown number of packs per day), Type II diabetes, a permanent pacemaker, an anterior MI, and a right-sided stroke 20 years ago with no deficits.**

   Three days ago, Gertrude had a hypotensive episode; her BP dropped to 82/48, and her heart rate was 70. The hospitalist ordered dobutamine and the blood pressure increased until the MAP was 72.

   Today, Gertrude remains on the dobutamine at 2 mcg/kg/min. Her BP is 108/60, MAP 76, heart rate 70. Attempts at weaning dobutamine have failed—her blood pressure drops precipitously if the dobutamine dosage is lowered.

   What do you think is the cause of Gertrude's initial hypotensive episode?
   A. Hypovolemic shock
   B. Previous MI
   C. Rapid rewarming postoperatively
   D. Cell mediated response

124. Continuing with the scenario in Question 123, which additional action could be taken to improve Gertrude's cardiac output and help wean her from dobutamine?
    A. Initiate a fluid challenge
    B. Start dopamine
    C. Place a pulmonary artery catheter
    D. Turn up the rate on the pacemaker

125. What does the acronym AICD stand for?
    A. Automated internal cardiac defibrillator
    B. Autocardiac internal converting defibrillator
    C. Automated implantable cardioverter/defibrillator
    D. Automatic implanted coronary defibrillator

126. Matthew has had an AICD for 6 months. He has been admitted to your unit for syncope. You notice his pulse is very irregular, and he complains of getting "zapped" often. On his monitor, the rhythm is sinus bradycardia with numerous pacemaker spikes. What could be wrong?
    A. Matthew's AICD has a faulty lead.
    B. Matthew has had a myocardial infarction.
    C. The battery in Matthew's AICD is losing power.
    D. Matthew has experienced a generator failure of his AICD.

127. Which physical finding is significant for carotid stenosis?
    A. Heberden's nodules
    B. Systolic murmur Grade IV/VI
    C. Carotid bruit
    D. Broussard's nodules

128. Barry has Wolf–Parkinson–White syndrome. He is experiencing increasing bouts of tachycardia. It has been decided to utilize overdrive pacing. How do you explain this type of pacemaker to a new orientee?
    A. The pacemaker is set at a constant rate of 70 bpm and is synchronized.
    B. The pacemaker or AICD is set on demand mode and is asynchronous.
    C. The pacemaker or AICD is set on demand mode and is synchronous.
    D. The pacemaker or AICD is set on inhibit mode and is synchronous.

129. Which pacemaker/AICD program code would you expect for a patient with complete heart block?
    A. VVI
    B. DDD
    C. VVT
    D. DDI

130. Gene had a DDD pacemaker inserted 3 years ago. He has been admitted for pacemaker syndrome. Which symptoms do you expect to see?
    A. Fatigue, agitation, dyspnea
    B. Fatigue, dizziness, confusion
    C. Fatigue, agitation, forgetfulness
    D. Fatigue, dizziness, syncope

131. **Georgia, a 49-year-old woman with an acute myocardial infarction, suddenly develops complete heart block. Her blood pressure drops, her heart rate is 27, and her color is ashen. What should you do?**
   A. Apply an external pacemaker and notify the physician.
   B. Wait for the physician to return your call and give atropine 4 mg intravenously.
   C. Apply a transvenous pacemaker, medicate the patient, and notify the physician.
   D. Call a Code Blue and prepare to start CPR.

132. **Your acute myocardial infarction patient waited for 16 hours before coming to the hospital. He has a right bundle branch block and a left anterior fascicular block. What is the significance of his condition?**
   A. He has extensive myocardial damage.
   B. He needs a pacemaker as soon as possible.
   C. He needs to be transferred to a facility that can perform a heart transplant.
   D. This problem will resolve itself over the next few weeks.

133. **Thomas has had an anterolateral myocardial infarction. Where do you expect to see changes on the 12-lead EKG?**
   A. V_1, V_2, I, AVL
   B. V_2, V_3, V_4, I, AVL
   C. V_2, V_3, V_4, II, III, AVF
   D. V_1, V_2, II, III, AVF

134. **What do abnormal Q waves signify on a 12-lead EKG?**
   A. Nothing—they are of no significance
   B. Repolarization of the myocardium
   C. Complete-thickness infarction of myocardium
   D. Partial-thickness death of myocardium

135. **Mary Margaret has had an inferior wall MI. Where do you expect to see the changes on her 12-lead EKG?**
   A. II, III, AVF
   B. I, II, AVL
   C. I, III, AVF
   D. V_1, V_2

136. **Your patient has had an anteroseptal MI. Where do you expect to see changes on the 12-lead EKG?**
   A. V_1, V_2, V_3, V_4
   B. V_2, V_3, V_4, V_5, V_6
   C. V_1, V_2, II, III, AVF
   D. V_1, V_2, I, AVL

137. **Which parameter is measured by the vertical lines on the EKG paper?**
   A. Velocity
   B. Time
   C. Voltage
   D. Intensity

138. **Which parameter is measured by the horizontal lines on the EKG paper?**
    A. Velocity
    B. Time
    C. Voltage
    D. Intensity

139. **V_1 and V_2 show which type of bundle branch block?**
    A. Right
    B. Left
    C. Dual bundle
    D. V_1, and V_2 do not show bundle branch blocks

140. **What are the most valuable pieces of information evaluated with a 12-lead EKG?**
    A. Rate, arrhythmias, infarction
    B. Rate, rhythm, axis, hypertrophy, infarction
    C. Rate, bundle branch block, hypertrophy
    D. Rate, rhythm, arrhythmias

141. **Which of the following conditions are associated with ST/T wave abnormalities?**
    A. Ventricular hypertrophy, pericarditis, COPD
    B. COPD, axis deviation
    C. Atrial hypertrophy, axis deviation
    D. Pericarditis, axis deviation

142. **Which 12-lead EKG changes would you expect to see in a patient with COPD?**
    A. Low-voltage P waves, tachycardia
    B. Tall P waves, left ventricular hypertrophy
    C. Tall, peaked P waves, right ventricular hypertrophy, low-voltage QRS
    D. Low-voltage QRS, left atrial hypertrophy

143. **What are some common reasons for pacemaker insertion?**
    A. Tachycardia, Wenckebach, bradycardia
    B. Symptomatic bradycardia, overdrive pacing, acute MI with sinus dysfunction
    C. Complete heart block, Wenckebach, tachycardia
    D. Bundle branch block, Wenckebach, tachycardia

144. **Quinidine and hypomagnesemia can both lead to which condition?**
    A. Torsades de Pointes
    B. Ventricular tachycardia
    C. Ventricular fibrillation
    D. Atrial tachycardia

145. **Which condition is required for a diagnosis of hospital-acquired pneumonia (HAP)?**
    A. Recent common cold prior to admission
    B. Cigarette smoking
    C. Acute myocardial infarction
    D. Hospitalization for more than 2 days

114. A
115. B
116. A
117. D
118. B
119. C
120. B
121. B
122. B
123. C
124. A
125. A
126. A
127. C
128. C
129. B
130. A
131. C
132. A
133. B
134. B
135. C

136. C
137. B
138. B
139. A
140. A
141. A
142. B
143. C
144. A
145. D
146. A
147

146. **What is the most common causative organism in hospital-acquired pneumonia (HAP)?**
   A. Methicillin-resistant *Staphylococcus aureus* (MRSA)
   B. *Pseudomonas aeruginosa*
   C. *Streptococcus pneumoniae*
   D. *Acinobacter* species

147. **What are some risk factors for developing hospital-acquired pneumonia?**
   A. Altered level of consciousness, urinary catheter, sedation
   B. COPD, ill hospital staff, beta blockers
   C. H_2 blockers, age, history of smoking
   D. H_2 blockers, postpartum patient, age

148. **Millie is a 78-year-old patient admitted postoperatively 2 days ago after undergoing a colon resection for cancer. She has a nasogastric tube through which she is receiving routine doses of antacids. Her morning labs are as follows: WBCs 15.6, neutrophils 9,100. Her chest X-ray is inconclusive. What is Millie's problem?**
   A. Pulmonary embolism
   B. Hospital-acquired pneumonia
   C. Congestive heart failure
   D. Atelectasis

149. **How does hospital-acquired pneumonia (HAP) differ from ventilator-acquired pneumonia (VAP)?**
   A. There is no difference.
   B. Different causative organisms
   C. The VAP patient is intubated.
   D. Therapies differ.

150. **What does SVO_2 measure?**
   A. Oxygen saturation of blood in the brachial vein
   B. Oxygen saturation of the blood returning to the lungs
   C. Oxygen saturation of blood in the coronary sinus
   D. Oxygen saturation in the capillary bed

151. **Mannie is a 15-year-old victim of a gunshot wound to his left chest and has a pneumo-hemothorax. He has been stable all day with minimal chest tube drainage. Over the past four hours, his O_2 saturation has been decreasing. The physician orders mixed venous gases, and the results show an SVO_2 of 64%. What does this information tell you about the patient's condition?**
   A. The amount of shunting that is occurring
   B. CO_2 levels
   C. HCO_3 levels
   D. PO_2 level

152. **One hour later, Mannie's SVO_2 is 22%. What does this indicate about his condition?**
   A. It is a normal reading.
   B. His shunt is improving.
   C. His shunt is worsening.
   D. His shunt is stable.

153. **Promethazine is contraindicated with fluoroquinolone antibiotics for what reason?**
    A. This combination leads to increased sedation.
    B. This combination leads to QT prolongation and arrhythmias.
    C. Promethazine is inactivated by fluoroquinolones.
    D. The antibiotic is inactivated by promethazine.

154. **What is the infusion rate for Lasix (furosemide)?**
    A. It can be given as an intravenous push at any dose.
    B. 4 mg/min
    C. 1 mg/min
    D. It should always be given as a piggyback.

155. **Why is Lasix given slowly?**
    A. Rapid infusion can lead to nausea.
    B. Rapid infusion can lead to rash.
    C. Rapid infusion can lead to hyperkalemia.
    D. Rapid infusion can lead to hearing loss.

156. **Your patient has undergone an angiogram today with stent placement. He is to start Plavix, and you are teaching him about this medication. The patient takes numerous herbal remedies daily. Which ones should he avoid while he is taking Plavix?**
    A. Dong quai, gingko biloba, saw palmetto
    B. Aloe extract, bilberry
    C. Calendula, clove
    D. Fenugreek, licorice

157. **What history should you know before starting Reo Pro (abciximab)?**
    A. Chest pain
    B. Any bleeding history
    C. Previous myocardial infarction
    D. Family history

158. **Warfarin is indicated for which of the following conditions?**
    A. DVT, CHF, atrial fibrillation
    B. DVT, atrial fibrillation, heart valve replacement
    C. Pulmonary embolism, DVT, COPD
    D. Pulmonary embolism, atrial fibrillation, CHF

159. **You are teaching Anne about her Coumadin (warfarin) therapy. Part of your teaching must include foods to avoid while on this medication. Which of the following should be avoided?**
    A. Broccoli, soybean oil, spinach
    B. Olive oil, peanut butter, kale
    C. Avocado, broccoli, peas
    D. Broccoli, green beans, spinach

160. **Integrilin (eptifbatide) is indicated for which condition?**
    A. DVT
    B. Pulmonary embolism
    C. Acute coronary syndrome (ACS)
    D. Occlusive cerebrovascular accident

161. **You overhear your patient discussing his aortic stenosis with his family. He states, "It can't be that bad, because the murmur isn't that loud." Your best response is:**
    A. Do not say anything, it would be considered eavesdropping.
    B. Interrupt and say that nothing has been confirmed yet.
    C. Ask the patient if his doctor told him that or if he learned it by searching the Internet.
    D. Use the opportunity to teach the patient by asking if you can clarify his understanding of his disease process.

162. **The pain associated with aortic stenosis is caused by**
    A. Angina.
    B. Left ventricular hypertrophy.
    C. Decreased coronary artery flow.
    D. Increased aortic pressures.

163. **Mr. B. was admitted to your unit to rule out myocardial infarction two days ago. He has a history of GERD and stomach ulcers. He is due to be discharged today on digoxin and oral antacids. You review his A.M. labs prior to beginning your physical assessment. Lab results are as follows:**

WBC 11,000/mm^3	RBC 5.2 mil/mm^3	PLT 350,000/mm^3
Hgb 13 g/dL	Hct 48 mL/dL	
Potassium 4.5 mEq/L	Total calcium 13.5 mg/dL	Magnesium 1.87 mg/dL
Sodium 140 mEq/L	Chloride 104 mEq/L	

    You would probably expect to see which of the following signs and symptoms during your assessment of Mr. B.?
    A. Hypotension, prolonged QT interval, junctional tachycardia
    B. Bradycardia, confusion, hypertension, decreased grasp strength
    C. Muscle spasms, hypertonicity, ventricular tachycardia
    D. Second-degree Type 2 heart block, shortened QT interval, hypotension

164. **You are caring for a 7-day postoperative CABG patient. He remains severely hypocalcemic despite calcium supplementation. Which of the following complications is this patient at greatest risk for developing?**
    A. Bleeding
    B. Muscle tetany
    C. Flattened T waves
    D. Deep vein thrombosis

165. You are preparing to flush Mr. N.'s Hep-locked PICC line with 1 mL of heparin. As you examine the vial, you note that its concentration is 10,000 units/mL. If administered at this dosage, which clotting factors would heparin impair?
    A. I, V, VIII
    B. VIII
    C. II
    D. II, VII, IX, X, XI

166. Carl was initially admitted to your unit with a diagnosis of congestive heart failure. After further study, it was determined that he has restrictive cardiomyopathy. A common cause of restrictive cardiomyopathy is
    A. Unknown etiology.
    B. Glycogen storage disease.
    C. History of diabetes.
    D. Viral infection.

167. The type of cardiomyopathy that is characterized by replacement of normal cells by fatty tissue is known as
    A. Hypertrophic.
    B. Dilated.
    C. Arrhythmogenic.
    D. Restrictive.

168. Which of the following hemodynamic effects would be seen in a patient with hypertrophic cardiomyopathy?
    A. Decreased CO, decreased ejection fraction
    B. Normal CO, increased ejection fraction
    C. Increased CO, increased ejection fraction
    D. Decreased CO, increased ejection fraction

169. Dilated cardiomyopathy is characterized by dilation of the ventricles and impaired systolic function. Common causes are valvular heart disease and ischemic heart disease. Other causes are idiopathic. The most common cause of idiopathic dilated cardiomyopathy is
    A. Alcohol.
    B. Familial.
    C. Genetic.
    D. Autoimmune.

170. Peripartum cardiomyopathy is a form of
    A. Restrictive cardiomyopathy.
    B. Hypertropic cardiomyopathy.
    C. Viral cardiomyopathy.
    D. Dilated cardiomyopathy.

171. Your patient was admitted for ascites, orthopnea, paroxysmal nocturnal dyspnea, and excessive fatigue. On physical examination, you note S_3 and S_4 gallops, basilar crackles, and the EKG shows sinus tachycardia. These symptoms are usually indicative of which type of cardiomyopathy?

A. Dilated

B. Restrictive

C. Alcohol induced

D. Hypertrophic

172. **The most common new-onset dysrhythmias seen in a patient with pulmonary edema is**

A. Supraventricular tachycardia.

B. RBBB.

C. Ventricular tachycardia.

D. Atrial fibrillation.

173. **Your patient will be having an LVAD placed this evening and will subsequently be cared for in your unit. Family members are quite anxious to learn more about the device and to participate in the patient's care. An important point when teaching caregivers is to make certain they understand which changes in the patient's condition should be reported immediately to the staff. A complication that should be reported immediately would be**

A. Irritation or redness at the incision site.

B. A temperature of 99.6°F.

C. Any change in the mentation of the patient.

D. A rise in blood pressure of more than 10 mm Hg.

174. **Stan is a 40-year-old construction worker who was seen in the ED after falling into a trench. He sustained a left fractured tibia and fibula and a fractured left scapula. Stan required a splenectomy and was just admitted to your care. The nursing supervisor tried to get a bed in the ICU, but none was available. Your initial assessment results are as follows:**

EKG: ST at 126 with isolated PVC

BP 84/50

Skin pale, cool, clammy

RR 26, breath sounds clear, slightly diminished RLL

O_2 2 L/min via NC

Mentation: Responds to questions slowly, oriented to self and time

CVP 4

Which of the following conditions do you believe this patient is developing?

A. Cardiogenic shock

B. Hypovolemic shock

C. Septic shock

D. Left ventricular failure

175. **You are preparing to give Mrs. D. her 0900 dose of Coumadin as part of her atrial fibrillation management. You are reviewing her A.M. labs prior to administration of the medication. Which lab result would cause alarm?**

A. PTT 72 seconds

B. PLT 180,000/mm^3

C. APTT 38 seconds

D. PT 28 seconds

176. **Which of the following medications would you anticipate using to improve the pumping action of the heart when a patient is developing cardiogenic shock?**
    A. Dobutamine
    B. Epinephrine
    C. Diltiazem
    D. Isoproterenol

177. **Yesterday, Warren was shoveling snow when he became short of breath and felt diffuse chest discomfort. When he went inside for lunch, the pain disappeared. Warren later resumed shoveling snow and felt more fatigued than ever. Today, he was admitted to your unit with orthopnea and profound dyspnea. He is constantly saying, "I'm 56 years old and have been outside all my life. I'm not sick enough to be in here." His girlfriend reports that over the past three weeks, Warren has been more tired than usual, even when performing small tasks around the house.**
    EKG: Borderline ST at 100 with rare PACs
    Manual cuff BP 142/74
    Skin warm, pale
    Capillary refill 4 seconds, 2+ pitting edema (pretibial)
    RR 20, breath sounds: crackles in posterior lobes
    O_2 2 L/min via NC
    ABGs were drawn, but results are unavailable
    Mentation: Alert, oriented $\times$ 4

    Warren has probably developed
    A. Mild pericarditis.
    B. Pulmonary edema (noncardiac).
    C. Chylothorax.
    D. Left ventricular failure.

178. **Nancy is 64 years old and has a history of COPD. Today, she was admitted with an inferior wall MI. About 30 minutes ago, she complained of increasing shortness of breath. When Nancy changed her position, the dyspnea abated. She is again complaining of dyspnea, and you perform a 12-lead EKG because your unit monitor allows monitoring of only leads II and MCL1. The EKG shows lead V_1–V_4 ST-segment depression. Other physical and laboratory findings are as follows:**
    EKG: Sinus arrhythmia at 93
    Manual cuff BP 102/60
    Skin pale, cool, clammy; sacral edema, pedal and pretibial edema
    RR 22, breath sounds: bilateral crackles
    O_2 2 L/min via NC
    ABGs: pH 7.38, pCO_2 48, paO_2 66, HCO_3 34
    Mentation: Alert, oriented $\times$ 4

    What is the interpretation of the ABGs?
    A. Uncompensated metabolic acidosis
    B. Compensated respiratory acidosis
    C. Uncompensated metabolic alkalosis
    D. Compensated respiratory alkalosis

179. **Continuing with the scenario from Question 178, Nancy is probably developing**
    A. Pulmonary effusion.
    B. Left ventricular failure.
    C. Pericarditis.
    D. Congestive heart failure.

180. **Approximately what percentage of coronary artery blockage is needed to cause angina?**
    A. 45%
    B. 60%
    C. 75%
    D. 90%

181. **Which of the following lead changes will identify a lateral MI?**
    A. II, III, aVF
    B. V_1–V_4
    C. V_2–V_6
    D. I, aVL, V_5, V_6

182. **Garrett was admitted to your unit about six hours ago with an inferior MI. He has been medicated for pain and is resting comfortably at this time. His wife is visiting when she approaches you and says Garrett is dizzy and cannot catch his breath. His EKG now shows a sinus bradycardia with multifocal PVCs at four per minute. Other findings include:**
    EKG: Sinus bradycardia at 52 with rare multifocal PVCs
    Manual cuff BP 82/46 (previous BP 110/76 30 minutes ago)
    Skin pale, cool, clammy
    RR 28
    O_2 2 L/min via NC
    Mentation: Anxious, oriented $\times$ 4
    Garrett's current arrhythmia will probably be
    A. Permanent, asymptomatic.
    B. Transient, possibly symptomatic.
    C. Permanent, symptomatic.
    D. Transient, asymptomatic.

183. **Joanne had a VVI pacemaker inserted. What does the first V in this acronym stand for?**
    A. Paced, ventricular
    B. Paced, inhibited
    C. Ventricular inhibited
    D. Ventricular

184. **What does the second V in the acronym for a VVI pacemaker stand for?**
    A. Ventricular paced
    B. Ventricular inhibited
    C. Ventricular sensed
    D. Ventricular programmed

185. **Maria is 60 years old. She was alert and active last evening, but was found this morning sitting in her kitchen, hardly able to move. At first, it was thought she had suffered a stroke. Maria was admitted because her EKG showed large R waves in leads V_1 and V_2. Physical parameters include the following data:**

    EKG: SR at 92, no ectopy

    Manual cuff BP 94/62

    Skin pale, cool, clammy

    RR 18, breath sounds clear, slightly diminished LLL

    O_2 2 L/min via NC

    Moderate jugular venous distention, no bruits

    CVP 18

    Mentation: Lethargic

    An expected diagnosis for Maria would be

    A. Aortic insufficiency.
    B. LV hypertrophy.
    C. RV infarction.
    D. Pericarditis.

186. **Pete was working on his roof yesterday when he slipped and fell, impaling his leg on a piece of rebar. The rebar was removed and he is now being cared for in your unit. Today, you note the following parameters and symptoms:**

    EKG: ST at 120 without ectopy

    Manual cuff BP 90/64

    Skin warm, dry

    Capillary refill 2 seconds

    RR 22, breath sounds: clear

    O_2 3 L/min via NC

    Temp 100.8°F

    Mentation: Alert, oriented × 4

    Pete is probably developing

    A. A pericardial tamponade.
    B. Left heart failure.
    C. Distributive shock.
    D. Septic shock.

187. **Mona was flying cross country and ate the snack provided by the airline. After about five minutes, she began to wheeze and her respirations became labored. A physician on board administered epinephrine, and the symptoms abated. The physician did not explain the reason for the reaction to Mona.**

    Two days later, Mona was sharing some of her snack mix with her nephew when she again began wheezing. She became severely tachypneic and was transported to the ED. She required treatment with epinephrine and steroids. She was stabilized and then sent to your unit. Mona is eight months pregnant. She is currently exhibiting the following signs and symptoms:

    EKG: ST at 128 without ectopy

    Manual cuff BP 88/58

Skin cool, pale

Capillary refill 4 seconds

RR 30, breath sounds: LLL crackles

Temp 99.4°F (oral)

Mentation: Awake, restless

Mona is probably developing
- A. Anaphylactic shock.
- B. Cardiogenic shock.
- C. Hypovolemic shock.
- D. Distributive shock.

188. **Your patient is a 45-year-old ironworker. He was admitted for cardiomyopathy. His initial ejection fraction was 21%, and he has been confused most of the time since his admission yesterday. On admission, his EKG showed ST depression in leads V_1–V_4. He has been more dyspneic and is getting restless. Current vital signs and parameters are as follows:**

EKG: ST at 116

Manual cuff BP 102/70

Skin pale, cool

Temp 99°F

Bilateral pretibial and pedal edema

Sacral edema also present

RR 30, breath sounds clear, slightly diminished RLL

O_2 4 L/min via mask

Mentation: Oriented to self, confused at times

From which condition does this patient appear to be suffering at this time?
- A. An anterior MI
- B. Inferior wall MI
- C. Biventricular failure
- D. Right ventricular failure

189. **Daniel was involved in a gang fight last week, during which he was stabbed several times in the anterior chest and twice in the abdomen. He has undergone two surgeries and is now post splenectomy, small bowel repair, and repair of a small laceration to the left subclavian artery. Daniel has received multiple units of blood and blood products. He was extubated this morning, but is now complaining of increasing shortness of breath. He is easily fatigued and his pulse oximeter reading is 0.94, down from 0.97. His A.M. CXR shows "bilateral widespread infiltrates." Other lab results and parameters are as follows:**

EKG: ST at 114, isolated PACs

Manual cuff BP 114/76

Skin warm

Temp 101°F

RR 30, breath sounds clear, slightly diminished RLL

O_2 4 L/min via mask

ABGs: pH 7.32, $PaCO_2$ 29, paO_2 70, HCO_3 19

Mentation: Oriented × 4 most of time, two episodes of confusion, easily reoriented

Which condition do you believe Daniel is developing?

A. ARDS

B. Pneumonia

C. Pulmonary emboli

D. Sepsis

190. Your patient has been prescribed paroxetine (Paxil) 50 mg PO/day. Your patient and family teaching should include side effects such as

A. Agitation, headaches, and insomnia.

B. Anaphylaxis, rash, and seizure activity.

C. Abdominal cramps, nausea, and diarrhea.

D. Dizziness, drowsiness, and blurred vision.

191. Your patient is placed on an EKG monitor. The rhythm is a sinus rhythm, rate of 78 with isolated PVCs, and a depressed ST segment. The ST depression might be indicative of

A. An MI in progressive infarction.

B. Ischemia.

C. Prolonged ventricular depolarization.

D. Hyperkalemia.

192. The type of myocardial infarction that involves the entire thickness of myocardium in a region is called

A. Subendocardial.

B. Anterioseptal.

C. Transmural.

D. Inferior wall.

193. In myocarditis, which medication is typically used to treat ventricular failure by improving myocardial contractility and reducing ventricular rate?

A. Inderal

B. Imuran

C. Amiodarone

D. Digoxin

194. Your patient has undergone a mitral valve repair with reconstruction of the valve leaflets and the annulus. This procedure is called a(n)

A. Valvuloplasty.

B. Annuloplasty.

C. Mitral commissurotomy.

D. Mitral valve replacement.

This concludes the Cardiovascular Questions section.

ANSWERS

1. **Correct Answer: B**
Normal cardiac output (CO) should be 4 to 8 L/min. The formula for calculating this value is CO = HR × SV. The answer will be in milliliters (mL), which should then be changed to liters.

2. **Correct Answer: B**
Atrial kick is a term that represents the amount of the total cardiac output that is supplied via atrial contraction. If the patient has a condition or dysrhythmia that impairs or eliminates the atrial contraction, the patient may be compromised.

3. **Correct Answer: A**
The ejection fraction should be more than 50%. It represents the amount of blood ejected from the left ventricle compared to the total amount available, expressed as a percentage. For example, if the ventricle contains 90 mL of blood and 50 mL are ejected, the amount would be represented as a percentage, in this case 55%. An ejection fraction of 35% or less indicates a problem with contractility, outflow, or filling.

4. **Correct Answer: B**
The change in quality, frequency, and duration indicates unstable angina and may indicate that the patient is at increased risk for a myocardial infarction. This patient should be closely monitored for EKG changes and rhythm disturbances. In addition, extensive teaching should begin with the family and patient on how to identify a myocardial infarction and how to perform basic CPR should the patient go into a cardiac arrest outside the hospital.

5. **Correct Answer: C**
Answer A gives the components of afterload. Answers B and D are mixed components of cardiac output.

6. **Correct Answer: D**
It is believed that the reflex exists to speed up the heart rate if the right side becomes overloaded, thereby helping to equalize pressures in both sides.

7. **Correct Answer: B**
Some people believe that the heart is virtually static during diastole.
During this period, the cardiac vessels and chambers fill—a process that takes up two-thirds of the time necessary to complete the cardiac cycle.

8. **Correct Answer: A**
The MAP is a mean pressure that takes into account the fact that the diastolic phase accounts for two-thirds of the cardiac cycle. The formula for calculating the MAP is MAP = 2(DBP) + (SBP) / 3. If you took the average of the two pressures, it would not account for the importance of the diastolic phase. The heart rate does not enter into this calculation. Patients should maintain a MAP of at least 60 to ensure adequate perfusion to the brain and kidneys. This calculation is incredibly simple to do and will provide you with early trending information related to your patient.

9. **Correct Answer: C**

   The cardiac index (CI) is a more specific indicator of hemodynamic status than is cardiac output (CO). The CO has a broad range of 4–8 L/min. To make the numbers specific to an individual, their body surface area (BSA) is entered into the equation. Then the normal range becomes 2.5–4.5 L/min/m^2. To perform this calculation, you must first calculate the CO. Then, use the following equation to calculate the CI:

$$CI = CO / BSA$$

10. **Correct Answer: D**

    This pressure represents a mean pressure in the systemic vasculature. The higher the resistance, the harder the heart has to work against it. For example, cold temperatures will cause vasoconstriction; the heart then has to pump harder to deliver blood through the narrowed vasculature.

11. **Correct Answer: B**

    Although the patient may want to be compliant with his plan of care, financial limitations may prohibit him from receiving expensive treatments, medications and support services. If the patient is to start an antiplatelet medication, request from the physician that over-the-counter medications be considered before the use of more expensive brand-name drugs if the patient cannot afford to continue drugs that are started while he is in the hospital. The patient may be better able to afford and continue "baby aspirin" therapy versus Plavix. If brand-name and generic drugs are required, attempt to contact the drug manufacturer and ask about discounts or special programs for low-income patients. Home visits would be paid for by the patient. Follow-up phone calls by the unit staff or case management may prove cost-effective in verifying patient compliance and in answering any questions that the patient has. A cardiology appointment would likely be scheduled earlier than 3 months after discharge to ensure that the patient's plan of care is effective and appropriate for his needs. Although exercise is beneficial, the cost of a gym membership might be prohibitive. Instead, suggest starting a walking club with other friends or neighbors to slowly increase activity while limiting costs. The companionship will improve the patient's physical, psychological, and social health.

12. **Correct Answer: D**

    The exercise stress test requires that the patient walk on a treadmill or ride a stationary bike for at least 30 to 60 minutes. For this patient, that level of activity would be difficult, if not impossible, owing to his decreased mobility and pain. The best choice is to first inform the physician of the patient's stated limitations and request an alternative test. The stress echocardiography uses dobutamine to stress the cardiac tissues without requiring the patient to walk or ride. The Weight-lift test does not exist.

13. **Correct Answer: C**

    Anginal pain usually occurs when approximately 75% of the artery's diameter becomes occluded. Pain is more pronounced with exertion or emotional distress, when oxygen demand by cardiac tissue cannot be met by oxygen supply via the occluded arteries. The severity of pain may be compounded with vasospasms that further restrict blood flow through the coronary arteries.

14. **Correct Answer: D**
S_1 and S_2 are normal sounds. S_3 is associated with fluid status. S_4 is associated with compliance.

15. **Correct Answer: C**
This is the best lead to monitor for RBBB.

16. **Correct Answer: C**
The PR interval may become prolonged. Also, if the potassium level is greater than 8, a wide-complex tachycardia may result. Keep in mind that low levels of calcium or sodium may potentiate the cardiac effects. A low pH may also potentiate the cardiac effects.

17. **Correct Answer: B**
Vecuronium is a paralytic and will prevent shivering. If the patient shivers, her temperature will rise.

18. **Correct Answer: D**
Myocarditis can also present with inspiratory pain. The pain when supine is a cardinal sign of myocarditis. Other findings can include symptoms that are consistent with a respiratory infection and an S_3, S_4, and pericardial friction rub may also be present.

19. **Correct Answer: A**
An endomyocardial biopsy is the only definitive way to diagnose myocarditis.

20. **Correct Answer: B**
Although 50–75 mL is certainly a small amount, the pressure in the intrapericardial space may equal or exceed atrial and ventricular diastolic pressures, causing an acute tamponade.

21. **Correct Answer: D**
Tachycardia is an early sign of tamponade. A narrowed pulse pressure occurs, and fluid cannot be ejected from the heart. The muffled heart sounds occur because the fluid in the sac minimizes the transmission of sound waves.

22. **Correct Answer: B**
Because the heart cannot adequately fill or eject its contents adequately, stroke volume decreases and causes a decreased cardiac output. Contractility decreases because the muscle cannot adequately stretch and, therefore, cannot contract effectively.

23. **Correct Answer: A**
The vena cava is dilated because blood cannot empty into the right atrium. JVD would not be visible on a CXR. The mediastinum would be widened. A CXR will not show delineation of the pericardium or epicardium.

24. **Correct Answer: D**
These symptoms could be caused by mitral stenosis, an ischemic left ventricle, or failure of a left ventricle. The S_3 and S_4 sounds suggest both a fluid problem and a pressure problem.

25. **Correct Answer: C**
Quincke's sign is elicited by pressing down on the fingertip; a visible pulsation is seen in the nail bed. This sign results from a pulse with a rapid, initial hard pulsation, followed by a sudden collapse as blood flows back through an incompetent valve.

26. **Correct Answer: B**

    Hill's sign reflects the rapid rise in pulsation. DeMusset's sign is also found in aortic insufficiency; it consists of the bobbing of the head in time with the forceful pulse. Answers C and D are not diagnostic signs.

27. **Correct Answer: D**

    Treadmill stress testing may miss as many as 40% of cases of single-vessel disease. LV dysfunction may be diagnosed via a thallium test (myocardial scintigraphy). A positive treadmill test may not be positive for CAD.

28. **Correct Answer: C**

    The parameters in answers A, B, and D are all increased.

29. **Correct Answer: A**

    Leads I and aVL will show damage to the higher areas of the lateral wall. Leads V_1 and V_2 will show septal wall damage. Leads V_5 and V_6 will show damage to the apical area.

30. **Correct Answer: D**

    Leads V_4 and R indicate right ventricular damage. Leads V_5 and V_6 indicate apical injury. Leads V_7–V_9 are specific to the posterior wall.

31. **Correct Answer: D**

    Pulsus alternans occurs when a weakened myocardium cannot maintain an even pressure with each contraction. The pulses alternate between strong and weak. This phenomenon is also seen in CHF.

32. **Correct Answer: C**

    The mitral valve is the most common site affected by infective endocarditis. The aortic valve is the next most common valve affected. The valve least likely to be affected by infective endocarditis is the pulmonic valve. The tricuspid valve is often involved secondarily as a result of IV drug abuse.

33. **Correct Answer: D**

    Answers A, B, and C are the effects of beta-adrenergic sympathetic stimulation.

34. **Correct Answer: B**

    Minute changes in the partial pressure of oxygen, pH, and the partial pressure of carbon dioxide result in changes in the heart and respiratory rates. These changes are initiated by the chemoreceptors located in the carotid and aortic bodies.

35. **Correct Answer: C**

    Answer A is the pulmonic area, answer B is the location of the mitral valve, and answer D is the tricuspid area.

36. **Correct Answer: C**

    A body mass index of more than 30 indicates obesity. A BMI in the range of 25–30 means the patient is overweight. In addition, a waist circumference of less than 36 inches is considered normal for females; a waist circumference of less than 41 inches is considered normal for males. To calculate the BMI, use this formula:

    $$\text{BMI} = [(\text{weight in pounds}) \div (\text{height in inches})^2] \times 703$$

37. **Correct Answer: C**
Answers A, B, and D are symptoms of left-sided heart failure. When the right side of the heart fails, it is often due to left-sided failure. The right ventricle cannot adequately pump blood out, so filling pressures rise and the blood backs up, resulting in hepatomegaly. As a consequence, the CVP is elevated. Additional symptoms may include splenomegaly, ascites, abdominal pain, S_3, S_4, and weight gain.

38. **Correct Answer: C**
Nonsteroidal anti-inflammatory drugs (NSAIDs) cause fluid retention and can contribute to renal insufficiency.

39. **Correct Answer: D**
Joe is presenting with chest wall pain, most likely as the result of his having undergone open-heart surgery. Although the pain is expected, to support his recovery and ensure the best possible outcome, the nurse will need to address his pain and discomfort. If left untreated, Joe may not perform deep-breathing exercises or participate fully in physical therapy, placing him at risk for other postoperative complications. Morphine and diazepam will treat both pain and muscle spasms. There is no indication of infection to the wound site, and the pain described by the patient is not consistent with another infarction. EKG changes would most likely be seen. The physician should be contacted if the pain and spasms do not resolve with morphine and diazepam administration or if the pain should present differently with EKG changes.

40. **Correct Answer: B**
The PQRST pain assessment method is used to collect assessment data regarding chest pain in a logical manner that ensures complete assessment data is gathered.
   - The P in the acronym stands for "provokes." Does any activity specifically provoke the pain?
   - Q represents the "quality of the pain." Typical adjectives used include sharp, stabbing, squeezing, pressure, tightness, dull, indigestion-like, and pulsating.
   - R is "radiation," meaning that pain starts at one location and ends at another location. For example, pain may radiate from the chest to the jaw, a specific arm, the back, and/or abdomen.
   - S stands for "severity of the pain." Some patients may have altered pain sensation from other disease processes such as diabetes, neuropathies, and multiple scleroses and may not present with typical symptoms for a myocardial infarction.
   - T stands for "time." The duration of the pain is important when considering antithrombolytics as treatment, as this is highly time sensitive and will impact success of the treatment.

41. **Correct Answer: A**
Answers B, C, and D are relative contraindications. Additional absolute contraindications include hypertension and bleeding disorders.

42. **Correct Answer: C**
Answers A, B, and D are effects of phenytoin, another Class 1B drug. Lidocaine may shorten the QT interval. Its side effects usually involve the CNS—slurred speech, drowsiness, confusion, paresthesias, seizures, and convulsions.

43. **Correct Answer: D**

    The high iodine content can actually exert an effect on the thyroid, thereby producing an antiarrhythmic action.

44. **Correct Answer: D**

    Amiodarone and quinidine are antiarrhythmics. Clonidine is an antihypertensive. Adenosine is a naturally occurring substance in the body and has a very short half-life (only a few seconds). Adenosine slows AV nodal conduction or can stop the conduction process altogether, potentially causing a transient AV block (seen as asystole). The patient may experience mild to moderate chest discomfort, slight hypotension, brady-cardia, and possibly flushing.

45. **Correct Answer: A**

    The QT interval may be prolonged by administration of tricyclic antidepressants, erythromycin, quinidine, or terfenidine. Magnesium acts on the processes by which calcium is transferred both across the cell membrane and within the cell itself. If high doses of magnesium are given, it may slow AV conduction.

46. **Correct Answer: B**

    Large-lumen vessels in the arterial system are affected. The advantage of this action is that both systolic and diastolic pressures are reduced and the patient will not have a pre-cipitous drop in blood pressure. The blood pressure may be lowered slightly and cause a reflex baroreceptor response to speed up the heart rate to maintain cardiac output.

47. **Correct Answer: C**

    The S_4 heart sound is also known as an atrial gallop. When the atria contract and fill the ventricle, there is naturally some resistance to that pressure, as the ventricle is already about 80% full. If the patient has a problem such as hypertension, an MI, an anginal episode, or aortic stenosis, the S_4 sound may become quite pronounced.

48. **Correct Answer: B**

    A heart murmur is a sound produced by turbulent blood flow. By definition, a systolic murmur would be heard during systole, when the ventricles are contracting. The mitral and tricuspid valves should be closed during this phase of the cardiac cycle. If these valves are incompetent (insufficiency), blood will flow back through the valve (regurgitation). Thus, pulmonic and aortic stenosis, and mitral and tricuspid insuffi-ciency, are systolic murmurs.

49. **Correct Answer: B**

    By definition, "pansystolic" means that the murmur is heard throughout systole. The only systolic murmur listed is tricuspid insufficiency. All the other answers are dias-tolic murmurs.

50. **Correct Answer: B**

    Pericarditis results in inflamed layers of the pericardial sac. Deep respirations, trunk rotation and flat positioning allow the parietal and visceral layers of the pericardial sac greater ability to rub against each other. Upright and forward positioning pulls the heart away from the diaphragmatic pleura of the lungs and eases the cardiac pain.

51. **Correct Answer: C**

    Systemic lupus erythematosus (SLE) is a chronic inflammatory autoimmune disease that affects the vascular and connective tissues within any body system and organ.

As a result of the disease, inflammation may be increased and the stress of injury would further exacerbate the SLE. Symptoms and conditions to monitor closely for include pericarditis, hypertension, diarrhea, thrombocytopenia, anemia, leucopenia, joint and muscle pain, vasculitis, proteinurea, seizures, depression, pneumonia, pleural effusions, nausea, and ulcers.

52. **Correct Answer: C**
Answers A, B, and D cause only a moderate rise in INR. Other drugs that significantly raise the INR include aspirin, sulfonamides, cimetidine, fluoroquinolones, and macrolide antibiotics.

53. **Correct Answer: B**
Answers A, C, and D decrease the INR only moderately. Other drugs that significantly decrease the INR include rifampin, phenobarbital, and glutethimide. Vitamin K is widely used as an antidote for warfarin, but can actually decrease the INR too much and increase warfarin resistance, so careful monitoring is critical. Warfarin breakdown is also accelerated by barbiturates.

54. **Correct Answer: B**
Necrotic tissue cannot conduct an impulse. Ischemic tissue may impair conduction. If the patient were hypokalemic, the energy level (mA) would have to be raised because a low potassium level depresses the myocardium.

55. **Correct Answer: D**
The MI has impaired the heart's ability to pump effectively. The cardiac output falls and the body reacts by vasoconstricting peripheral circulation and increasing the heart rate. Tachycardia is also the result of catecholamine release, and the myocardial oxygen consumption increases. The left ventricle works harder, but has been compromised by the MI. Preload increases because fluid cannot be pumped out of the chambers effectively. The S_3 is a signal of increased preload. Pulmonary congestion occurs due to increased left heart pressures.

56. **Correct Answer: C**
A new holosystolic murmur at the lower left sternal border means that turbulent blood flow is occurring there. The turbulence is caused by a hole that is allowing blood to flow through a previously closed area. The SvO_2 will increase due to the mixing of blood. This condition must be corrected surgically.

57. **Correct Answer: A**
The CXR will probably show a pericardial effusion. The elevated sed rate and WBCs indicate infection. In pericarditis, leaning forward often relieves chest pain, whereas lying supine makes it worse. If the pain worsens on inspiration, it is because the lungs expand and come in contact with the pericardium. The patient will probably also have a fever. It is necessary to assess for any signs of cardiac tamponade and to make certain anticoagulants are discontinued.

58. **Correct Answer: C**
New evidence suggests that an ejection fraction of 35% or less may predispose an individual to sudden cardiac death. A low ejection fraction and existing CAD mean the likelihood of a cardiac event is increased. Generally, if an individual has disease in the left main artery, any three vessels, or the proximal LAD with one additional vessel, he

or she is a candidate for a CABG. Emergent conditions for a CABG include MI with shock or refractory pain or unstable angina. Patients who dissect during a stent placement require immediate surgery.

59. **Correct Answer: A**
The new AHA guidelines specify that ventilation should occur every 6 to 8 seconds. The compressions should continue at a rate of 100. The recommended ventilation rate approximates a normal adult rate and allows for cardiac fill. Ventilating too fast raises intrathoracic pressure and interferes with cardiac fill.

60. **Correct Answer: D**
Two hundred joules on a biphasic defibrillator is as effective as 360 joules on a monophasic defibrillator. The purpose of defibrillation is to deliver enough electricity to cause a large enough mass of myocardium to depolarize simultaneously. If that occurs, it is then possible for a normal rhythm to reemerge or become the primary rhythm. It is important to identify the initial cause of the dysrhythmia and treat it, if possible, to prevent recurrence.

61. **Correct Answer: B**
Acute pericarditis is usually self-limiting within 2 to 6 weeks after its onset. Treatment includes bed rest, oxygen therapy, antiviral, antifungal, or antibacterial agents. In addition, drainage and management of cardiac tamponade may be necessary. The classic presentation of chronic pericarditis (also known as constrictive pericarditis) demonstrates fibrous pericardial thickening. Treatment may include the extreme measure of pericardiotomy (removal of the pericardium).

62. **Correct Answer: B**
Wellen's syndrome is a type of angina that occurs when the LAD is stenosed proximally. The ST segment is not elevated more than 1 mm in leads V_1–V_3, there is mild T wave inversion in leads V_2–V_3, and Q waves are not pathologic (greater than 25% of the total length). Because of the location of the stenosis, surgery is required emergently.

Variant angina is another name for Prinzmetal's angina; in this type of angina, the pain occurs at rest and is associated with vasospasm. Crescendo angina means that over time it takes less to initiate the pain and the pain lasts longer.

63. **Correct Answer: D**
Nitroglycerin is a vasodilator for both arterial and venous systems. Sometimes the diseased coronary vessels are stiff and calcified. If the patient has good collateral circulation, oxygen and blood can reach the ischemic areas. Nitroglycerin is now available in a metered-dose oral spray, in addition to pressed tablets, paste, and intravenous (nitroprusside) formulations.

64. **Correct Answer: B**
An infarct in the left main coronary artery is an ominous sign. Sudden death may occur, along with heart blocks and atrial and ventricular dysrhythmias.

65. **Correct Answer: D**
In a chronic condition, as much as 2,000 mL of fluid may collect in the pericardial sac before symptoms appear. This fluid buildup is usually due to a chronic pleural effusion or uremia. Acute tamponade may occur when as little as 50 mL of fluid collects in the pericardial sac.

66. **Correct Answer: B**

    The classic description of the CXR associated with pericardial effusion is the "water bottle" silhouette. QRS amplitude is decreased, as is diastolic filling.

67. **Correct Answer: A**

    Hypovolemia and sepsis decrease afterload, as does aortic insufficiency. Aortic stenosis increases afterload, as do peripheral vasoconstriction and hypertension.

68. **Correct Answer: C**

    A pressure of at least 50 mm Hg is required to maintain auto-regulatory control.

69. **Correct Answer: D**

    Renin (a protease) will be secreted if the sodium concentration falls, sympathetic output increases, or blood pressure decreases. Blood pressure may be lowered by diuretics, hemorrhage, dehydration, or sodium depletion. Something as simple as NG tube drainage can decrease blood pressure, so in any setting it is critical to maintain accurate intake and output.

70. **Correct Answer: C**

    Pulsus paradoxus may be present in conjunction with asthma, emphysema, cardiac tamponade, restrictive pericarditis, or hemorrhagic shock. Pulse pressure is the difference between systolic and diastolic blood pressure. Pulsus parvus means a small or weak pulse. Pulsus alternans means the upstroke is more powerful than the downstroke—that is, the stroke alternates in strength.

71. **Correct Answer: B**

    Visitation policies vary by institution. However, it is best to identify one person as the point of contact. HIPAA regulations require limitations on the release of any medical information be set by the patient if the patient is able to communicate his or her wishes. If the patient is unable to make this decision, the next of kin can act as a contact person.

72. **Correct Answer: A**

    The best response would be to respond collaboratively and interact with other professionals.

73. **Correct Answer: D**

    The religious preference of the patient must be respected. The only acceptable form of transfusion in this case is via auto-transfusion.

74. **Correct Answer: B**

    Utilizing the internal mammary artery means grafts do not have to come from the saphenous veins in the leg, minimizing the risk for infection from another site. In the graft procedure, the internal mammary artery is separated at only one end and reanastomosed to the affected coronary artery distal to the affected area. The patency of the resulting graft is generally quite good. After 10 years, approximately 90% of grafts are still patent.

75. **Correct Answer: A**

    Iodine dye is used and will cause a rash, itching, swelling, and can also lead to laryngospasm and anaphylaxis in some patients. It is imperative to determine whether the patient is allergic to iodine, shellfish, or horses prior to initiating the procedure.

76. **Correct Answer: A**

    Along with acute ST elevation, another indicator of necrosis would be an abnormal Q wave. If the Q wave appears within about six hours of a transmural MI, it is an ominous sign. If the Q wave is more than 0.04 seconds long, it is a sign of necrosis. In an inferior MI, the Q wave should not exceed 0.03 seconds or it is indicative of necrosis.

77. **Correct Answer: C**

    The antagonist for morphine or other opioids is Narcan (naloxone). Generally, the naloxone dose is 0.4 mg IV. This dose can be repeated about every 3 to 4 minutes for a total of three times. When you give Narcan, you must always be alert for the patient to relapse once the dose wears off. Administering multiple follow-up doses is not uncommon.

78. **Correct Answer: A**

    Answers B, C, and D are complications of an intra-aortic balloon pump (IABP). Additional complications that are commonly seen with VADs include infection and bleeding.

79. **Correct Answer: B**

    Prolonged cardiac arrest, especially with neurological damage, is a contraindication to use of a VAD. Extensive organ damage is another contraindication. VADs are not indicated for dysrhythmias. Other indications for a VAD include use as a bridge to transplant, treatment of cardiogenic shock, and inability to wean from cardiopulmonary bypass. Always be aware of the possibility of device failure.

80. **Correct Answer: C**

    Pneumonia secondary to immobility is the primary reason for infection with VADs. There may also exist a need for some type of ventilatory support. Just the fact that tubes are placed into the body is a potential source of infection, but this is usually minimized by good hand washing and aseptic technique.

81. **Correct Answer: D**

    The left ventricular assist device is the most commonly used because left heart failure is more common and usually precedes right ventricular failure.

82. **Correct Answer: C**

    Quite often, the patient develops cardiogenic shock and requires emergent placement of a VAD. If the nurse is able to at least explain the function of the device, it can be a great relief to the family.

83. **Correct Answer: B**

    The patient is approaching crisis and may feel hopeless. The nurse should take the time to fully explore and validate the patient's feelings, then decide on the appropriate course of action.

84. **Correct Answer: D**

    If the patient is bleeding, the blood may settle into the lumbar area. Blood is heavy and will flow into the retroperitoneal area because of gravity. More than an hour may pass and several hundred milliliters of blood may be lost before vital signs are affected.

85. **Correct Answer: D**

    The aortogram is the established standard for definitive diagnosis of aortic dissection and is the only invasive procedure listed as an option for this question. This test is sometimes called an aortic angiogram with (radiopaque) contrast dye.

86. **Correct Answer: B**
    Men (70%) definitely have more aneurysms than women (30%). Aortic regurgitation is often a cause for an aneurysm, not stenosis. Advanced age contributes to mortality, with younger patients having a better chance of survival.

87. **Correct Answer: A**
    Quite often the patient will describe a ripping or tearing sensation and severe pain. Hypotension may be present as the dissection progresses. Warning signs include hypertension, a new murmur (aortic insufficiency), weak peripheral pulses, and possible deterioration of level of consciousness. Aneurysms that dissect downward radiate pain to the lower abdomen, lower back, and legs.

88. **Correct Answer: B**
    Any aortic aneurysm that extends over 4 cm will need surgical repair. Other criteria for immediate repair include impending rupture, limb ischemia, uncontrolled pain, cardiac tamponade, and increasing size.

89. **Correct Answer: A**
    The inner layer of the vessel becomes separated, and blood enters the area under pressure.

90. **Correct Answer: B**
    The abdominal area is most commonly affected and usually offers good surgical access. Aneurysms in the aortic arch are sometimes not accessible surgically and may pose a high risk of dissection during procedures intended to mitigate them.

91. **Correct Answer: C**
    The P wave represents depolarization of the atrium and the QRS the depolarization of the ventricles; the size difference is related to the muscle mass involved in the polarization. The P wave's amplitude represents the amount or size of the muscle mass involved in the depolarization of the atrium. The QRS wave represents the amount or size of the muscle mass involved in the depolarization of the ventricles. The greater the muscle mass, the greater the change in amplitude. Non-patient-related factors that may affect these waves' amplitude include gain setting, lead placement, and interference. Patient-related factors may include electrolyte imbalances, hypertrophy, and cardiac injury.

92. **Correct Answer: A**
    Obstructive jaundice may lead to cardiac changes, including sinus bradycardia.

93. **Correct Answer: B**
    Patients with heart transplants do not feel cardiac pain because the heart has been denervated.

94. **Correct Answer: D**
    Rheumatic fever remains the most common cause of acquired valvular disease. The valves are a perfect place for bacteria to colonize, and blood is a perfect medium for bacterial growth. The causative organism is beta-hemolytic *Streptococcus.*

95. **Correct Answer: B**
    When the heart is denervated, it has no connection to the autonomic nervous system, so a reflexive response does not occur. A sympathetic stimulant must be used to provide this response. If no other complications occur, the ventricle will eventually adjust to not receiving autonomic input.

96. **Correct Answer: C**

    All of the other conditions listed as options may contribute to an aneurysm, but hypertension remains the primary cause of dissecting aneurysms. Constant pressure on the vessel walls will weaken the vessel over time.

97. **Correct Answer: A**

    Pain is a cardinal sign of an arterial obstruction. The nurse should check for pallor, other signs of an arterial blockage, sensation, and quality of pulses. If the obstruction is venous, the limb may exhibit cyanosis.

98. **Correct Answer: D**

    The pericardial sac usually contains 20–25 mL of pericardial fluid. This fluid is secreted and reabsorbed, acting as a lubricant between the parietal and visceral pericardial layers.

99. **Correct Answer: B**

    Reperfusion rhythms such as ventricular tachycardia, sinus bradycardia, accelerated idioventricular rhythm, and underlying sinus rhythms with ventricular ectopy may occur. The patient should experience less chest pain. The CPK isoenzymes may temporarily become elevated as blood flows freely through newly opened arteries. CHF is not a result of this therapy.

100. **Correct Answer: C**

    Family members are probably quite used to providing care for this patient. Do not ignore the patient. There is no point in speaking slowly unless the caregiver or the patient has difficulty understanding your instructions. Teaching quickly is counterproductive and may be considered rude and unprofessional. Allow time for a return demonstration of skills and allow for questions.

101. **Correct Answer: C**

    You should feel only a mild tingling sensation. You should not fear this device to the point of not performing CPR, and CPR should not be delayed in any event. If the ICD fires, anyone touching the patient at that moment may feel the tingling sensation.

102. **Correct Answer: D**

    Biphasic defibrillation works by sending electricity from cathode to anode, and then reversing the current. It takes less energy to cause mass depolarization of the myocardium. Cardioversion is much more successful as well. Both defibrillation and cardioversion take less energy to convert patients. Be certain to follow the latest American Heart Association guidelines when using these devices.

103. **Correct Answer: A**

    The ICD should be set 10 joules above the defibrillation threshold on at least two successive attempts. The threshold varies from patient to patient and depends on the patient's current catecholamine levels. The standard is to set the ICD to 10 joules above the defibrillation threshold. Some physicians routinely set the ICD to 10 joules below the maximum output. This practice saves time, but does not really fine-tune the ICD to the patient.

104. **Correct Answer: B**

    The magnet is used to inhibit the shocking (tachy) feature of the ICD. It can shut down a malfunctioning ICD. Patient teaching includes letting the patient know the dangers of being in proximity to large magnets. Most ICDs have a warning tone built in so that if the patient comes too near a magnet, the tone is emitted. The type of tone produced varies with the device's manufacturer.

105. **Correct Answer: B**
These waves actually heat the tissue around the active sites and prevent reentry loop. Once the temperature reaches 50°C, cell damage and death occur. The continuing heat creates a lesion approximately 2–5 mm in diameter. This "burned" area causes necrosis and will not conduct electricity.

106. **Correct Answer: D**
Ibutilide is a relatively new Class III/IV medication. It must be used at the time of the cardioversion and will be ineffective if used prior to the cardioversion.

107. **Correct Answer: A**
Chronic pericarditis presents as chronic right-sided heart failure caused by increased systemic venous pressures, fluid retention, ascites, and hepatomegaly. Many of the symptoms relate to restrictive cardiac tamponade accompanied by decreased forward blood flow and altered cardiac contraction.

108. **Correct Answer: C**
Renal failure and sepsis may lead to pericarditis, so A.M. lab results should show an increased WBC, increased ESR, cardiac tissue involvement, and an elevated CK-MB level. An additional lab test would focus on detecting uremia. Assessment would also include checking for ST-segment elevation, arrhythmias, and pleural effusions on echocardiography.

109. **Correct Answer: A**
Coxsackievirus is the most common cause of myocarditis, although any bacterial, viral, or fungal pathogen may be the initial infectious agent.

110. **Correct Answer: C**
If the catheter is in the right ventricle and touches the myocardium, PVCs can result. Occasionally, the physician will insert the catheter a bit too far, causing PVCs. In this case, the catheter simply has to be withdrawn to a better position in the right atrium. This is a rare occurrence. If the patient's catheter was left in the right ventricle, the V-tach might continue and the patient might suffer cardiac arrest.

111. **Correct Answer: C**
Silent infarcts account for approximately 20% of myocardial infarctions. Silent infarcts are often seen in patients who present atypically, such as elderly individuals and persons with diabetes.

112. **Correct Answer: A**
The circumflex coronary artery feeds the left atrium and left ventricle. Infarctions as a result of occlusion of this artery result in lateral or left-sided heart damage. The left anterior descending artery and the circumflex artery both branch off from the left coronary artery.

113. **Correct Answer: B**
New-onset or acute mitral valve regurgitation is often a result of myocardial infarction of the left anterior descending and circumflex arteries. These arteries feed the papillary muscles, which in turn support mitral valve function. Prolonged ischemia causes the

papillary and/or chordae tendinae of the mitral valve to rupture and prevent full closure of the mitral valve during systole. As the blood flows back into the left atrium, the murmur can be auscultated.

114. **Correct Answer: A**

Gina has endocarditis. It is thought that microvascular clots form in the heart and pass through the microcirculation and impede peripheral circulation, sometimes causing necrosis (i.e., Janeway lesions, Osler's nodes, and Roth spots). Janeway lesions are flat and painless erythematous areas typically found on the palms and soles of the feet. Osler's nodes are small, painful nodules found on the fingers and toes. Roth spots are rounded, white spots seen when examining the retina. Pella's sign is not a medical term.

115. **Correct Answer: B**

Stage I disease (pathological arterial changes) produces no symptoms. Stage II is representative of a 75% occlusion and the patient will exhibit intermittent claudication. Stage III represents a 90–95% occlusion and the patient will have pain at rest. Stage IV is a 99–100% occlusion that will result in necrosis if not treated.

116. **Correct Answer: C**

Patients with peripheral vascular disease are often hypothermic because of poor circulation. Healing is also slowed because of the decrease in circulation. The nurse should provide proper alignment without impeding circulation and monitor the patient's peripheral pulses for presence and quality. The color and temperature of the extremity should be monitored and results charted.

117. **Correct Answer: B**

A primary goal in cardiogenic shock is to improve the pumping action of the heart (improve myocardial contractility), reduce the workload of the heart, reduce oxygen demand, and improve cardiac output. If possible, systemic vascular resistance should be decreased and the left ventricle augmented with an inotrope. Nitroprusside will reduce preload and afterload. The cardiac workload and the myocardial oxygen demand should decrease.

118. **Correct Answer: C**

Mitral valve stenosis presents with a low-pitched murmur that can be heard during diastole and that does not radiate. Mitral valve regurgitation presents with a high-pitched murmur that is heard during systole that may radiate to the left arm. If severe, both conditions present with symptoms of pulmonary edema, low cardiac output, and heart failure.

119. **Correct Answer: C**

The first step is to check the sensitivity control. Even though most of these pacemakers have a cover, the dial may have been moved and indicate that a fixed rate is set. If the pacer continues to fire, it may cause R-on-T phenomenon and cause ventricular tachycardia or fibrillation. If the patient has an adequate rhythm, you can turn off the pacer and notify the physician. If the patient has a non-sustaining rhythm, try positioning the patient on the left side to see if the wire will come in contact with the myocardium. You can also try turning up the mA level. Either way, the physician must be notified and vital signs carefully monitored until the physician can reposition the electrodes.

120. **Correct Answer: C**
During ventricular diastole, both the aortic and pulmonic valves close. If a valve is incompetent, the blood will flow backward through the valve, creating turbulent blood flow—that is, a murmur.

121. **Correct Answer: B**
During diastole, the tricuspid and mitral valves close just prior to systole. If the valve is stenotic, it will not close completely. When the atria contract, a murmur is heard as blood goes through this narrow opening.

122. **Correct Answer: A**
The injuries to the patient's chest may have caused a pulmonary artery laceration or a cardiac contusion (the latter condition is more likely). His blood pressure is low and the EKG shows ST-segment elevation in the anterior leads. If the myocardium is contused, it will react the same way as if an MI had occurred. The ST elevation may be the result of a physiologic insult to a coronary artery, and an area of the myocardium may be ischemic. If so, the pumping function of the myocardium will be compromised and may need additional support with inotropes. The patient may undergo angiography and/or surgery. Volume replacement may be necessary. This patient is probably in the first stage of cardiogenic shock.

123. **Correct Answer: D**
Approximately 24 hours after a surgical procedure, the release of inflammatory cell mediators can lead to vasodilation. Gertrude has a permanent pacemaker, but apparently her heart rate cannot compensate for the drop in blood pressure. The cardiac output did not increase as a result of the reduced systemic resistance. Her pacemaker did not allow the heart rate to climb above 70. The dobutamine acted on the pump and increased the heart's contractility. Gertrude also has a history of a previous MI.

124. **Correct Answer: D**
Turning up the rate should allow for weaning off dobutamine. This patient is also in the beginning stage of cardiogenic shock, but she can easily be helped by simply changing the rate on the pacemaker. We are noticing that more progressive care areas are using dobutamine, but at this time its use is not emphasized on the PCCN exam. Even so, you should be knowledgeable about this drug and the process of weaning.

125. **Correct Answer: C**
AICDs may be implanted in patients with recurrent ventricular tachycardia. They can also be programmed to act as pacemakers.

126. **Correct Answer: A**
Matthew has probably dislodged a lead, or the lead may have been damaged on insertion. Either way, Matthew needs either a new AICD or new leads.

127. **Correct Answer: C**
Carotid bruit is the significant physical finding associated with carotid stenosis. Heberden's nodules and Broussard's nodules are both seen with arthritis. The systolic murmur is an indication of a valvular problem.

128. **Correct Answer: B**
This patient needs a pacemaker or AICD that can deliver a more powerful impulse. The asynchronous mode will override Barry's internal pacemaker.

129. **Correct Answer: B**

    A dual-lead pacemaker/AICD is necessary to maintain the atrial kick. Single-chamber pacing can lead to pacemaker syndrome. The letters on pacemaker modes are interpreted as follows:

Chamber Paced	Chamber Sensed	Mode of Response	Programmability, Rate Modulation	Anti-tachycardia/ Anti-arrhythmia Function
V = Ventricle	V = Ventricle	I = Inhibit	P = Simple programmable	P = Pacing
A = Atrium	A = Atrium	T = Triggered	M = Multi-programmable	S = Shock
D = Dual chamber	D = Dual chamber	D = Dual (T & I)	R = Rate modulation	Dual = Dual (P & S)

130. **Correct Answer: C**

    Pacemaker syndrome is caused by a loss of atrial kick or regurgitation against a closed A-V valve. Gene's atrial lead may be damaged or may have failed.

131. **Correct Answer: A**

    The most important action is to improve the cardiovascular status of this patient. A patient with a transcutaneous pacemaker must be sedated for comfort. The physician must be notified for a possible transvenous or permanent pacemaker insertion. It would be acceptable to give the patient atropine for this condition, but not at the dose listed in answer B.

132. **Correct Answer: B**

    Because your patient has lost two of the three main fascicles that innervate the heart, he is at great risk for sudden death. He needs a pacemaker as soon as possible.

133. **Correct Answer: B**

    Changes in leads V_2, V_3, V_4, I, and AVL are indicative of an anterolateral MI. The MI could also be detected in V_5, and V_6, which are also lateral leads.

134. **Correct Answer: C**

    When tissue dies as a result of myocardial infarction, it becomes electrically dead, causing the opposing energy to become the dominant feature. Partial-thickness myocardial death would be classified as a non-Q wave MI.

135. **Correct Answer: A**

    You would identify an inferior wall MI in leads II, III, and AVF.

136. **Correct Answer: A**

    An anteroseptal MI is seen in leads V_1, V_2, V_3, and V_4. The septal leads are V_1 and V_2. The anterior leads, which overlap, are V_2, V_3, and V_4.

137. **Correct Answer: B**

    The vertical lines on the EKG graph paper represent time. When conduction defects occur, the tracings are wider because it takes more time to travel the same distance.

138. **Correct Answer: C**

Voltage is measured by the horizontal lines on the EKG graph paper. If a ventricle is enlarged, a larger voltage will be apparent on the 12-lead EKG.

139. **Correct Answer: A**

Leads V_1 and V_2 show right bundle branch blocks. A simple way to remember the type of bundle branch block with a QRS wider than 0.12 seconds is to think of the turn signals on your car. For a right turn, you must push the lever up; for a left turn, you must push the lever down. So, when looking at leads V_1, and V_2, if the QRS is upright, then there is a right bundle branch block. If V_1, and V_2 are downward in force, then the patient has a left bundle branch block.

140. **Correct Answer: B**

Rate, rhythm, axis, hypertrophy, and infarction are the most valuable areas examined in a 12-lead EKG.

141. **Correct Answer: A**

Ventricular hypertrophy, pericarditis, and COPD all create ST/T wave abnormalities on the 12-lead EKG.

142. **Correct Answer: C**

COPD causes changes in the 12-lead EKG due to the workload for the right side of the heart. Changes commonly seen in patients with COPD include tall, peaked P waves, right axis deviation, right ventricular hypertrophy, and low-voltage QRS.

143. **Correct Answer: B**

There are multiple reasons for pacemaker insertion—for example, symptomatic bradycardia, bradycardia with escape beats, overdrive pacing, bradycardia/arrest, acute MI with sinus dysfunction, Mobtiz type II, complete heart block, and development of a new bundle branch block.

144. **Correct Answer: A**

Quinidine and hypomagnesemia can lead to Torsades de Pointes—a recurrent ventricular tachycardia that turns on its axis every 6 to 8 beats, giving the EKG a twisting or "turning on point" look. Hypomagnesemia can occur when the patient receives total parenteral nutrition.

145. **Correct Answer: D**

Hospitalization for more than 2 days is required for a diagnosis of hospital-acquired pneumonia (HAP). If pneumonia occurs prior to 2 days' stay in the hospital, the infection is considered to be a community-acquired pneumonia. HAP is especially dangerous in a cardiac patient, but can be prevented most of the time via hand washing and aseptic technique.

146. **Correct Answer: B**

Pseudomonas aeruginosa is the organism most commonly implicated in HAP. Methicillin-resistant *Staphylococcus aureus* is the second most common cause of HAP. Cardiac patients are usually already quite compromised and susceptible to these organisms.

147. **Correct Answer: C**

Factors associated with higher risk of HAP include altered level of consciousness, placement of a nasogastric tube, the elderly, COPD, postoperative patients, use of H_2 blockers, antacids, periodontal work, and acute illness or injury.

148. **Correct Answer: B**

Millie's age, time in the hospital, nasogastric tube, and use of antacids are all risk factors for HAP. The fact that her chest x-ray is inconclusive is not unusual with elderly patients. Elderly patients often have other underlying diseases that make it difficult to identify pneumonia.

149. **Correct Answer: C**

The major difference between HAP and VAP is that the patient who develops VAP is intubated. Both types of pneumonia are caused by the same organism, *Pseudomonas aeruginosa.*

150. **Correct Answer: B**

SVO_2 measures the oxygen saturation of venous blood as it returns to the lungs for oxygenation. Normal SVO_2 is in the range of 60–80%. This percentage decreases as lung function worsens, meaning the blood leaving the left ventricle has less oxygen to deliver in the first place.

151. **Correct Answer: A**

The SVO_2 shows shunting. There is a normal 5% physiologic shunt due to blood in the bronchial, pleural and Thebesian veins. When there is infection, trauma, or ARDS, blood is shunted at a higher rate, which is seen as a lower SVO_2 level.

152. **Correct Answer: C**

The patient's shunt is worsening. A chest x-ray should also be done to assess his pneumo-hemothorax for possible increase in size. His chest tube drainage system should be examined for the possibility of clots blocking drainage. The patient will probably be transferred to the ICU and placed on a ventilator.

153. **Correct Answer: B**

Concomitant use of promethazine and fluoroquinolones is contraindicated because their combination can produce prolongation of the QT interval and increase the patient's risk of arrhythmias.

154. **Correct Answer: B**

The infusion rate should not exceed 4 mg/min. A rate faster than 4 mg/min may result in tinnitus or hearing loss.

155. **Correct Answer: D**

Too-rapid infusion of Lasix can cause tinnitus and hearing loss.

156. **Correct Answer: A**

Dong quai, gingko biloba, and ginseng can all increase bleeding times. Saw palmetto decreases the effectiveness of Plavix.

157. **Correct Answer: B**

Reo Pro, like any platelet inhibitor, requires that the patient be carefully questioned about any bleeding history.

158. **Correct Answer: B**

DVT, atrial fibrillation, heart valve replacements, and myocardial infarction are conditions that require the use of warfarin. Patients with DVT, atrial fibrillation, and heart valve replacements will take warfarin on a chronic basis. By comparison, MI patients may be weaned off warfarin in 3 to 4 months.

159. **Correct Answer: A**
Many foods must be avoided when the patient is taking warfarin. Specifically, patients must avoid foods that have high vitamin K: broccoli, Brussels sprouts, cabbage, spinach, turnip greens, endive, scallions, parsley, red leaf lettuce, watercress, soybean, canola, and salad oils. All of these foods decrease the effectiveness of warfarin.

160. **Correct Answer: C**
Integrilin (eptifbatide) is used primarily for patients with acute coronary syndrome to inhibit platelet aggregation.

161. **Correct Answer: D**
If the conversation is not hushed and you overhear the statement as part of your regular duties, it would be appropriate to clarify or correct misinformation if it would not involve diagnosing the patient's disease process. In this case, the patient provides you an opportunity to teach him about his cardiac murmur. Aortic stenosis will cause a murmur, but the harshness or degree of auscultation is not directly correlated with the degree of severity or risk to the patient. Based on his statement, he may not understand what a diagnosis of aortic stenosis entails. By asking about his comprehension, you will be able to determine what his degree of understanding is, which knowledge you may correct or clarify, and to what degree his physician may need to discuss his prognosis or plan of care.

162. **Correct Answer: C**
Aortic stenosis is directly caused by decreased blood flow to the coronary arteries during systole due to the stenotic valve. Prolonged resistance to blood flow via the stenotic aortic valve results in left ventricular hypertrophy and left-sided heart failure. The prognosis is poor unless the aortic valve is replaced.

163. **Correct Answer: B**
Mr. B. would exhibit signs and symptoms of hypercalcemia, confirmed by his lab value of 13.5 mg/dL. Signs and symptoms would include smooth-muscle relaxation, lethargy, confusion, shortened QT interval, bradycardia, heart blocks, bundle branch blocks, and hypertension. Symptoms can be further compounded by the effects of digitalis and, possibly, digitalis toxicity.

164. **Correct Answer: A**
Due to the decreased availability of calcium essential to the coagulation phase (used within the intrinsic, extrinsic and common pathways), the patient will not have formed permanent clots. The platelet plugs formed over damaged vessels initially after surgery may be dislodged by blood flow, leading to recurrent bleeding at postoperative days 7 to 10.

165. **Correct Answer: C**
Heparin impairs Factor II in the clotting cascade. The vial provided by pharmacy is more than 100 times the normal dose for a heparin lock flush (the normal dose is 10 units/mL or 100 units/mL). It is imperative that the order be compared to the medication received prior to administration to prevent serious medication errors. A heparin overdose may result in cardiac arrhythmias, seizures, coma, agitation, fever, thermal fluctuations, blood pressure instability, and severe bleeding. Factors I, V, and VIII are impaired in DIC and fibrinolysis. Factor VIII complications are related to autoimmune disorders. Impaired Factors II, VII, IX, X, and XI are seen with vitamin K deficiencies and Coumadin (warfarin) administration.

166. **Correct Answer: B**
Amyloidosis is another cause of restrictive cardiomyopathy. The myocardium (especially the left ventricle) becomes rigid from fibrosis, which results in inadequate left ventricular filling and increased atrial dilatation. Left ventricular diastolic dysfunction occurs, but systolic function remains normal in this type of cardiomyopathy. Fluid backs up into the lungs, and the patient looks as if he or she has congestive heart failure. There is no cure for restrictive cardiomyopathy; instead, symptoms are treated as they occur.

167. **Correct Answer: C**
"Arrhythmogenic" is a relatively new classification for cardiomyopathy. In this condition, the normal myocardial cells are replaced by fatty tissue and fibrous tissue. The right ventricle is primarily affected. Conduction cannot occur normally, so the patient will have multiple ventricular arrhythmias and right ventricular failure. Young people with arrhythmogenic cardiomyopathy are at risk for sudden death. The cause of this condition is unknown, but some research has shown a possible link to an autosomal dominant gene.

168. **Correct Answer: B**
In hypertrophic cardiomyopathy, the myocardium thickens, but it is not symmetrical. Specifically, there is more thickening of the ventricular septum than of the ventricle. If you were to look at a heart with this condition, it could appear normal externally. When the septum is thicker, it creates a hyperdynamic state by increasing contractility, so the ejection fraction is increased. In rare conditions where the septum is asymmetrically thickened, then the left ventricular outflow will be impaired, so the cardiac output will be decreased.

169. **Correct Answer: A**
The exact causes of this condition are unknown, but a large number of alcoholics develop dilated cardiomyopathy. Three possible reasons for this link have been identified:
  • The alcohol itself, or the metabolites, may have a toxic effect.
  • Alcohol sometimes contains additives, such as cobalt.
  • The cause may be nutritional in origin, such as a thiamine deficiency.
New research shows that a viral link between chronic alcoholism and dilated cardiomyopathy may exist.
Interestingly, this type of cardiomyopathy may potentially reverse itself if the drinking is stopped. Other types of cardiomyopathy are not reversible.

170. **Correct Answer: D**
Peripartum cardiomyopathy develops during the first three to four months after completion of pregnancy. Sometimes the cause is myocarditis.

171. **Correct Answer: A**
Dilated cardiomyopathy causes systolic dysfunction. As a result, you will hear S_3 and S_4 gallops and the EKG may show atrial fibrillation, ventricular dysrhythmias, or sinus tachycardia most of the time. The patient may have a systolic murmur of the AV valves. In addition, the patient will probably have peripheral edema or ascites, hepatomegaly, and pale, cool extremities. Changes in mentation are possible as well. Hypertrophic and restrictive cardiomyopathies are diastolic dysfunctions.

172. **Correct Answer: D**

Atrial fibrillation is the result of the constant stretching and disruption of normal pathways in the atrium due to increased preload produced by the pulmonary congestion.

173. **Correct Answer: C**

The nurse would monitor the patient's vital signs. This family is so eager to help the patient, and they would probably have someone at the bedside many hours during the day. Any change in mentation is very significant, and the family can help monitor the patient when the nurse is away from the room. The family will be ready to embrace learning and assume more tasks as time passes if they are positively reinforced for their efforts.

174. **Correct Answer: B**

The blood pressure and CVP are low. The respiratory rate is low, and the patient's mentation is diminished. These values indicate hypovolemic shock.

175. **Correct Answer: D**

Coumadin (warfarin) blocks vitamin K coagulation factors of II, VII, IX, X, and XI of the extrinsic pathway. Normal PT is in the range of 11.2 to 13. 2 seconds. A PT of 28 seconds indicates severe risk of bleeding and the Coumadin dose should be held and the physician notified immediately. Many laboratories and physicians will use the INR value for purposes of Coumadin titration, as it is more reliable and standardized. The PT value must still be obtained to determine the INR calculation. The INR target is 2 to 3.5. INR values > 4.5 indicate that the patient is at increased risk for bleeding, and a value > 6 indicates the need for vitamin K administration.

176. **Correct Answer: A**

Dobutamine is an inotrope and will improve the pumping action of the heart. This alpha-, beta$_1$-, and beta$_2$-agonist will increase contractility and cardiac output, with little or no concomitant increase in myocardial oxygen consumption. Dobutamine has a very mild vasodilatory effect, though high doses can cause ischemia.

177. **Correct Answer: D**

Warren has increased exercise intolerance, edema, and dyspnea, all of which are signs of left ventricular failure. The crackles are probably the result of fluid buildup in the lungs. Because the left heart cannot pump effectively, the fluid backs up.

178. **Correct Answer: B**

The pH is normal (compensated), the CO_2 level is high (respiratory acidosis), and the HCO_3 level is normal.

179. **Correct Answer: D**

Nancy's intolerance for activity and crackles indicate pulmonary congestion. Edema indicates third spacing. All of these symptoms are cardinal signs of CHF.

180. **Correct Answer: C**

Anginal pain usually occurs when approximately 75% of the artery becomes occluded. Pain is more pronounced with exertion or emotional distress when oxygen demand by cardiac tissue cannot be met by the oxygen supply via the occluded arteries. The severity of pain may be compounded by vasospasms that further restrict blood flow through the coronary arteries.

181. **Correct Answer: D**
A lateral MI is identified by changes in leads I, aVL, V_5, and V_6.

182. **Correct Answer: B**
Because the RCA perfuses the SA node in slightly more than half the population, and supplies the proximal bundle of His and the AV node in more than 90% of individuals, conduction defects may occur, but will probably be transient.

183. **Correct Answer: A**
Using ICHD nomenclature, the first "V" is the chamber paced.

184. **Correct Answer: C**
Using ICHD nomenclature, the second "V" is the chamber sensed.

185. **Correct Answer: C**
Of the options presented here, the problem is in the right ventricle. The CVP is high and there is some jugular distention. These findings indicate a problem with the right ventricle—it cannot pump effectively. The lethargy may be unrelated and needs to be evaluated because it is a significant change for this patient.

186. **Correct Answer: D**
Pete is in the hyperdynamic ("warm") stage of septic shock. The endotoxins are causing an increase in metabolism and act as vasodilators. His temperature is increased because of the increased metabolism and infection. Hypotension occurs because of vasodilation, and the heart rate increases to compensate. Urine output should be quite high. Pete needs immediate treatment with large quantities of fluids, vasopressors, antibiotics, and anti-endotoxins.

187. **Correct Answer: D**
Mona was admitted for anaphylactic shock. She is eight months pregnant, and the baby is probably pressing on her aorta and vena cava. A simple change of position might fix the problem. In anaphylactic shock, the blood pressure would be low in the initial stages because of vasodilation. Mona probably has a mild form of distributive shock, and her symptoms will probably resolve quickly once this problem is eliminated.

188. **Correct Answer: C**
The heart cannot pump the fluid out and the lungs are congested (dyspnea). Edema is a sign of pump failure. The patient will probably develop ascites and hepatomegaly.

189. **Correct Answer: D**
Daniel has all the classic signs of sepsis: He has a low-grade fever, his respiratory rate is increased, and he has subtle changes in mentation.

190. **Correct Answer: A**
Agitation, headaches, and insomnia are common side effects of paroxetine. Additional side effects to monitor for include exacerbation of manic symptoms, seizures, tremors, nervousness, confusion, vertigo, risk of suicide, hallucinations, hypertonia, dry mouth, constipation, rectal hemorrhage, and anemia.

191. **Correct Answer: B**
Depression of the ST segment is indicative of myocardial ischemia: Electrical conduction through the heart is altered as cardiac tissue dies. Dead or necrotic myocardial tis-

sue is unable to conduct electricity, so the electrical impulse must go around the tissue and is seen as a depression on the cardiac monitor.

192. **Correct Answer: C**

    "Transmural" describes the full thickness of the myocardial wall. "Subendocardial" indicates that the infarction has not affected the full thickness of the myocardium. The anterioseptal and inferior walls are potential locations of the myocardial infarction.

193. **Correct Answer: D**

    Digoxin is often used to treat ventricular failure because it improves myocardial contractility and reduces the ventricular rate. Use this drug with caution when patients have myocarditis because digoxin's cardiac side effects are more likely to occur.

194. **Correct Answer: B**

    In annuloplasty, the mitral valve is repaired through reconstruction of the valve leaflets and the annulus. This technique may also be used to repair the tricuspid valve. A prosthetic ring may or may not be used.

BIBLIOGRAPHY

Abraham, W. T., & Hayes, D. L. (2003). Cardiac resynchronization therapy for heart failure. *Circulation, 108*(21), 2596–2603.

Adams-Hamoda, M. G., & Pelter, M. M. (2003). Heart blocks. *American Journal of Critical Care, 12*(1), 77–78.

Ahrens, T. (2006). *Critical care nursing certification.* Columbus, OH: McGraw-Hill.

Albert, N. M. (2003). Cardiac resynchronization therapy through biventricular pacing in patients with heart failure and ventricular dyssynchrony. *Critical Care Nurse, 23*(3 suppl), 2–16.

Allocca, G., Slavich, G., Nucifora, G., Slavich, M., Frassani, R., Crapis, M., et al. (2007). Successful treatment of polymicrobial multivalve infective endocarditis: Multivalve infective endocarditis. *International Journal of Cardiovascular Imaging, 23*(4), 501.

Alpert, J. S. (2003). Defining myocardial infarction: "Will the real myocardial infarction please stand up?" *American Heart Journal, 146*(3), 377–379.

American Association of Critical-Care Nurses. (2004, May). *Practice alert: Pulmonary artery pressure measurement.* Retrieved July 16, 2008 from http://www.aacn.org/WD/Practice/Docs/PAP_Measurement_05-2004.pdf

American Association of Critical-Care Nurses. (2004, August). *Practice alert: ST segment monitoring.* Retrieved July 16, 2008 from http://www.aacn.org/WD/Practice/Docs/ST_Segment_Monitoring_04-2008.pdf

American Association of Critical-Care Nurses (AACN). (2006). *Core curriculum for critical care nursing* (6th ed.). Philadelphia: Saunders.

American Association of Critical-Care Nurses (AACN). (2007). *AACN certification and core review for high acuity and critical care* (6th ed.). Philadelphia: Saunders.

American Heart Association. (2005). *Guidelines 2005 for cardiopulmonary resuscitation and emergency cardiovascular care.* Retrieved July 16, 2008 from http://circ.ahajournals.org/content/vol112/24_suppl

Anavekar, N. S., McMurray, J. J. V., Velazquez, E. J., Solomon, S. D., Kober, L., Rouleau, J. L., et al. (2004). Relation between renal dysfunction and cardiovascular outcomes after myocardial infarction. *New England Journal of Medicine, 351*(13), 1285–1295.

Anderson, R. H., Razavi, R., & Taylor, A. M. (2004). Cardiac anatomy revisited. *Journal of Anatomy, 205*(3), 159–177.

Antezano, E. S., & Hong, M. (2003). Sudden cardiac death. *Journal of Intensive Care Medicine, 18*(6), 313–329.

Antzelevitch, C., Brugada, P., Borggrefe, M., Brugada, J., Brugada, R., Corrado, D., et al. (2005). Brugada syndrome: Report of the Second Consensus Conference. Endorsed by the Heart Rhythm Society and the European Heart Rhythm Association. *Circulation, 111*(5), 659–670.

Archbold, R. A., & Schilling, R. J. (2004). Atrial pacing for the prevention of atrial fibrillation after coronary bypass graft surgery: A review of the literature. *Heart, 90,* 129–133.

Ariyan, C. E., & Sosa, J. A. (2004). Assessment and management of patients with abnormal calcium. *Critical Care Medicine, 32*(4 suppl), S146–S154.

Aronow, W. S. (2003). Homocysteine: The association with atherosclerotic vascular disease in older persons. *Geriatrics, 58*(2), 22–24, 27–28.

Aurigemma, G. P., & Gaasch, W. H. (2004). Clinical practice: Diastolic heart failure. *New England Journal of Medicine, 351*(11), 1097–1105.

Barrett, M. J., Lacey, C. S., Sekara, A. E., Linden, E. A., & Gracely, E. J. (2004). Mastering cardiac murmurs: The power of repetition. *Chest, 126*(2), 470–475.

Barter, P. J., Nicholls, S., Rye, K., Anantharamaiah, G. M., Navab, M., & Fogelman, A. M. (2004). Antiinflammatory properties of HDL. *Circulation Research, 95*(8), 764–772.

Baur, L. H. B. (2008). Three dimensional echocardiography: A valuable tool to assess left atrial function in non-compaction cardiomyopathy. *International Journal of Cardiovascular Imaging, 24*(3), 243.

Berdajs, D., Patonay, L., & Turina, M. I. (2003). The clinical anatomy of the sinus node artery. *Annals of Thoracic Surgery, 76*(3), 732–735.

Birnbaum, Y., & Drew, B. J. (2003). The electrocardiogram in ST elevation acute myocardial infarction: Correlation with coronary anatomy and prognosis. *Postgraduate Medical Journal, 79*(935), 490–504.

Blake, G. J., & Ridker, P. M. (2003). C-reactive protein and other inflammatory risk markers in acute coronary syndromes. *Journal of the American College of Cardiology, 41*(4 suppl S), 37S–42S.

Bollinger, K., & Sader, A. M. (2003). Care and management of the patient with right heart failure secondary to diastolic dysfunction: An advanced practice perspective and case review. *Critical Care Nursing Quarterly, 26*(1), 22–27.

Bolno, P. B., & Kresh, J. Y. (2003). Physiologic and hemodynamic basis of ventricular assist devices. *Cardiology Clinics, 21*(1), 15–27.

Booker, K. J., Holm, K., Drew, B. J., Lanuza, D. M., Hicks, F. D., Carrigan, T., et al. (2003). Frequency and outcomes of transient myocardial ischemia in critically ill adults admitted for noncardiac conditions. *American Journal of Critical Care, 12*(6), 508–516.

Callahan, H. E. (2003). Families dealing with advanced heart failure: A challenge and an opportunity. *Critical Care Nursing Quarterly, 26*(3), 230–243.

Cannon, C. P. (2003). Small molecule glycoprotein IIb/IIIa receptor inhibitors as upstream therapy in acute coronary syndromes. *Journal of the American College of Cardiology, 41*(4 suppl S), 43S–48S.

Canto, J. G., & Iskandrian, A. E. (2003). Major risk factors for cardiovascular disease: Debunking the "only 50%" myth. *Journal of the American Medical Association, 290*, 947–949.

Cardenas, G. A., Lavie, C. J., & Milani, R. V. (2004). Importance and management of low levels of high-density lipoprotein cholesterol in older adults: Part I: Role and mechanism. *Geriatrics and Aging, 7*(3), 40–45.

Cardenas, G. A., Lavie, C. J., & Milani, R. V. (2004). Importance and management of low levels of high-density lipoprotein cholesterol in older adults: Part II: Screening and treatment. *Geriatrics and Aging, 7*(3), 41–48.

Carmona, I. T., Dios, P. D., & Scully, C. (2007). Efficacy of antibiotic prophylactic regimens for the prevention of bacterial endocarditis of oral origin. *Journal of Dental Research, 86*(12), 1142.

Chen, E. W., Canto, J. G., Parsons, L. S., Peterson, E. D., Littrell, K. A., Every, N. R., et al. (2003). Relation between hospital intra-aortic balloon counterpulsation volume and mortality in acute myocardial infarction complicated by cardiogenic shock. *Circulation, 108*(8), 951–957.

Chiu, C., & Sequeira, I. B. (2004). Diagnosis and treatment of idiopathic ventricular tachycardia. *AACN Clinical Issues, 15*(3), 449–461.

Chobanian, A. V., Bakris, G. L., Black, H. R., Cushman, W. C., Green, L. A., Izzo, J. L. Jr., et al. (2003). The seventh report of the Joint National Committee on prevention, detection, evaluation and treatment of high blood pressure: The JNC 7 report. *Journal of the American Medical Association, 289*, 2560–2572.

Chun, A. A., & McGee, S. R. (2004). Bedside diagnosis of coronary artery disease: A systematic review. *American Journal of Medicine, 117*(5), 334–343.

Cianci, P., Lonergan-Thomas, H., Slaughter, M., & Silver, M. A. (2003). Current and potential applications of left ventricular assist devices. *Journal of Cardiovascular Nursing, 18*(1), 17–22.

Coffey, M., Crowder, G. K., & Cheek, D. J. (2003). Reducing coronary artery disease by decreasing homocysteine levels. *Critical Care Nurse, 23*(1), 25–29.

Cohen, M. (2003). The role of low-molecular-weight heparin in the management of acute coronary syndromes. *Journal of American College of Cardiology, 41*(4 suppl S), 55S–61S.

Colbert, K., & Greene, M. H. (2003). Nesiritide: A new treatment for acutely decompensated congestive heart failure. *Critical Care Nursing Quarterly, 26*(1), 40–44.

Conover, M. B. (2003). *Understanding electrocardiography* (8th ed.). St. Louis, MO: Mosby/Elsevier.

Constantine, G., Shan, K., Flamm, S. D., & Sivananthan, M. U. (2004). Role of MRI in clinical cardiology. *Lancet, 363*(9247), 2162–2171.

Conti, R., Fuster, V., & Badimon, J. J. (2003). Pathogenic concepts of acute coronary syndromes. *Journal of the American College of Cardiology, 41*(4 suppl S), 37S–42S.

Copstead, L., & Banasik, J. L. (2000). *Pathophysiology: Biological and behavioral perspectives* (2nd ed.). Philadelphia: W. B. Saunders/Elsevier.

Coulthwaite, L., & Verran, J. (2007). Potential pathogenic aspects of denture plaque. *British Journal of Biomedical Science, 64*(4), 180.

Coviello, J. S., & Nystrom, K. V. (2003). Obesity and heart failure. *Journal of Cardiovascular Nursing, 18*(5), 360–366.

Crawford, M. H., DiMarco, J. P., & Paulus, W. J. (Eds.). (2004). *Cardiology* (2nd ed.). Philadelphia: Mosby.

Criddle, L. M. (2003). Rhabdomyolysis: Pathophysiology, recognition, and management. *Critical Care Nurse, 23*(6), 14–28.

Cripe, L., Andelfinger, G., Martin, L. J., & Benson, D. W. (2004). Bicuspid aortic valve is heritable. *Journal of American College of Cardiology, 44*(1), 138–143.

Crystal, E., & Connolly, S. J. (2004). Atrial fibrillation: Guiding lessons from epidemiology. *Cardiology Clinics, 22*(1), 1–8.

Curley, M. A. Q. (1998). Patient–nurse synergy: Optimizing patients' outcomes. *American Journal of Critical Care, 7,* 64–72.

Davidson, M. B., Thakkar, S., Hix, J. K., et al. (2004). Pathophysiology, clinical consequence, and treatment of tumor lysis syndrome. *American Journal of Medicine, 116*(8), 546–554.

D'Avila, A., Scanavacca, M., Sosa, E., Ruskin, J. N., & Reddy, V. Y. (2003). Pericardial anatomy for the interventional electrophysiologist. *Journal of Cardiovascular Electrophysiology, 14*(4), 422–430.

Darovic, G. O. (2002). *Hemodynamic monitoring: Invasive and noninvasive clinical application* (3rd ed.). Philadelphia: Saunders.

Deaton, C., Dunbar, S. B., Moloney, M., Sears, S. F., & Ujhelyi, M. R.. (2003). Patient experiences with atrial fibrillation and treatment with implantable atrial defibrillation therapy. *Heart and Lung, 32*(5), 291–299.

De Rosa, F. G., Cicalini, S., Canta, F., Audagnotto, S., Cecchi, E., & Di Perri, G. (2007). Infective endocarditis in intravenous drug users from Italy: The increasing importance in HIV-infected patients. *Infection, 35*(3), 154.

Diercks, D. B., Shumaik, G. M., Harrigan, R. A., Brady, W. J., & Chan, T. C. (2004). Electrocardiographic manifestations: Electrolyte abnormalities. *Journal of Emergency Medicine, 27*(2), 153–160.

Dimick, J. B., Swoboda, S., Talamini, M. A., Hendrix, C. W., & Lipsett, P. A. (2004). Risk of colonization of central venous catheters: Catheters for total parenteral nutrition vs. other catheters. *American Journal of Critical Care, 12*(4), 328–335.

Diskerson, R. N., Alexander, K. H., Minard, G., Croce, M. A., & Brown, R. O. (2004). Accuracy of methods to estimate ionized and "correct" serum calcium concentrations in critically ill multiple trauma patients receiving specialized nutrition support. *Journal of Parenteral and Enteral Nutrition, 28*(3), 133–141.

Drazner, M. H., Rame, J. E., & Dries, D. L. (2003). Third heart sound and elevated jugular venous pressure as markers of the subsequent development of heart failure in patients with asymptomatic left ventricular dysfunction. *American Journal of Medicine, 114*(6), 431–437.

Drew, B. J., Califf, R. M., Funk, M., Kaufman, E. S., Krucoff, M. W., Laks, M. M., et al. (2004). Practice standards for electrocardiographic monitoring in hospital settings. *Circulation, 110*(17), 2721–2746.

Eagle, K. A., Kline-Rogers, E., Goodman, S. G., Gurfinkel, E. P., Avezum, A., Flather, M. D., et al. (2004). Adherence to evidence-based therapies after discharge for acute coronary syndromes: An ongoing prospective, observational study. *American Journal of Medicine, 117*(2), 73–81.

Edwards, D. F. (1999). The Synergy Model: Linking patient needs to nurse competencies. *Critical Care Nurse, 19*(1), 88–98.

Emergency Nurses Association & Newberry, L. (2003). *Sheehy's emergency nursing: Principles and practice* (5th ed.). St. Louis, MO: Mosby/Elsevier.

Enriquez-Sarano, M., Schaff, H. V., & Frye, R. L. (2003). Mitral regurgitation: What causes the leakage is fundamental to the outcome of valve repair. *Circulation, 108,* 253–256.

Epstein, A. E. (2004). An update on implantable cardioverter–defibrillator guidelines. *Current Opinion on Cardiology, 19*(1), 23–25.

Eremeeva, M. E., Gerns, H. L., Lydy, S. L., Goo, J. S., Ryan, E. T., Mathew, S. S., et al. (2007). Bacteremia, fever, and splenomegaly caused by a newly recognized *Bartonella* species: Brief report. *New England Journal of Medicine, 356*(23), 2381.

Everett, T. H., & Olgin, J. E. (2004). Basic mechanism of atrial fibrillation. *Cardiology Clinics, 22*(1), 9–20.

Faybush, E. M., & Fass, R. (2004). Gastroesophageal reflux disease in noncardiac chest pain. *Gastroenterology Clinics of North America, 33*(1), 41–54.

Fields, L. E., Burt, V. L., Cutler, J. A., Hughes, J., Roccella, E. J., & Sorlie, P. (2004). The burden of adult hypertension in the United States 1999 to 2000: A rising tide. *Hypertension, 44*(4), 398–404.

Finkelmeier, B. A. (2000). *Cardiothoracic surgical nursing* (2nd ed.). Philadelphia: Lippincott, Williams & Wilkins.

Finta, B., & Haines, D. E. (2004). Catheter ablation therapy for atrial fibrillation. *Cardiology Clinics, 22*(1), 127–145.

Fox, C. S., Evans, J. C., Larson, M. G., Kannel, W. B., & Levy, D. (2004). Temporal trends in coronary heart disease mortality and sudden cardiac death from 1950 to 1999: The Framingham Heart Study. *Circulation, 110*(5), 522–527.

Franklin, K., Goldberg, R. J., Spencer, F., Klein, W., Budaj, A., Brieger, D., et al. (2004). Implications of diabetes in patients with acute coronary syndromes: The Global Registry of Acute Coronary Events. *Archives of Internal Medicine, 164*(13), 1457–1463.

Frey, N., Katus, H. A., Olson, E. N., & Hill, J. A. (2004). Hypertrophy of the heart: A new therapeutic target? *Circulation, 109*(13), 1580–1589.

Frishman, W. H., Sonnenblick, E. H., & Sica, D. A. (Eds.). (2004). *Cardiovascular pharmacotherapeutics* (2nd ed.). New York: McGraw-Hill.

Garber, A. J., Moghissi, E. S., Bransome, Jr., E. D. Clark, N. G., Clement, S., Cobin, R. H., et al. (2004). American College of Endocrinology position statement on inpatient diabetes and metabolic control. *Endocrinology Practice, 10*(1), 37–82.

Goldman, L., & Ausiello, D. (2004). *Cecil textbook of medicine* (22nd ed.). Philadelphia: Mosby.

Goldstein, J. A. (2004). Cardiac tamponade, constrictive pericarditis, and restrictive cardiomyopathy. *Current Problems in Cardiology, 29*(9), 503–567.

Graham, L. (2008). AHA releases updated guidelines on the prevention of infective endocarditis. *American Family Physician, 77*(4), 538.

Greenland, P., Knoll, M. D., Stamler, J., Neaton, J. D., Dyer, A. R., Garside, D. B., et al. (2003). Major risk factors as antecedents of fatal and nonfatal coronary heart disease events. *Journal of the American Medical Association, 290,* 891–897.

Greig, J., O'Sullivan, C. E., Adam, O., Klein, H. H., & Schäfers, H. J. (2007). Intraaortic vegetations and infective endocarditis. *New England Journal of Medicine, 356*(23), 2430.

Grif Alspach, J. (Ed.). (2006). *Core curriculum for critical care nursing* (6th ed.). St. Louis, MO: Saunders.

Grundy, S. M., Cleeman, J. I., Merz, C. N., Brewer, H. B. Jr., Clark, L. T., Hunninghake, D. B., et al. (2004). Implications of recent clinical trials for the National Cholesterol Education Program Adult Treatment Panel III. *Circulation, 110*(2), 227–239.

Hallstrom, A. P., Ornato, J. P., Weisfeldt, M., Travers, A., Christenson, J., McBurnie, M. A., et al. (2004). Public-access defibrillation and survival after out-of-hospital cardiac arrest. *New England Journal of Medicine, 351*(7), 637–646.

Halperin, J. L., & Fuster, V. (2003). Meeting the challenge of peripheral arterial disease. *Archives of Internal Medicine, 28,* 877–878.

Hardin, S. R., & Kaplow, R. (Eds.). (2004). *Synergy for clinical excellence: The AACN Synergy Model for Patient Care.* Sudbury, MA: Jones and Bartlett.

Haskell, W. L. (2003). Cardiovascular disease prevention and lifestyle interventions: Effectiveness and efficacy. *Journal of Cardiovascular Nursing, 18*(4), 245–255.

Henry, L. B. (2003). Left ventricular systolic dysfunction and ischemic cardiomyopathy. *Critical Care Nursing Quarterly, 26*(1), 16–21.

Hickey, J. V. (2002). *The clinical practice of neurological and neurosurgical nursing* (5th ed.). Philadelphia: Lippincott, Williams & Wilkins.

Hill, E. E., Vanderschueren, S., Verhaegen, J., Herijgers, P., Claus, P., Herregods, M. C., et al. (2007). Risk factors for infective endocarditis and outcome of patients with *Staphylococcus aureus* bacteremia. *Mayo Clinic Proceedings, 82*(10), 1165.

Hirsh, J., Heddle, N., & Kelton, J. G. (2004). Treatment of heparin-induced thrombocytopenia: A critical review. *Archives of Internal Medicine, 164*(4), 361–369.

Holmes, E. C. (2003). Outpatient management of long-term assist devices. *Cardiology Clinics, 21,* 91–99.

Horstkotte, D., Follath, F., Gutschik, E., Lengyel, M., Oto, A., Pavie, A., et al. (2004). Guidelines on prevention, diagnosis and treatment of infective endocarditis: Executive summary. The Task Force on Infective Endocarditis of the European Society of Cardiology. *European Heart Journal, 25*(3), 267–276.

Houterman, S., Verchuren, W. M., & Kromhout, D. (2003). Smoking, blood pressure, and serum cholesterol: Effects on 20-year mortality. *Epidemiology, 14*(1), 24–29.

Irwin, M. E. (2004). Cardiac pacing device therapy for atrial dysrhythmias. *AACN Clinical Issues, 15*(3), 377–390.

Jacobs, A. K., Leopold, J. A., Bates, E., Mendes, L. A., Sleeper, L. A., White, H., et al. (2003). Cardiogenic shock caused by right ventricular infarction: A report from the SHOCK registry. *Journal of the American College of Cardiology, 41*(8), 1273–1279.

James, T. N. (2003). Structure and function of the sinus node, AV node and His bundle of the human heart: Part II: Function. *Progress in Cardiovascular Disease, 45*(3), 327–360.

Jessup, M., & Brozena, S. C. (2003). Epilogue: Support devices for end stage heart failure. *Cardiology Clinics, 21,* 135–139.

Jesurum, J. (2004). Protocols for practice: SvO$_2$ monitoring. *Critical Care Nurse, 24*(4), 73–76.

Kang, N., Smith, W., Greaves, S., & Haydock, D. (2007). Pulmonary-valve endocarditis. *New England Journal of Medicine, 356*(2), 2224.

Kawasaki, T., Akakabe, Y., Yamano, M., Miki, S., Kamitani, T., Kuribayashi, T., et al. (2008). R-wave amplitude response to myocardial ischemia in hypertrophic cardiomyopathy. *Journal of Electrocardiology, 41*(1), 68.

Kellen, J. C. (2004). Implementations for nursing care of patients with atrial fibrillation: Lessons learned from the AFFIRM and RACE studies. *Journal of Cardiovascular Nursing, 19*(2), 128–137.

Keller, K. B., & Lemberg, L. (2004). Prinzmetal's angina. *American Journal of Critical Care, 13*(4), 350–354.

Kern, L. S. (2004). Postoperative atrial fibrillation: New directions in prevention and treatment. *Journal of Cardiovascular Nursing, 19*(2), 103–115.

Khurana, R. K. (2008). Takotsubo cardiomyopathy in a patient with postural tachycardia syndrome. *Clinical Autonomic Research, 18*(1), 43.

Khot, U. N., Khot, M. B., Bajzer, C. T., Sapp, S. K., Ohman, E. M., Brener, S. J., et al. (2003). Prevalence of conventional risk factors with coronary heart disease. *Journal of the American Medical Association, 290,* 898–904.

Krahn, A. D., Mason, P. K., Wood, M. A., & Yee, R. (2003). Use of the implantable loop recorder in evaluation of patients with unexplained syncope. *Journal of Cardiovascular Electrophysiology, 14*(9 suppl), S70–S73.

Krajinovic, V., Andrasevic, A. T., & Barsic, B. (2007). Tricuspidal valve endocarditis due to *Yersinia enterocolitica. Infection, 35*(3), 203.

Krinsley, J. S. (2003). Test-ordering strategy in the intensive care unit. *Journal of Intensive Care Medicine, 18*(6), 330–339.

Lang, C., Sauter, M., Szalay, G., Racchi, G., Grassi, G., Rainaldi, G., et al. (2008). Connective tissue growth factor: A crucial cytokine-mediating cardiac fibrosis in ongoing enterovirus myocarditis. *Journal of Molecular Medicine, 86*(10), 49.

Lefler, L. L., & Bondy, K. N. (2004). Women's delay in seeking treatment with myocardial infarction: A meta-synthesis. *Journal of Cardiovascular Nursing, 19*(4), 251–268.

Lin, J. C., Apple, F. S., Murakami, M. M., & Luepker, R. V. (2004). Rates of positive cardiac troponin I and creatine kinase MB mass among patients hospitalized for suspected acute coronary syndromes. *Clinical Chemistry, 50*(2), 333–338.

Lipson, J. G., Dibble, S. L., & Minarik, P. A. (Eds.). (1996). *Culture and nursing care: A pocket guide.* San Francisco, CA: UCSF Nursing Press.

Lloyd-Jones, D. M., Wang, T. J., Leip, E. P., Larson, M. G., Levy, D., Vasan, R. S., et al. (2004). Lifetime risk for development of atrial fibrillation: The Framingham Heart Study. *Circulation, 110*(9), 1042–1046.

López, J., Revilla, A., Vilacosta, I., Villacorta, E., González-Juanatey, C., Gómez, I., et al. (2007). Definition, clinical profile, microbiological spectrum, and prognostic factors of early-onset prosthetic valve endocarditis. *European Heart Journal, 28*(6), 760.

Maalouf, M., Moon, W., Leers, S., Papasavas, P. K., Birdas, T., & Caushaj, P. F. (2007). Mycotic aneurysm of the infrarenal aorta after drainage of an infected chronic pancreatic pseudocyst: Case report and review of the literature. *American Surgeon, 73*(12), 1266.

Maisch, B., Seferovic, P. M., Ristic, A. D., Erbel, R., Rienmüller, R., Adler, Y., et al. (2004). Guidelines on the diagnosis and management of pericardial diseases executive summary: The Task Force on the Diagnosis and Management of Pericardial Diseases of the European Society of Cardiology. *European Heart Journal, 25*(7), 586–610.

Malinoski, D. J., Slater, M. S., & Mullins, R. J. (2004). Crush injury and rhabdomyolysis. *Critical Care Clinics, 20*(1), 171–192.

McGuire, D. K., Newby, L. K., Bhapkar, M. V., Moliterno, D. J., Hochman, J. S., Klein, W. W., et al. (2004). Association of diabetes mellitus and glycemic control strategies with clinical outcomes after acute coronary syndromes. *American Heart Journal, 147*(2), 246–252.

McKay, R. G. (2003). Ischemic guided versus early invasive strategies in the management of acute coronary syndromes/non–ST-segment elevation myocardial infarction. *Journal of the American College of Cardiology, 41*(4 suppl S), 96S–102S.

McQuillan, K. A., Von Rueden, K. T., Hartsock, R. L., Flynn, M. B., & Whalen, E. (Eds.). (2002). *Trauma nursing: From resuscitation through rehabilitation* (3rd ed.). Philadelphia: W. B. Saunders/Elsevier.

McSweeney, J. C., Cody, M., O'Sullivan, P., Elberson, K., Moser, D. K., & Garvin, B. J. (2003). Women's early warning symptoms of acute myocardial infarction. *Circulation, 108*(21), 2619–2623.

Medina, J., & Puntillo, K. (2006). *AACN protocols for practice: Palliative care and end-of-life issues in critical care.* Sudbury, MA: Jones and Bartlett.

Mehta, L. S. R., & Yusuf, S. (2003). Short- and long-term oral antiplatelet therapy in acute coronary syndromes. *Journal of the American College of Cardiology, 41*(4 suppl S), 79S–88S.

Menon, T., Nandhakumar, B., Jaganathan, V., Shanmugasundaram, S., Malathy, B., & Nisha, B. (2008). Bacterial endocarditis due to Group C *Streptococcus*. *Journal of Postgraduate Medicine, 54*(1), 64.

Mosca, L., Appel, L. J., Benjamin, E. J., Berra, K., Chandra-Strobos, N., Fabunmi, R. P., et al. (2004). Evidence based guidelines for cardiovascular disease prevention in women. *Circulation, 109*(5), 672–693.

Nemes, A., Anwar, A. M., Caliskan, A. K., Soliman, O. I., van Dalen, B. M., Geleijnse, M. L., et al. (2008). Evaluation of left atrial systolic function in noncompaction cardiomyopathy by real-time three-dimensional echocardiography. *International Journal of Cardiovascular Imaging, 24*(3), 237.

Newby, L. K., Goldmann, B. U., & Ohman, E. M. (2003). Troponin: An important prognostic marker and risk-stratification tool in non–ST-segment elevation acute coronary syndromes. *Journal of the American College of Cardiology, 41*(4 suppl S), 31S–36S.

Niebauer, J. (2008). Effects of exercise training on inflammatory markers in patients with heart failure. *Heart Failure Reviews, 13*(1), 39.

Nikolsky, E., Mehran, R., Halkin, A., Aymong, E. D., Mintz, G. S., Lasic, Z., et al. (2004). Vascular complications associated with arteriotomy closure devices in patients undergoing percutaneous coronary procedures: A meta-analysis. *Journal of the American College of Cardiology, 44*(6), 1200–1209.

Nishimura, R. A., Ommen, S. R., & Tajik, A. J. (2003). Hypertrophic cardiomyopathy: A patient perspective. *Circulation, 108,* e133–e135.

Novis, D. A., Jones, B. A., Dale, J. C., Walsh, M. K., & College of American Pathologists. (2004). Biochemical markers of myocardial injury test turnaround time: A College of American Pathologists Q-Probes study of 7020 troponin and 4368 creatine kinase-MB determinations in 159 institutions. *Archives of Pathology and Laboratory Medicine, 128*(2), 158–164.

Olivery, H. E., Compton, L. A., & Barnett, J. V. (2004). Coronary vessel development the epicardium delivers. *Trends in Cardiovascular Medicine, 14*(6), 246–251.

Paelinck, B., & Dendale, P. A. (2003). Images in clinical medicine: Cardiac tamponade in Dressler's syndrome. *New England Journal of Medicine, 248*(23), e8.

Pagana, K. D., & Pagana, J. (2005). *Mosby's manual of diagnostic and laboratory tests* (3rd ed.). St. Louis, MO: Mosby/Elsevier.

Palmer, B. F. (2004). Managing hyperkalemia caused by inhibitors of the renin–angiotensin–aldosterone system. *New England Journal of Medicine, 351*(6), 585–592.

Patel, H., & Pagani, F. D. (2003). Extracorporeal mechanical circulatory assist. *Cardiology Clinics, 21*(1), 29–41.

Paterick, T. E., Paterick, T. J., Nishimura, R. A., & Steckelberg, J. M. (2007). Complexity and subtlety of infective endocarditis. *Mayo Clinic Proceedings, 82*(5), 615.

Patten, R. D., & Soman, P. (2004). Prevention and reversal of LV remodeling with neurohormonal inhibitors. *Current Treatment Options in Cardiovascular Medicine, 6*(4), 313–325.

Paul, S. (2003). Ventricular remodeling. *Critical Care Nursing Clinics of North America, 15*(4), 407–411.

Peel, D. A. (2007). Endocarditis due to a nutritionally variant *Streptococcus:* A lesson in recognition and isolation. *British Journal of Biomedical Science, 64*(4), 175.

Pelter, M. M., Adams, M. G., & Drew, B. J. (2003). Transient myocardial ischemia is an independent predictor of adverse in-hospital outcomes in patients with acute coronary syndromes treated in the telemetry unit. *Heart and Lung, 32*(2), 71–78.

Perez-Lugones, A., McMahon, J. T., Ratliff, N. B., Saliba, W. I., Schweikert, R. A., Marrouche, N. F., et al. (2003). Evidence of specialized conduction cells in human pulmonary veins of patients with atrial fibrillation. *Journal of Cardiovascular Electrophysiology, 14*(8), 803–809.

Pope, J. H., Ruthazer, R., Kontos, M. C., Beshansky, J. R., Griffith, J. L., & Selker, H. P. (2004). The impact of electrocardiographic left ventricular hypertrophy and bundle branch block on the triage and outcome of ED patients with a suspected acute coronary syndrome: A multicenter study. *American Journal of Emergency Medicine, 22*(3), 156–163.

Prabhakar, N. R., & Peng, Y. J. (2004). Peripheral chemoreceptors in health and disease. *Journal of Applied Physiology, 96*(1), 359–366.

Prahash, A., & Lynch, T. (2004). B-type natriuretic peptide: A diagnostic, prognostic, and therapeutic tool in heart failure. *American Journal of Critical Care, 13*(1), 46–55.

Pyle, W. G., & Solaro, R. J. (2004). At the crossroads of myocardial signaling: The role of Z-discs in intracellular signaling and cardiac function. *Circulation Research, 94*(3), 296–305.

Reinhart, K., Kuhn, H., Hartog, C., & Bredle, D. L. (2004). Continuous central venous and pulmonary artery oxygen saturation monitoring in the critically ill. *Intensive Care Medicine, 30*(8), 1572–1578.

Richard, C., Warszawski, J., Anguel, N., Deye, N., Combes, A., Barnoud, D., et al. (2003). Early use of the pulmonary artery catheter and outcomes in patients with shock and acute respiratory distress syndrome: A randomized controlled trial. *Journal of the American Medical Association, 290*(20), 2713–2720.

Robicsek, F., Thubrikar, M. J., Cook, J. W., & Fowler, B. (2003). The congenitally bicuspid aortic valve: How does it function? Why does it fail? *Annals of Thoracic Surgery, 77*(1), 177–185.

Roden, D. M. (2004). Drug-induced prolongation of the QT interval. *New England Journal of Medicine, 350*(10), 1013–1022.

Rudisill, P. T., Kennedy, C., & Paul, S. (2003). The use of beta-blockers in the treatment of chronic heart failure. *Critical Care Nurse of North America, 15*(4), 439–446.

Sandham, J. D., Hull, R. D., Brant, R. F., Knox, L., Pineo, G. F., Doig, C. J., et al. (2003). A randomized, controlled trial of the use of pulmonary artery catheters in high-risk surgical patients. *New England Journal of Medicine, 348*(1), 5–14.

Saul, L., & Shatzer, M. (2003). B-type natriuretic peptide testing for detection of heart failure. *Critical Care Nursing Quarterly, 26*(1), 35–59.

Schwarz, K. A., & Elman, C. S. (2003). Identification of factors predictive of hospital readmissions for patients with heart failure. *Heart and Lung, 32*(3), 88–99.

Schwert, D. W., & Vatikus, P. (2003). Drug-eluding stents to prevent re-blocking of coronary arteries. *Journal of Cardiovascular Nursing, 18*(1), 11–16.

Sealey, B., & Lui, K. (2004). Diagnosis and management of vasovagal syncope and dysautonomia. *AACN Clinical Issues, 15*(3), 449–461.

Segal, B. L. (2003). Valvular heart disease, part 2: Mitral valve disease in older adults. *Geriatrics, 58*(10), 26–31.

Shadman, R., Criqui, M. H., Bundens, W. P., Fronek, A., Denenberg, J. O., Gamst, A. C., et al. (2004). Subclavian artery stenosis: Prevalence, risk factors, and association with cardiovascular diseases. *Journal of the American College of Cardiology, 44*(3), 618–623.

Shak, P. K. (2003). Mechanisms of plaque vulnerability and rupture. *Journal of the American College of Cardiology, 41*(4 suppl S), 15S–22S.

Shan, K., Constantine, G., Sivananthan, M., & Flamm, S. D. (2004). Role of cardiac magnetic resonance imaging in the assessment of myocardial viability. *Circulation, 109*(11), 1328–1334.

Sharis, P. J., & Cannon, C .P. (2003). *Evidence-based cardiology* (2nd ed.). Philadelphia: Lippincott, Williams & Wilkins.

Singer, D. E., Albers, G. W., Dalen, J. E., Go, A. S., Halperin, J. L., & Manning, W. J. (2004). Antithrombotic therapy in atrial fibrillation: The Seventh ACCP Conference on Antithrombotic and Thrombolytic Therapy. *Chest, 126*(3 suppl), 429S–456S.

Skidmore-Roth, L. (2004). *Mosby's 2004 nursing drug reference.* St. Louis, MO: Mosby/Elsevier.

Smeltzer, S., & Bare, B. G. (2003). *Brunner and Suddarth's textbook of medical–surgical nursing* (10th ed.). Philadelphia: Lippincott, Williams & Wilkins.

Smith, S. W., Tibbles, C. D., Apple, F. S., & Zimmerman, M. (2004). Outcome of low-risk patients discharged home after a normal cardiac troponin I. *Journal of Emergency Medicine, 26*(4), 401–406.

Sneed, N. V., & Paul, S. C. (2003). Readiness for behavioral changes in patients with heart failure. *American Journal of Critical Care, 12*(5), 444–453.

Sohail, M. R., Uslan, D. Z., Khan, A. H., Friedman, P. A., Hayes, D. L., Wilson, W. R., et al. (2008). Infective endocarditis complicating permanent pacemaker and implantable cardioverter–defibrillator infection. *Mayo Clinic Proceedings, 83*(1), 46.

Sole, M. L., Hartshorn, J., & Lamborne, M. L. (2001). *Introduction to critical care nursing* (3rd ed.). Philadelphia: W. B. Saunders/Elsevier.

Stuart-Shor, E. M., Buselli, E. F., & Carroll, D. L. (2003). Are psychosocial factors associated with pathogenesis and consequences of cardiovascular disease in the elderly? *Journal of Cardiovascular Nursing, 18*(3), 169–183.

Swami, A., & Spodick, D. H. (2003). Pulsus paradoxus in cardiac tamponade: A pathophysiologic continuum. *Clinical Cardiology, 26*(5), 215–217.

Szekendi, M. K. (2003). Compliance with acute MI guidelines lowers inpatient mortality. *Journal of Cardiovascular Nursing, 18*(5), 356–359.

Taubert, K. A. (2008). Endocarditis prophylaxis: An evolution of change. *American Family Physician, 77*(4), 421.

Thohan, V., Torre-Amione, G., & Koerner, M. M. (2004). Aldosterone antagonism and congestive heart failure: A new look at an old therapy. *Current Opinions in Cardiology, 19*(4), 301–308.

Tilley, P., & Petersen, D. (2003). Pulling axis together. *Dimensions of Critical Care Nursing, 22*(5), 210–215.

Timothy, P. R., & Rodeman, B. J. (2004). Temporary pacemakers in critically ill patients: Assessment and management strategies. *AACN Clinical Issues, 15*(3), 305–325.

Tleyjeh, I. M., & Baddour, L. M. (2007). *Staphylococcus aureus* bacteremia and infective endocarditis: Old questions, new answers? *Mayo Clinic Proceedings, 82*(10), 1163.

Topol, E. J. (2003). A guide to therapeutic decision-making in patients with non–ST-segment elevation in acute coronary syndromes. *Journal of the American College of Cardiology, 41*(4 suppl S), 123S–129S.

Topol, E. J. (Ed.). (2004). *Textbook of interventional cardiology* (4th ed.). Philadelphia: Saunders.

Trotman-Dickenson, B. (2003). Radiology in the intensive care unit (Part I). *Journal of Intensive Care Medicine, 18*(4), 198–210.

Trotman-Dickerson, B. (2003). Radiology in the intensive care unit (Part II). *Journal of Intensive Care Medicine, 18*(4), 239–252.

Tsai, T., Chen, H., Hsia, H., Zei, P., Wang, P., & Al-Ahmad, A. (2007). Cardiac device infections complicated by erosion. *Journal of Interventional Cardiac Electrophysiology, 19*(2), 133.

Tung, P., Kopelnik, A., Banki, N., Ong, K., Ko, N., Lawton, M. T., et al. (2004). Predictors of neurocardiogenic injury after subarachnoid hemorrhage. *Stroke, 35*(2), 548–551.

Urden, L. D., Stacy, K. M., & Lough, M. E. (2007). *Thelan's critical care nursing: Diagnosis and management* (5th ed.). St. Louis, MO: Mosby.

Wang, K., Asinger, R. W., & Marriott, H. J. (2003). ST-segment elevation in conditions other than acute myocardial infarction. *New England Journal of Medicine, 349*(22), 2128–2135.

Wessels, M. W., De Graaf, B. M., Cohen-Overbeek, T. E., Spitaels, S. E., de Groot-de Laat, L. E., Ten Cate, F. J., et al. (2008). A new syndrome with noncompaction cardiomyopathy, bradycardia, pulmonary stenosis, atrial septal defect and heterotaxy with suggestive linkage to chromosome 6p. *Human Genetics, 122*(6), 595.

Wiegand, D. J. L., & Carlson, K. K. (Eds.). (2005). *AACN procedure manual for critical care* (5th ed.). Philadelphia: Elsevier.

Wong, W. M., & Fass, R. (2004). Noncardiac chest pain. *Current Treatment Options in Gastroenterology, 7*(4), 273–278.

Woods, S., Sivarajan Froelicher, E. S., & Motzer, S. U. (2000). *Cardiac nursing* (4th ed.). Philadelphia: Lippincott, Williams & Wilkins.

Wu, L. A., & Nishimura, R. A. (2003). Images in clinical medicine: Pulses paradoxus. *New England Journal of Medicine, 349*(7), 666.

Yasuma, F., & Hayano, J. (2004). Respiratory sinus arrhythmia: Why does the heartbeat synchronize with respiratory rhythm? *Chest, 125*(2), 683–690.

Zhang, J. (2003). Sudden cardiac death: Implantable cardioverter defibrillations and pharmacological treatments. *Critical Care Nursing Quarterly, 26*(1), 45–49.

Zhang, S., Younis, G., Hariharan, R., Ho, J., Yang, Y., Ip, J., et al. (2004). Lower loop reentry as a mechanism of clockwise right atrial flutter. *Circulation, 109*(13), 1630–1635.

Zile, M. R., Baicu, C. F., & Gaasch, W. H. (2004). Diastolic heart failure: Abnormalities in active relaxation and passive stiffness of the left ventricle. *New England Journal of Medicine, 350*(19), 1953–1959.

Zimetbaum, P. J., Constantine, G., Sivananthan, M., Fisher, J. D., Hafley, G. E., Lee, K. L., et al. (2004). Electrocardiographic predictors of arrhythmic death and total mortality in the multicenter unsustained tachycardia trial. *Circulation, 110*(7), 776–769.

Pulmonary

QUESTIONS

1. Your patient had an exacerbation of COPD. The rapid response team was called and is currently intubating the patient and preparing him for transfer to the ICU. When the family visits, they are shocked to see the people working with the patient. No one had told them the patient had deteriorated and required intubation. After the patient is intubated and is being wheeled past them, family members try to communicate verbally with the patient, but he does not respond except to gesture. The nurse should tell family members:
   A. They must leave the area because they are exciting the patient.
   B. The tube used for breathing prevents the patient from speaking.
   C. They must speak with the doctor, who will explain why the patient cannot speak.
   D. The patient is very sick and may die.

2. Ben was just transferred to your progressive care unit. He had been in the ICU two weeks. Ben was intubated for a time because of his ARDS. On arrival in your unit, you note that he is tachycardic and restless. Ben states, "I can't be here now. What if something like this happens to me again?" The nurse's best response would be:
   A. "The nurses in our unit can take care of you."
   B. "We are not very far away at the nurses' station."
   C. "Your insurance will not cover another day there."
   D. "You sound concerned about leaving our ICU."

3. Continuing with the scenario in Question 2, a set of blood gases drawn just prior to Ben's transfer shows the following results: pH 7.52, $PaCO_2$ 31, HCO_3 22, PaO_2 87. These results would indicate
   A. Respiratory acidosis.
   B. Respiratory alkalosis.
   C. Metabolic acidosis.
   D. Metabolic alkalosis.

4. Continuing with the scenario in Questions 2 and 3, Ben is finally released from the hospital. He plans to visit his family in Denver. Part of the patient teaching for Ben should include information on the effects of high altitude on his ability to oxygenate effectively. Which of the following changes would be expected on his blood gas results?
   A. The pH would decrease.
   B. No effect
   C. The O_2 saturation would decrease.
   D. The PaO_2 would increase.

5. SaO$_2$ values account for what percentage of oxygen (O$_2$) carried within the bloodstream?
   A. 2–3%
   B. 10–24%
   C. 97–98%
   D. 100%

6. Hypoxemia is best defined as:
   A. A decrease in oxygen at the cellular level
   B. A decrease in oxygen levels in arterial blood
   C. A decrease in oxygen levels in venous blood
   D. A decrease in oxygen levels from the brain

7. Your patient has been diagnosed with pulmonary hypertension. Which of the following compensatory mechanisms would be expected if the patient suffered from chronic hypoxia?
   A. Polycythemia
   B. Hypoplasia of the pulmonary vasculature
   C. Thinning of blood vessels in the lungs
   D. Cor pulmonale

8. Type II alveolar cells produce
   A. Macrocytes.
   B. Phagocytes.
   C. Surfactant.
   D. CO$_2$.

9. If you hear faint breath sounds on the left side of the chest and normal sounds on the right side immediately after your patient has been intubated, most likely
   A. The patient has a tumor.
   B. The physician has intubated the esophagus.
   C. The ET is at the carina.
   D. The right mainstem has been intubated.

10. John is a 32-year-old engineer that has been on hemodialysis for three years. He missed his last two treatments. He is lethargic, lacks stamina, and is very edematous. His ABGs show the following results: pH 7.30, PaCO$_2$ 32, HCO$_3$ 17, PaO$_2$ 90. John's results indicate
    A. Metabolic alkalosis.
    B. Respiratory acidosis.
    C. Metabolic acidosis.
    D. Respiratory alkalosis.

11. You ask a fellow nurse to carry a newly drawn ABG specimen to the lab. She does not place the sample on ice. What effect will the lack of icing have on the sample?
    A. None
    B. It will invalidate the sample.
    C. The pH will rise.
    D. The PaO$_2$ will rise.

12. Your patient must have an arterial blood gas sample drawn. The respiratory therapist says he is out of prepared syringes, so he obtains a syringe into which he places heparin. What effect will too much heparin have on the sample, if any?
    A. Decreased bicarbonate
    B. No effect
    C. Increased $PaCO_2$
    D. Totally prevent clotting

13. While the respiratory therapist is attempting to draw an arterial blood gas sample, you note that he is exerting a lot of force to move the cylinder of the syringe. What effect will this high-friction syringe have on blood gas results, if any?
    A. It will put the artery into spasm
    B. Increase the $PaCO_2$
    C. Decrease the PaO_2
    D. No effect on results

14. The respiratory therapist asks if the patient has a fever. The possibility of fever will have what effect on the sample?
    A. The HCO_3 will be elevated.
    B. The PaO_2 will rise.
    C. Fever has no effect.
    D. The pH will rise.

15. Familial emphysema is a condition that results in a deficiency in
    A. Adenosine monophosphate.
    B. Ability to produce mucus.
    C. Alveoli.
    D. Serum alpha-antitrypsin.

16. People who have emphysema develop chronic hypoxia. Which potential imbalance would be expected with this condition?
    A. Hypokalemia
    B. Hypochloremia
    C. Decreased bicarbonate levels
    D. Hyponatremia

17. Sherie is a 20-year-old admitted to your unit with status asthmaticus. She has been taking Accolate, Allegra, and has been using a Proventil HFA rescue inhaler at home. Today Sherie was working in her garden when she found that she could not catch her breath. Her bronchospasms worsened, and she was transported to the ED. In the ED she received albuterol, oxygen and epinephrine without significant improvement. On auscultation, inspiratory and expiratory wheezing with a prolonged expiratory phase is heard throughout the lung fields. Sherie is using accessory muscles for respiration and is tachycardic and tachypneic. She is placed on O_2 at 2 L/min via NC and ABGs are drawn. Blood gas results are as follows: pH 7.52, PaO_2 106 mm Hg, $PaCO_2$ 27 mm Hg, HCO_3 24 mEq/L. These blood gas results show
    A. Uncompensated respiratory acidosis.
    B. Compensated metabolic alkalosis.
    C. Compensated metabolic acidosis.
    D. Uncompensated respiratory alkalosis.

18. Continuing with the scenario in Question 17, the hospitalist now orders Inderal (propanolol) for Sherie. As a nurse, you know that propanolol is contraindicated for asthmatics because
    A. It will exacerbate the tachycardia.
    B. It will lead to a severe respiratory acidosis.
    C. Pneumonia may result.
    D. Bronchospasm may worsen.

19. Continuing with the scenario in Questions 17 and 18, the most probable cause of Sherie's acid–base imbalance would be
    A. An adverse effect of albuterol.
    B. A side effect of theophylline.
    C. Hyperventilation.
    D. Hypoventilation.

20. Continuing with the scenario in Questions 17–19, Sherie's O_2 was increased to 5 L/min via mask. On auscultation, you note that the wheezing is barely audible. This finding may indicate
    A. Improvement.
    B. Need to lower O_2.
    C. A need for epinephrine.
    D. A worsening condition.

21. A possible treatment to best improve air flow in status asthmaticus is
    A. Bromex.
    B. Heliox.
    C. Norepinephrine.
    D. Nebulizer treatments.

22. Continuing with the scenario in Questions 17–20, Sherie now needs to be immediately intubated, placed on mechanical ventilation, and then transferred to the ICU. The physician uses pancuronium bromide (Pavulon) to paralyze the respiratory muscles. Which of the following drugs will counteract the effects of Pavulon?
    A. Atropine
    B. Narcan
    C. Neostigmine
    D. Regitine

23. Hugh, a 47-year-old patient with severe bronchitis, has been treated with a nonrebreather mask for five days. He is exhibiting increased distress with chest discomfort, restlessness, a dry hacking cough with dyspnea, and numbness in his extremities. Pulmonary function tests (PFTs) indicate a decreased vital capacity (VC), decreased compliance, and decreased functional residual capacity (FRC). As the nurse caring for this patient, you should
    A. Prepare for intubation with 100% FiO_2 (fraction of inspired oxygen).
    B. Administer Lasix 40 mg IV.
    C. Take the patient for a CT scan and prepare to give tPA.
    D. Check the pulse oximeter correlation with an arterial blood gas and decrease the FiO_2.

24. Eileen, a 30-year-old female, was admitted three days ago with a right fractured femur and fractures of two ribs. She has been on O_2 at 60% since admission. During your assessment, you note a temperature of 100°F, heart rate of 120, respiratory rate of 30, increased cough, and decreased breath sounds on the right side without tracheal deviation. You suspect her symptoms are the result of
    A. Pulmonary edema.
    B. Atelectasis.
    C. Pneumothorax.
    D. Sepsis.

25. As patients age, chest wall compliance decreases. One of the reasons for this change is that
    A. Total lung capacity decreases.
    B. Costal cartilage degenerates.
    C. Arterial oxygen tension increases.
    D. Residual volume decreases.

26. The cells that are responsible for forming a barrier for alveoli are
    A. Macrophages.
    B. Type II alveolar epithelial cells.
    C. Type I alveolar epithelial cells.
    D. Cilia.

27. Anatomic dead space is referred to as
    A. Minute ventilation.
    B. Wasted ventilation.
    C. Physiologic dead space.
    D. Conducting airways.

28. The oxyhemoglobin dissociation curve is
    A. A graphic representation showing the relationship between dissolved oxygen and the affinity for oxygen by the hemoglobin molecule.
    B. A graphic representation of carbon dioxide content versus oxygen content in arterial blood.
    C. A measure of methemoglobin.
    D. A way to calculate gas transport across the alveoli.

29. If the oxyhemoglobin curve shifts to the right, one factor that will affect this shift is
    A. A decrease in CO_2.
    B. A decrease in pH.
    C. A decrease in temperature.
    D. A decrease in 2,3-DPG.

30. If the oxyhemoglobin dissociation curve shifts to the left, which of the following would precipitate this change?
    A. Increased temperature
    B. Increased $PaCO_2$
    C. Increased 2,3-DPG
    D. Increased pH

31. Your patient has pulmonary hypertension. The physician has been utilizing diuretics without much effect. Which of the following therapies might be effective?
    A. Digitalis
    B. Increased hydration
    C. Nitric oxide
    D. Neostigmine

32. Chronic hypoxia usually results in which of the following electrolyte imbalances?
    A. Decreased chloride
    B. Decreased potassium
    C. Decreased calcium
    D. Decreased bicarbonate

33. If you are auscultating lung sounds and you can clearly hear the patient's spoken word through the stethoscope, this is known as
    A. Egophony.
    B. A friction rub.
    C. Whispered pectroliloquy.
    D. Bronchophony.

34. What is the interpretation for the following arterial blood gas?
    pH 7.22
    PO_2 93 mm Hg
    $PaCO_2$ 52 mm Hg
    HCO_3 23 mEq/L
    A. Uncompensated respiratory acidosis
    B. Compensated metabolic acidosis
    C. Uncompensated metabolic alkalosis
    D. Compensated respiratory acidosis

35. Your patient had 1,250 mL of pleural effusion removed via thoracentesis and immediately began coughing and was dyspneic. You believe he has developed
    A. A pneumothorax.
    B. Reexpansion pulmonary edema.
    C. Cardiac tamponade.
    D. Hemothorax.

36. Falsely low readings on a pulse oximeter may be due to
    A. Electronic interference from hemodialysis.
    B. Fever.
    C. Vascular dyes.
    D. Polycythemia.

37. Joseph's tracheostomy tube cuff has been requiring increasing pressures all shift to maintain a good air seal. What is a possible complication?
    A. Tracheal stenosis
    B. Air embolus
    C. Tracheal atresia
    D. Erosion of the innominate artery

38. **A contraindication for use of a nasal trumpet would include**
    A. Use as an alternative to oral intubation.
    B. Basilar skull fracture.
    C. Use with unconscious patients.
    D. A situation in which the nasal trumpet might be easily dislodged.

39. **The respiratory therapist tells you he is covering another unit and cannot perform postural drainage on your patient. He says your patient needs the left upper lobes drained if possible. The correct position to help this patient is**
    A. Semi-reclining.
    B. Flat with hips elevated.
    C. Supine.
    D. Flat on left side.

40. **The respiratory therapist has just given your patient an aerosol treatment. Which of the following conditions is contraindicated for this treatment?**
    A. Pleural effusions
    B. Head injury
    C. Asthma
    D. Stridor

41. **BiPAP is somewhat useful in acute respiratory distress syndrome (ARDS) because**
    A. BiPAP decreases cardiac output.
    B. BiPAP decreases venous return so lungs drain more effectively.
    C. BiPAP prevents barotrauma.
    D. BiPAP can open collapsed alveoli.

42. **Patients at risk for thrombosis formation have been classified by a trio of factors known as**
    A. Beck's triad.
    B. Belchod's triad.
    C. Virchow's triad.
    D. Goodman's triad.

43. **An example of a beta$_2$-adrenergic agonist would be:**
    A. Brethine
    B. Mucomyst
    C. Alupent
    D. Atrovert

44. **During a cardiopulmonary arrest, you note that the patient is being forcefully ventilated by the respiratory therapist using a bag-valve mask device. You know this patient is at risk for**
    A. Alveolar collapse.
    B. Barotrauma.
    C. Cardiac tamponade.
    D. Hemothorax.

45. Signs and symptoms of a pulmonary embolus can include
    A. A normal EKG or sinus bradycardia.
    B. Pleuritic chest pain and decreased cardiac output.
    C. ABGs showing respiratory acidosis and increased respiratory rate.
    D. Decreased pulmonary pressures.

46. Your patient is undergoing a cardiopulmonary arrest. The patient is being ventilated with a bag-valve mask device and an oropharyngeal airway in place. A continuous end-tidal CO_2 (PET CO_2) device is built into the BVM. The physician suspects the patient has suffered a pulmonary embolism. An expected change in parameters would include
    A. Increased PaO_2.
    B. Decreased CVP.
    C. Decreased PET CO_2.
    D. Increased $PaCO_2$.

47. On an EKG, an extensive pulmonary embolism may show
    A. Tall, peaked T waves in leads II, III, and AVF.
    B. Sinus bradycardia.
    C. Inverted T waves in leads V_6–V_9.
    D. Complete heart block.

48. Hannah was admitted to the ICU with a fever of 102.3°F, headache, dyspnea, dry cough, and chills. Her lab results indicate a low white blood cell count, low platelets, and raised C-reactive protein levels. Hannah's history includes a recent trip to a remote Chinese village within the past two weeks. You suspect Hannah may have
    A. Pneumonia.
    B. SARS.
    C. Influenza.
    D. Pericarditis.

49. Which of the following statements is true about a pulmonary embolism?
    A. Respiratory acidosis will occur.
    B. Heparin is used to dissolve clots.
    C. Normal D-dimer results can rule out a pulmonary embolism.
    D. Metabolic alkalosis will develop.

50. Gail was admitted to the progressive care unit following a fall from a stepstool. She complains of stabbing substernal pain each time she changes her position. Gail has been diagnosed with pneumomediastinum. A common significant finding with this diagnosis is
    A. Cullen's sign.
    B. Grey–Turner's sign.
    C. Hamman's sign.
    D. Handes' sign.

51. Severe carbon monoxide poisoning occurs when carboxyhemoglobin levels are higher than which of the following percentages?

A. 10–15%

B. 20–40%

C. 40–50%

D. 50–60%

52. Carbon monoxide has an affinity for hemoglobin thought to be 200–300 times greater than that of oxygen. Elimination of carbon monoxide occurs via the
   A. Kidneys.
   B. Liver.
   C. Spleen.
   D. Lungs.

53. Bernard lost his home to a fire this morning. He was burned on the chest and neck while trying to put out the fire. He is dyspneic and has soot on his face, and his eyebrows and nares are singed. The priority during treatment is to
   A. Maintain cardiac output.
   B. Maintain airway patency.
   C. Treat burned areas.
   D. Obtain ABGs and a carboxyhemoglobin level.

54. Increases in lung compliance occur with
   A. Pulmonary edema.
   B. Pleural effusions.
   C. Obesity.
   D. Emphysema.

55. Which of the following statements about laryngeal mask airways is true?
   A. A laryngeal mask airway may be inserted by any nurse.
   B. A laryngeal mask airway may cause hoarseness after removal.
   C. The patient must have an absent gag reflex.
   D. A laryngeal mask airway eliminates the risk of aspiration.

56. Which of the following drugs would be considered a mucolytic agent?
   A. Atropine
   B. Terbutaline
   C. Acetyl-cysteine
   D. Albuterol

57. Side effects of acetyl-cysteine include
   A. Bronchospasm.
   B. Headache.
   C. Hypertension.
   D. Red urine.

58. One of the most effective ways to relieve bronchospasm is to administer
   A. Adrenalin.
   B. An antihistamine.
   C. Prednisone.
   D. A B_2-receptor agonist.

59. **Which of the following drugs is a methylzanthine?**
    A. Prednisone
    B. Theophylline
    C. Atropine
    D. Accolate

60. **To determine whether your patient has a genetic predisposition for malignant hyperthermia, which of the following drugs might be used?**
    A. Halothane
    B. Caffeine
    C. Accolate
    D. Singulair

61. **During a cardiac arrest, your patient aspirated gastric contents. Which of the following statements is true regarding this type of aspiration?**
    A. If the pH of the material is < 2.5, necrosis will be minimal.
    B. The patient will always develop ARDS.
    C. Onset of symptoms occurs gradually.
    D. There is little danger of atelectasis.

62. **Devin was admitted for abrupt-onset fever, chills, vomiting, diarrhea, and headache that developed in the past 24 hours. Devin had recently been on a cruise to Barbados. Devin is probably suffering from**
    A. A *Pseudomonas* infection.
    B. Influenza.
    C. A *Klebsiella* infection.
    D. Legionnaire's disease.

63. **Placement of a central line via a subclavian vein may cause**
    A. Cardiac tamponade.
    B. An open pneumothorax.
    C. A tension pneumothorax.
    D. Limb pain.

64. **When the resident attempts to place a central line, air is accidentally introduced into the line when the IV tubing becomes disconnected. The best position to place this patient to minimize the venous air embolism is**
    A. Reverse Trendelenburg.
    B. On the right side.
    C. Trendelenburg with left decubitus tilt.
    D. On the left side.

65. **The definitive study for determination of thrombolic emboli is**
    A. Pulmonary ventilation–perfusion scan.
    B. Mixed venous oxygen saturation.
    C. Pulmonary angiography.
    D. PAWP.

66. **Risk factors for thrombolic emboli include**
    A. A patient who is one week postpartum.
    B. Carcinoma.
    C. Long bone fractures.
    D. Heparin administration.

67. **A venous air embolism may be caused by**
    A. Hemodialysis.
    B. Pulmonary artery catheter.
    C. Radial arterial catheter.
    D. Peritoneal dialysis.

68. **Blood gases you would expect to see with thrombotic emboli are**
    A. pH 7.42, PaO_2 88, $PaCO_2$ 28, and HCO_3 22.
    B. pH 7.50, PaO_2 74, $PaCO_2$ 52, and HCO_3 24.
    C. pH 7.32, PaO_2 86, $PaCO_2$ 29, and HCO_3 26.
    D. pH 7.32, PaO_2 90, $PaCO_2$ 30, and HCO_3 24.

69. **Barbara was admitted for multiple fractures and contusions following a motor vehicle accident this evening. She complains of dyspnea and petechiae are noted. Barbara probably has**
    A. A pulmonary embolus.
    B. Thrombocytopenia.
    C. A venous air embolus.
    D. A fat embolus.

70. **The best position for a patient with ARDS is**
    A. Prone.
    B. On the right side.
    C. On the left side.
    D. Supine.

71. **Fluid therapy in ARDS is directed toward**
    A. Keeping a high cardiac output state.
    B. Maintaining a low protein content.
    C. Maintaining hyponatremia.
    D. Maintaining a low circulating fluid volume.

72. **Pulmonary hypertension is usually defined by the level of the mean pulmonary artery pressure (MPAP). A diagnosis of pulmonary hypertension can be made if the MPAP is**
    A. 3–5 mm Hg.
    B. 5–9 mm Hg.
    C. 10–20 mm Hg.
    D. >20 mm Hg.

73. **The hallmark sign of asthma is**
    A. PEFR 100–125.
    B. FEF of 80%.
    C. Decreased FEV_1.
    D. Wheezing.

74. **When assessing a patient with a chest tube drainage system, which of the following statements would be correct?**
    A. Check for subcutaneous emphysema around the insertion site by auscultation.
    B. If using a Pleur-Evac with auto-transfusion connection, make certain all clamps are open.
    C. The average chest tube size for an adult is 20 Fr.
    D. If using a chest tube drainage system with a one-way valve and suction, water is required to maintain a seal.

75. **The oxyhemoglobin dissociation curve may be shifted to the right by**
    A. Alkalosis, hyperthermia, hypercapnia.
    B. Acidosis, hypercarbia, hyperthermia.
    C. Acidosis, hypocarbia, hypothermia.
    D. Alkalosis, hypothermia, hypercapnia.

76. **Which statement about esophageal detection devices (EDDs) is true?**
    A. An EDD reduces silent aspiration.
    B. An EDD will have a beige color when gas exchange is adequate.
    C. An EDD is more reliable than a CO_2 detector in a pulseless patient.
    D. A false-positive result may occur if the patient recently ingested a carbonated beverage.

77. **Research has shown that use of normal saline does not thin secretions and may cause which of the following adverse effects?**
    A. Anxiety
    B. Depression
    C. Decreased mean arterial pressure
    D. Bronchodilation

78. **Your patient is receiving an antibiotic intravenously for pneumonia. The antibiotic is mixed as 1 g in 100 mL of D_5W. You need to administer the medication over 40 minutes. The only IV tubing you have delivers 15 gtts/mL. How many drops per minute should you set your infusion pump to deliver?**
    A. 38 gtts/min
    B. 16 gtts/min
    C. 32 gtts/min
    D. 19 gtts/min

79. **Which of the following conditions will decrease the production of 2,3-DPG?**
    A. Hypothyroidism
    B. Hypoxemia
    C. Congenital heart disease
    D. Anemia

80. **Central cyanosis is usually seen when the Hgb level is**
    A. 2 g/dL.
    B. 5 g/dL.
    C. 8 g/dL.
    D. 10 g/dL.

81. **A side effect of succinylcholine is**
    A. Hypokalemia.
    B. Malignant hypothermia.
    C. Hypotension.
    D. Cardiac arrest.

82. **Vecuronium (Norcuron) is eliminated primarily via the**
    A. Renal glomerulus.
    B. Spleen.
    C. Hepatic/biliary system.
    D. Hoffman elimination.

83. **Asthma patients may receive steroids and neuromuscular blocking agents, so these patients are at increased risk for**
    A. Renal failure.
    B. Hypertension.
    C. Hepatic failure.
    D. Prolonged muscle weakness.

84. **The FiO$_2$ for a nasal cannula set at a flow rate of 6 L/min is**
    A. 24%.
    B. 30%.
    C. 21%.
    D. 40%.

85. **A non-rebreathing mask can deliver what percentage of oxygen when the O$_2$ flow rate is 10–15 L?**
    A. 30–40%
    B. 24–40%
    C. 60–80%
    D. 50–60%

86. **Pulse oximetry readings are considered unreliable when oxygen saturation falls below**
    A. 60%.
    B. 90%.
    C. 55%.
    D. 70%.

87. **A factor that increases pulmonary vascular resistance is**
    A. Prostaglandin therapy.
    B. Sepsis.
    C. Hypoxia.
    D. Hypovolemia.

88. A cause of decreased SVO_2 would be
    A. An increased metabolic rate.
    B. Sedation.
    C. A decreased metabolic rate.
    D. An increased cardiac output.

89. When an oral ETT is properly positioned in an adult, the centimeter mark will usually be _____ for women at the front teeth.
    A. 14 cm
    B. 21 cm
    C. 23 cm
    D. 25 cm

90. The normal anterior–posterior diameter of the thorax ratio to the lateral diameter is a ratio of
    A. 1:1.
    B. 2:5.
    C. 2:3.
    D. 1:2.

91. A common site for the placement of electrodes for a peripheral nerve is on the
    A. Posterior tibial.
    B. Medial nerve.
    C. Temporal nerve.
    D. Radial nerve.

92. Muscles will stop moving in the following order in response to neuromuscular blocking agents:
    A. Abdomen, glottis, extremities, face, eyes
    B. Glottis, extremities, face, abdomen, eyes
    C. Eyes, face, extremities, abdomen
    D. Glottis, intercostals, extremities, neck

93. The usual goal for a patient having neuromuscular blockade during mechanical ventilation is one to two twitches, indicating _____ to _____ block.
    A. 85%, 90%
    B. 60%, 70%
    C. 40%, 50%
    D. 25%, 40%

94. Analyze the following arterial blood gas results. Use the provided space to the right side to assist in interpretation by writing acidosis or alkalosis, compensated or uncompensated.
    pH 7.38
    CO_2 27
    HCO_3 16

    A. Normal

    B. Compensated respiratory acidosis

    C. Compensated metabolic acidosis

    D. Uncompensated respiratory alkalosis

95. **Analyze the following arterial blood gas results. Use the provided space to the right side to assist in interpretation by writing acidosis or alkalosis, compensated or uncompensated.**

    pH 7.46

    CO_2 34

    HCO_3 24

    A. Normal

    B. Compensated respiratory acidosis

    C. Compensated metabolic acidosis

    D. Uncompensated respiratory alkalosis

96. **Analyze the following arterial blood gas results. Use the provided space to the right side to assist in interpretation by writing acidosis or alkalosis, compensated or uncompensated.**

    pH 7.18

    CO_2 40

    HCO_3 15

    A. Normal

    B. Compensated respiratory acidosis

    C. Uncompensated metabolic acidosis

    D. Uncompensated respiratory alkalosis

97. **Analyze the following arterial blood gas results. Use the provided space to the right side to assist in interpretation by writing acidosis or alkalosis, compensated or uncompensated.**

    pH 7.56

    CO_2 25

    HCO_3 34

    A. Uncompensated (mixed) respiratory/metabolic alkalosis

    B. Compensated respiratory acidosis

    C. Compensated metabolic acidosis

    D. Uncompensated respiratory alkalosis

98. **Analyze the following arterial blood gas results. Use the provided space to the right side to assist in interpretation by writing acidosis or alkalosis, compensated or uncompensated.**

    pH 7.42

    CO_2 36

    HCO_3 23

    A. Compensated respiratory acidosis

    B. Normal

    C. Compensated metabolic acidosis

    D. Uncompensated respiratory alkalosis

99. Analyze the following arterial blood gas results. Use the provided space to the right side to assist in interpretation by writing acidosis or alkalosis, compensated or uncompensated.

pH 7.49

CO_2 30

HCO_3 22

    A. Uncompensated metabolic alkalosis

    B. Compensated respiratory acidosis

    C. Compensated metabolic acidosis

    D. Uncompensated respiratory alkalosis

100. Analyze the following arterial blood gas results. Use the provided space to the right side to assist in interpretation by writing acidosis or alkalosis, compensated or uncompensated.

pH 7.37

CO_2 68

HCO_3 38

    A. Uncompensated metabolic alkalosis

    B. Compensated respiratory acidosis

    C. Compensated metabolic acidosis

    D. Uncompensated respiratory alkalosis

101. Analyze the following arterial blood gas results. Use the provided space to the right side to assist in interpretation by writing acidosis or alkalosis, compensated or uncompensated.

pH 7.11

CO_2 65

HCO_3 17

    A. Uncompensated (mixed) respiratory/metabolic acidosis

    B. Uncompensated metabolic alkalosis

    C. Compensated metabolic acidosis

    D. Uncompensated respiratory alkalosis

102. Analyze the following arterial blood gas results. Use the provided space to the right side to assist in interpretation by writing acidosis or alkalosis, compensated or uncompensated.

pH 7.43

CO_2 31

HCO_3 20

    A. Uncompensated metabolic alkalosis

    B. Compensated respiratory acidosis

    C. Compensated respiratory alkalosis

    D. Uncompensated respiratory alkalosis

103. Analyze the following arterial blood gas results. Use the provided space to the right side to assist in interpretation by writing acidosis or alkalosis, compensated or uncompensated.

pH 7.51

CO_2 40

HCO_3 35

    A. Uncompensated metabolic alkalosis

    B. Compensated respiratory acidosis

    C. Compensated metabolic acidosis

    D. Uncompensated respiratory alkalosis

104. **Analyze the following arterial blood gas results. Use the provided space to the right side to assist in interpretation by writing acidosis or alkalosis, compensated or uncompensated.**

pH 7.17

CO_2 55

HCO_3 20

    A. Uncompensated metabolic alkalosis

    B. Uncompensated (mixed) respiratory/metabolic acidosis

    C. Compensated metabolic acidosis

    D. Uncompensated respiratory alkalosis

105. **Analyze the following arterial blood gas results. Use the provided space to the right side to assist in interpretation by writing acidosis or alkalosis, compensated or uncompensated.**

pH 7.38

CO_2 38

HCO_3 22

    A. Uncompensated metabolic alkalosis

    B. Compensated respiratory acidosis

    C. Compensated metabolic acidosis

    D. Normal

106. **Analyze the following arterial blood gas results. Use the provided space to the right side to assist in interpretation by writing acidosis or alkalosis, compensated or uncompensated.**

pH 7.30

CO_2 61

HCO_3 25

    A. Uncompensated metabolic alkalosis

    B. Compensated respiratory acidosis

    C. Compensated metabolic acidosis

    D. Uncompensated respiratory acidosis

107. **A disadvantage of closed catheter suctioning of a tracheally ventilated patient would be**

    A. The extra weight of the inline tubing.

    B. The patient does not receive oxygen during the procedure.

    C. The cost is higher with a single-use catheter.

    D. Closed catheter suctioning is cost-effective only if used sporadically.

108. **The function of a stoma stent is**
    A. To provide the ability for the patient to speak.
    B. To prevent aspiration.
    C. To avoid translaryngeal intubation.
    D. To keep the stoma tract open.

109. **Which of the following statements is true regarding the use of a laryngeal mask airway (LMA)?**
    A. Nurses routinely insert these airways.
    B. There is a low risk of aspiration.
    C. It is a temporary airway.
    D. The vocal cords must be visualized.

110. **Which of the following statements about silicone or plastic tracheostomy tubes is true?**
    A. The tubes offer a lower cost to the facility.
    B. Wire-reinforced tubes cannot be used during MRI imaging.
    C. A one-way speaking valve is easy to use.
    D. Silicone holds up to repeated cleaning.

111. **A complication of a tracheostomy tube would be that**
    A. It allows for right mainstem intubation.
    B. It increases airway resistance.
    C. It leaves a permanent scar.
    D. The airway is less stable.

112. **A complication/contraindication of a nasal endotracheal tube could be**
    A. The patient cannot drink.
    B. The tube offers easy access to the right mainstem bronchus.
    C. The tube cannot be used for a patient with a cervical injury.
    D. The tube may cause otitis.

113. **Your patient has just been intubated. Documentation of the procedure usually would not include**
    A. The amount of time the intubator took to complete the task.
    B. The depth of the tube.
    C. The size of the tube.
    D. CXR taken.

114. **Which of the following statements is true regarding the use of capnography to verify endotracheal tube placement?**
    A. $ETCO_2$ is a moderately reliable indicator of correct tube placement.
    B. It is not necessary to auscultate lung sounds when this device is used.
    C. It is a substitute for pulse oximetry.
    D. Placement of the device can be difficult to learn initially.

115. Sinusitis, hospital-acquired pneumonia (HAP), and ventilator-acquired pneumonia (VAP) pose many challenges for the progressive care nurse. Sometimes a patient will be transferred to your unit with an already-acquired infection, but then symptoms will become more pronounced. Which statement is true regarding these conditions?
    A. Good hand washing technique is effective for reducing VAP.
    B. Sinusitis can be prevented by using a smaller-diameter endotracheal tube.
    C. Nasogastric tubes are preferred to orogastric tubes.
    D. Oral tubes have a greater incidence of sinusitis.

116. Richard is a 61-year-old male with a significant history of emphysema. He started smoking when he was five years old, and until this admission he continued to smoke as many as five packs of cigarettes a day. In addition, he has uncontrolled diabetes and peripheral vascular disease. Three days ago, Richard had a major stroke when he was walking down the stairs. He suffered a broken pelvis and fractured his left radius. He has been comatose since his admission, with a flat-line EEG study. His wife has agreed that Richard should be placed on a do not resuscitate (DNR) status. She has also agreed to discontinue ventilatory support. His physician recommends that the patient receive morphine as a comfort measure during this process. Richard's wife has been informed that the morphine will make him more comfortable, but may decrease his ability to ventilate and, in fact, may hasten his demise. This type of ethical dilemma is known as
    A. A null ethical principle.
    B. Double effect.
    C. Slippery slope.
    D. Palliative principle.

117. A patient with a suspected diagnosis of active tuberculosis has been admitted to your care. The type of protective face mask you should use is the
    A. N95 respirator.
    B. Particulate mask.
    C. TB face mask.
    D. Hood mask.

118. You watch a fellow nurse administer a TB skin test. She appears to place the needle too deep under the skin. As a nurse, you know that the test may be affected because
    A. It may produce a false-positive result.
    B. Subcutaneous injection will nullify the result.
    C. Necrosis will result.
    D. Ulceration will result.

119. The volume of gas that is inspired and expired with normal effort is known as
    A. Lung capacity.
    B. Tidal volume.
    C. Inspiratory versus expiratory ventilation.
    D. Minute volume.

120. Ian was driving his car through an intersection when he was T-boned by another car. Ian suffered a fractured pelvis and was stabilized in the ED, then transferred to your unit to await surgical fixation of the fracture. When auscultating lung sounds, you hear what you believe to be bowel sounds in his chest. Ian states he has moderate shoulder pain on the left side, and he is mildly tachypneic. Ian will probably be diagnosed with
    A. A fractured scapula.
    B. Diaphragmatic rupture.
    C. Hemothorax.
    D. Bowel rupture.

121. Continuing with the scenario in Question 120, the immediate priority for Ian's treatment is now
    A. To ensure adequate oxygenation.
    B. Immediate surgery.
    C. Locate additional injuries.
    D. Insert a chest tube.

122. Which of the following conditions mandates the use of pain control?
    A. Hemothorax
    B. ARDS
    C. Flail chest
    D. Pulmonary contusion

123. Your patient has a confirmed flail chest. Which alteration in acid–base balance would you expect?
    A. Metabolic alkalosis
    B. Metabolic acidosis
    C. Respiratory acidosis
    D. Respiratory alkalosis

124. One of the factors to be considered when assessing a patient for possible aspiration and chemical/aspiration pneumonitis is
    A. The possibility of using syrup of ipecac.
    B. pH.
    C. The type of infiltrates on CXR.
    D. ABG results.

125. What is the proper location of a chest tube for evacuation of a hemothorax?
    A. Second intercostal space, midclavicular line
    B. Second intercostal space, midaxillary line
    C. Fifth intercostal space, midaxillary line
    D. Fifth intercostal space, midclavicular line

126. The hypoxemic type of respiratory failure is defined as
    A. Increased dead air space.
    B. $PaO_2 < 60$ mm Hg while person is at rest, at sea level, on room air.
    C. ARDS.
    D. COPD.

127. A term for a patient who has been diagnosed with right ventricular hypertrophy caused by pulmonary hypertension caused by lung disease is
    A. Hyperplasia.
    B. Thrombotic syndrome.
    C. Cor pulmonale.
    D. ARDS.

128. Multiple organ dysfunction (MODS) may be directly caused by
    A. Venous thrombosis.
    B. Shunting.
    C. Oral estrogen therapy.
    D. Pulmonary embolism.

129. Pulmonary embolism is actually considered a complication of deep venous thrombosis. To assess for deep venous thrombosis, which of the following signs should be assessed?
    A. Moses'
    B. Davis'
    C. Corrigan's
    D. Hamman's

130. Your 50-year-old patient was admitted with a complaint of a history of a cough that occurred predominately in the morning for the past four years. The severity of the cough has increased over the past three days and wheezing is present, and the patient is dyspneic with mild exercise. The patient has been a smoker since he was a teenager. Your patient is probably suffering from
    A. Asthma.
    B. A pulmonary embolus.
    C. COPD.
    D. Pneumonia.

131. A 34-year-old male is admitted to your unit with a history of ETOH use and multiple previous admissions. He is now in severe end-stage hepatic failure. He is currently sedated and is in restraints for self-protection. Vital signs are as follows:
    RR 16
    BP 140/84
    EKG ST at 112
    SpO_2 96%

    The patient's wife visits and you inform her about the need for the restraints and the patient's need to sleep. She acknowledges this information and says she will sit quietly at the patient's bedside. About five minutes later, you find the patient extubated and very agitated. His wife states she released the restraints because she felt they were, "too tight." Your priority in the care of this patient is
    A. Immediate sedation for the agitation.
    B. Remove the wife from the unit.
    C. Notify the charge nurse.
    D. Place the patient on a 40% mask and observe his response.

132. **You are teaching your COPD patient about his treatment plan. Which of the following statements would indicate that the patient understands his disease and his treatment plan?**
     A. "I should limit my fluid intake to one liter per day."
     B. "I should use my Serevent inhaler as a rescue inhaler."
     C. "I should elevate and cross my legs while watching television."
     D. "I should avoid drinking or ingesting dairy products."

133. **Expected pharmacologic treatment for your patient with COPD would include**
     A. Sedatives.
     B. Antihistamines.
     C. Steroids.
     D. Beta blockers.

134. **Where does the hypoxemic drive to breathe originate?**
     A. Cerebellum
     B. Aortic and carotid arteries
     C. Hypothalamus
     D. Medulla

135. **The functional residual capacity is**
     A. The amount of gas that can be forcefully exhaled after a maximum inspiration.
     B. The amount of air left in the lungs after a normal expiration.
     C. The amount of gas normally exhaled after a maximum inhalation.
     D. The amount of gas left in the lungs after a maximum exhalation.

136. **Subcutaneous emphysema usually occurs in the area of the**
     A. Head.
     B. Neck.
     C. Thorax.
     D. Abdomen.

137. **Pulse oximetry has not been shown to be affected by**
     A. Dark skin.
     B. Elevated bilirubin.
     C. Dark nail polish.
     D. Presence of hemoglobin.

138. **Pulse oximeters should never be used**
     A. To determine oxygen saturation values.
     B. During a cardiac arrest.
     C. As a determinant for predicting hemoglobin affinity for oxygen.
     D. To help determine a patient's activity tolerance.

139. **When setting alarm limits for a pulse oximeter, the oxygen saturation limit should be what percentage less than the patient's acceptable baseline?**

A. 2%

B. 5%

C. 8%

D. 10%

140. An SpO_2 value of 95% correlates with which of the following PaO_2 values?
   A. 95 mm Hg
   B. 80 mm Hg
   C. 90 mm Hg
   D. 75 mm Hg

141. What is the minimum number of staff required for use of the Vollman Prone Positioner (VPP) when providing manual pronation therapy for your patient?
   A. 2
   B. 3
   C. 4
   D. 5

142. Which of the following conditions would not be considered a contraindication for the use of pronation therapy?
   A. Pregnancy
   B. Weight of 160 kg
   C. Unstable pelvis
   D. Open abdomen

143. Nursing actions that should be performed prior to initiating pronation therapy would include
   A. Securing the EKG leads on the anterior chest with tape.
   B. Noting the amount of all drainage for colostomies and ileostomies.
   C. Utilizing capnography monitoring.
   D. Documenting existing drainage on any wound dressings.

144. To prevent complications with chest tube drainage systems, the suction level should not be higher than
   A. -20 cm/H_2O.
   B. -30 cm/H_2O.
   C. -40 cm/H_2O.
   D. -50 cm/H_2O.

145. Which of the following statements is true regarding chest tube drainage systems?
   A. Drainage of frank blood in amounts > 100 mL/h is not significant.
   B. Drainage tubing should be placed horizontally on the bed and down to the collection chamber.
   C. All drainage tubing should be dependent to the insertion site.
   D. Chest tube drainage from a mediastinal tube should not bubble in the water seal chamber.

146. Cayden is a 36-year-old patient originally admitted for a fractured femur and to rule out a coronary contusion following a skiing accident. While you are giving Cayden his discharge teaching, he suddenly complains of pain in his left chest. He immediately becomes tachypneic and tachycardic. As you lay Cayden back down in the bed, you note asymmetrical chest wall excursion and neck vein distention. He has absent breath sounds on the left side and his heart sounds are muffled. Cayden rapidly becomes dyspneic and cyanotic. Cayden's condition is likely due to
    A. Tension pneumothorax.
    B. Cardiac tamponade.
    C. Pulmonary embolism.
    D. Esophageal rupture.

147. Continuing with the scenario from Question 146, Cayden requires an immediate needle decompression for a left tension pneumothorax. The needle will be placed in
    A. The second intercostal space at the left midclavicular line.
    B. The third intercostal space at the left midaxillary line.
    C. The fourth intercostal space at the left midaxillary line.
    D. The fifth intercostal space at the left midclavicular line.

148. Which of the following would be considered a relative complication for performing a thoracentesis?
    A. Splenomegaly
    B. Coagulation disorder
    C. Previous pneumonectomy
    D. Pleural fluid protein to serum protein ratio greater than 0.5 g/dL

149. Physiologic PEEP is
    A. The same as plateau pressure.
    B. The same as static pressure.
    C. The positive pressure remaining in the alveoli.
    D. A factor that decreases the work of breathing.

150. A condition that increases lung compliance is
    A. Kyphoscoliosis.
    B. Emphysema.
    C. ARDS.
    D. Pulmonary edema.

151. A factor that would decrease lung resistance is
    A. Endotracheal tube size.
    B. Bronchospasm.
    C. Secretions.
    D. Albuterol administration.

152. Your patient's blood gas results indicate uncompensated metabolic acidosis. A probable cause for this result would be
    A. Anxiety.
    B. Nasogastric suction.
    C. Neuromuscular disorders.
    D. Diabetic ketoacidosis.

153. Your patient has emphysema. During chest percussion, you would expect which of the following types of sound to occur?
    A. Flat
    B. Dull
    C. Hyperresonant
    D. Resonant

154. Carol has chronic COPD. She has smoked for several years. Which physiological changes would you expect to see in a patient with COPD?
    A. Clubbed fingers
    B. Splenomegaly
    C. Left ventricular failure
    D. Hypotension

155. The most common cause of COPD is
    A. Pollution.
    B. Smoking.
    C. Heredity.
    D. Occupation.

156. The cardinal sign of respiratory failure includes all of the following except
    A. Tachypnea.
    B. Diaphoresis.
    C. Restlessness.
    D. Headache.

157. Surya is a construction worker who does not speak English; he was admitted to your unit with a pulmonary contusion and a flail chest after a fall at work. He will not let you assess him and you cannot determine what language he is speaking. Surya becomes quite anxious. ABGs are drawn by a respiratory therapist without incident. You would expect the results to show
    A. Respiratory acidosis.
    B. Metabolic alkalosis.
    C. Respiratory alkalosis.
    D. Metabolic acidosis.

158. Which of the following medications might cause a cough?
    A. Tylenol
    B. Ibuprofen
    C. ACE inhibitors
    D. Ampicillin

159. Early signs of impending respiratory failure include
    A. Tachypnea and agitation.
    B. Crackles and cough.
    C. Peripheral cyanosis and tachypnea.
    D. Restlessness and tachycardia.

160. **In ARDS, pulmonary capillaries leak from blood into the pulmonary interstitium. This phenomenon is due to**
    A. The alveolar-oxygen gradient.
    B. Colloid osmotic pressure.
    C. The A-a gradient.
    D. Diffusion.

161. **Carbon dioxide is carried in the blood as**
    A. Bicarbonate.
    B. Carbonic acid.
    C. Carbon anhydrase.
    D. Carbonalate-1.

162. **When correctly placed, a chest tube will be in**
    A. The intercostal space.
    B. The pleural space.
    C. The mediastinal space.
    D. Intrapleural space.

163. **Why is prednisone contraindicated in tuberculosis?**
    A. Prednisone masks the infection.
    B. Prednisone increases edema, leading to dyspnea.
    C. Prednisone decreases the effectiveness of isoniazid.
    D. Prednisone increases the effectiveness of isoniazid.

164. **Your patient is receiving chemotherapy for lung cancer. His labs show a WBC of 0.7. You anticipate he will receive which medication?**
    A. Epogen
    B. Antibiotics
    C. Plasmapheresis
    D. Neupogen

165. **After 3 doses of Neupogen, your patient complains of bone pain and muscle aches. What do you tell him?**
    A. These are common side effects of the medication.
    B. His bone cancer has metastasized.
    C. His arthritis has flared up.
    D. He has gout.

166. **Amanda is a 54-year-old secretary who was admitted to your unit with nonradiating chest pain. The pain was intermittent and occurred predominately on the right side, and changes of position or deep inhalation did not affect the quality of the pain. Amanda's V/Q scan showed the probability of a pulmonary embolism. Laboratory and physical findings are as follows:**
    Current ABGs: pH 7.24, $PaCO_2$ 32, HCO_3 17, PaO_2 97
    SpO_2 0.98
    Lactate 4.4

EKG: ST at 102 with isolated PVC

Cuff BP 98/60

Skin pale, cool

T 98.4°F

RR 26, breath sounds; crackles, RML, RLL

O_2 30% via mask

Mentation: Alert, oriented × 4

What is the interpretation of Amanda's ABGs?
   A. Respiratory acidosis, compensated
   B. Metabolic acidosis, compensated
   C. Respiratory alkalosis, uncompensated
   D. Metabolic acidosis, compensated respiratory alkalosis

167. **Continuing with the scenario in Question 166, what is your overall impression of Amanda's oxygenation status?**
   A. Oxygenation is adequate, and her O_2 and SpO_2 are normal.
   B. Oxygenation is inadequate because she needs a FiO_2 of 30%.
   C. Oxygenation is adequate, and the FiO_2 is irrelevant.
   D. Oxygenation is inadequate, the lactate is high, and pH and HCO_3 are low.

168. **A 42-year-old female was admitted to your progressive care unit following a fall down some patio stairs. She sustained a fracture of the fourth rib on the right and fractures of the fourth and fifth ribs on the left. She was medicated for pain and, while visiting with her husband, becomes dyspneic. Her respiratory rate increases to 36 from 16. The patient's trachea is noted to deviate to the left, and diminished breath sounds are heard throughout the left lung fields. You also note crepitus over the site of the fracture on the right side. She is probably developing**
   A. A pericardial tamponade.
   B. A pneumothorax.
   C. A hemothorax.
   D. A chylothorax.

169. **When a patient is being auto-transfused, what size filter is commonly used?**
   A. 10 mcg
   B. 40 mcg
   C. 50 mcg
   D. 20 mcg

170. **Your patient has a closed chest tube drainage system. When he turns slightly to the left, a large amount of dark red blood enters the pleural tube. This situation is probably due to**
   A. A ruptured effusion.
   B. Erosion into the intercostal vessels.
   C. Old blood dumping.
   D. A new hemothorax.

171. Which type of device can deliver precise, high flow rates of O_2?
    A. Partial rebreather mask
    B. Venturi mask
    C. Non-rebreathing mask
    D. Transtracheal catheter

This concludes the Pulmonary Questions section.

ANSWERS

1. **Correct Answer: B**
   This is a case where communication is clearly the problem. The family should have been informed by someone that the patient needed assistance with breathing and that they should expect a transfer. It should also have been mentioned how the patient might look in the ICU. In addition, it could have been communicated about the patient's inability to speak. Answers A, C, and D are all nontherapeutic responses. The family is clearly distressed, so a simple explanation is best.

2. **Correct Answer: D**
   Therapeutic communication occurs when the patient's feelings are validated. This response allows for the patient to express the concerns he has about the transfer. The other answers are closed and judgmental and do not allow for any expression of feeling from the patient.

3. **Correct Answer: B**
   Ben was quite anxious and tachycardic. His respiratory rate probably was increased because of both his anxiety and his condition. He would blow off CO_2. His pH is below normal, so it is uncompensated. The HCO_3 is low, indicating alkalosis. The interpretation would be uncompensated respiratory alkalosis.

4. **Correct Answer: C**
   At higher altitudes, there is decreasing atmospheric pressure to force oxygen into the lungs. To compensate for the lower pressure, the person must breathe faster. The percentage of oxygen remains the same, but the partial pressure of the oxygen decreases. Arterial PaO_2 decreases, as does O_2 saturation. The rapid breathing will result in hyperventilation, raising the pH and lowering the $PaCO_2$ level.

5. **Correct Answer: C**
   The percentage of total oxygen carried within the bloodstream attributed to the SaO_2 is 97–98%. SaO_2 is the arterial saturation of hemoglobin. The percentage corresponds to the percentage of hemoglobin on the red blood cells that carries O_2. Typically this percentage is documented as normal when within the range of 93–99%. PaO_2 is the percentage of oxygen within the bloodstream that is free or dissolved in the plasma. This value is documented in mmHg and is considered normal when within the range of 80–100 mm Hg.

6. **Correct Answer: B**
   Hypoxemia is a decreased oxygen level in the arterial blood or PaO_2 < 80 mm Hg. Hypoxia is defined as a decreased oxygen level at the cellular level. Decreased oxygen levels within the veins and the brain refer to PaO_2 < 50 mm Hg and $ScVO_2$ < 20%, respectively.

7. **Correct Answer: A**
   Effects of acute hypoxia are reversible. Chronic hypoxia causes permanent changes in the lungs and pulmonary vasculature (hyperplasia and hypertrophy). This will cause thickening of the blood vessels and will narrow the lumen. Polycythemia develops and the blood viscosity increases. The increased number of cells will be available to carry

oxygen, but the increased viscosity will increase pressure in the pulmonary vasculature and force the right ventricle to pump harder to maintain the CO level. The right ventricle will hypertrophy and eventually weaken, and the patient will develop right heart failure (cor pulmonale).

8. **Correct Answer: C**

Surfactant is a lipoprotein that functions by increasing surface tension of alveoli and allow alveoli to expand and contract. Some residual pressure should be present in the alveoli at the end of respiration to keep the alveoli open (physiologic PEEP). If surfactant production is impaired, the alveoli's ability to exchange O_2 is compromised. Type I cells line the outside of the alveoli.

9. **Correct Answer: D**

The right mainstem bronchus is somewhat wider and has less of an angle off the mainstem bronchus, so it is much more readily intubated.

10. **Correct Answer: C**

More specifically, these ABG results indicate an uncompensated metabolic acidosis. The pH is low, as is the $PaCO_2$.

11. **Correct Answer: B**

The $PaCO_2$ will rise approximately 3–10 mm Hg per hour. The PaO_2 and the pH will decrease.

12. **Correct Answer: A**

The heparin will have dilutional effects and will decrease the bicarbonate level and the $PaCO_2$.

13. **Correct Answer: C**

Using a vacutainer or a high-friction syringe will create a vacuum. When that occurs, dissolved gases come out of solution, which decreases PaO_2 and $PaCO_2$. The increased effort required to move the cylinder may cause the artery to spasm and make it more difficult to obtain the sample, but will not directly affect the results.

14. **Correct Answer: D**

Most ABG machines are calibrated to 37°C. If the patient has a fever, the oxyhemoglobin curve will be shifted to the right. More oxygen will be given off to the tissues, so the machine has to be calibrated to account for the higher temperature.

15. **Correct Answer: D**

Familial emphysema is extremely rare. Many references estimate the incidence of this condition at only 1–3%. It is believed that serum $alpha_1$-antitrypsin destroys lung tissue through enzymatic action. Usually Caucasians of European descent express this disease, which is associated with an autosomal recessive trait. Symptoms usually appear when the patient is a teenager—a characteristic that can assist in the diagnosis because most emphysema occurs in later years.

16. **Correct Answer: B**

Chronic hypoxia leads to chronic respiratory acidosis. The kidneys then retain bicarbonate in the form of sodium bicarbonate. The bicarbonate is exchanged for sodium chloride. Ammonia is an acid and excess amounts must be removed from the body. This is accomplished by releasing ammonium chloride. Chronic hypoxia is characterized by an increase in bicarbonate levels and a decrease in chloride levels. Other causes of hypochloremia include NG suction, vomiting, and diarrhea.

17. **Correct Answer: D**
The pH is elevated, indicating alkalosis. The HCO_3 is normal, but the $PaCO_2$ is decreased, indicating respiratory alkalosis.

18. **Correct Answer: D**
Propanolol may cause bronchospasm. It works by blocking beta-adrenergic effects of the sympathetic nervous system (like bronchodilation). Some beta blockers are cardioselective (e.g., atenolol), and newer agents, such as nebivolol, provide for cardioselective beta blockade with vasodilation.

19. **Correct Answer: C**
Sherie is probably very anxious and hyperventilating because she is unable to get enough oxygen due to bronchial constriction. Hypoventilation causes a buildup of CO_2, leading to respiratory acidosis. This patient has not received theophylline and Albuterol may cause tachycardia, but not an acid–base imbalance.

20. **Correct Answer: D**
It is unlikely that Sherie's condition is improving. The air becomes trapped in the alveoli and excessive mucus is produced. The patient struggles to breathe and may become exhausted. When the wheezing diminishes or stops altogether, it means air is not able to pass through an opening. This is a medical emergency, and the patient may need to be intubated. A lot of controversy surrounds the issue of intubating asthmatics, because this procedure may cause barotrauma, hyperinflation, and cardiac compromise.

21. **Correct Answer: B**
Norepinephrine is a vasoconstrictor. Nebulizers may also work, but if the patient's condition is compromised the effectiveness is minimal at best. Heliox is a helium–oxygen mixture that can help with delivery of inhaled medications, thereby decreasing the work of breathing.

22. **Correct Answer: C**
Neostigmine is an enzyme that prevents the breakdown of acetylcholine into its enzyme. This medication also improves impulse transmission. Sometimes neostigmine causes bradycardia and increases bronchial secretions, so atropine may be used with this agent to mitigate its effects. Narcan is an opioid antagonist.

23. **Correct Answer: D**
Hugh is exhibiting signs and symptoms of oxygen toxicity after five days of oxygen therapy at $> 50\%$ FiO_2. Non-rebreather masks provide a minimum of 60% FiO_2 at 6 L/min. An arterial blood gas would show an increased $PaO_2 > 100$ mm Hg, ruling out respiratory failure ($PaO_2 < 60$) that would require intubation. The dry, hacking cough rules out pulmonary edema and the need for Lasix. The numbness in the extremities results from the presence of oxygen radicals in the blood, rather than a neurologic impairment that would indicate the need for a CT scan with possible tPA administration.

24. **Correct Answer: B**
Three days of high FiO_2 has resulted in a nitrogen washout, resulting in atelectasis. Nitrogen's high partial pressure is necessary to maintain alveolar inflation. It is important to

titrate FiO_2 to maintain O_2 saturation within a prescribed range when oxygen therapy is utilized. Pulmonary edema would result in coarse breath sounds. With a unilateral pneumothorax, tracheal deviation might be observed. Sepsis would not necessarily present with diminished breath sounds, but additional findings could include increased purulent secretions, coarse breath sounds, and altered laboratory diagnostic results.

25. **Correct Answer: B**
Sometimes the costal cartilage becomes calcified with age. Vertebrae develop osteoporosis, and a degree of kyphosis can occur. Weight gain is common and posture is affected. The chest wall compliance decreases, as does vital capacity. Residual volume increases, PaO_2 decreases, and $PaCO_2$ increases.

26. **Correct Answer: C**
Type I cells line the outside of the alveoli. These cells, which maintain the blood–gas interface, are easily inflamed by inhaled toxins or heated air. Type II cells produce surfactant.

27. **Correct Answer: D**
Conducting airways are ventilated, but perfusion (gas exchange) does not take place. Wasted ventilation is the amount of ventilation that does not participate in gas exchange.

28. **Correct Answer: A**
The oxyhemoglobin dissociation curve reflects physiological circumstances and their effect on the hemoglobin's affinity for oxygen.

29. **Correct Answer: B**
A shift to the right means hemoglobin has less affinity for oxygen. 2,3-Diphosphoglyceride (2,3-DPG) is needed to help force O_2 off the hemoglobin molecule. If 2,3-DPG levels decrease, the hemoglobin will hang on to the O_2. If the temperature increases, the tissues need more O_2. Also, if the PCO_2 becomes elevated, the tissues need more oxygen.

30. **Correct Answer: D**
When the oxyhemoglobin dissociation curve shifts to the left, it means that hemoglobin holds on to the oxygen. In this circumstance, 2,3-DPG is lacking, CO_2 would be decreased, and temperature would be decreased. Tissues would not need as much O_2.

31. **Correct Answer: C**
Nitric oxide is a vasodilator and may be administered by mask, ET tube, or tracheostomy. The nitric oxide reduces blood pressure in the pulmonary circulation. This is a fairly new approach in the progressive care area.

32. **Correct Answer: A**
The kidneys try to correct the imbalance by retaining bicarbonate. Chronic hypoxia results in increased CO_2 (chronic respiratory acidosis). The bicarbonate exchanges for the chloride to maintain a balance.

33. **Correct Answer: D**
Normally, lung sounds are somewhat muffled. Sounds may be heard clearly if the lung is consolidated. If a whisper is transmitted, it is unusual and may also indicate consolidation. Egophony is a sound that changes in intensity; if the patient says "E," it is heard as "A."

34. **Correct Answer: A**
The pH shows that the patient's condition is uncompensated and acidotic (< 7.35), the elevated CO_2 indicates that the condition is respiratory (> 45 mm Hg), and the bicarbonate is normal (22–26 mm Hg). Hence the patient has uncompensated respiratory acidosis.

35. **Correct Answer: B**
Removal of large amounts of pleural fluid (>1000 mL) increases negative intrapleural pressure. Edema occurs when the lung does not reexpand. The patient develops a severe cough and dyspnea. If these symptoms occur during a thoracentesis, the procedure should be stopped.

36. **Correct Answer: C**
Certain dyes interfere with the sensor's ability to conduct red and infrared light. These dyes include methylene blue, fluroscein, indocyanine green, and indigo carmine.

37. **Correct Answer: D**
Erosion of the innominate artery is probable when the tip of the tube rubs against tissue or the stoma is too low. The trachea is somewhat oval, whereas the tube and cuff are circular. The tube may have been loose and allowed for more than the usual movement of the tube.

38. **Correct Answer: B**
The nasopharyngeal airway should not be used on patients with basilar skull fractures, sepsis, bleeding disorders, malformations or injuries to the nares, or nasal obstructions. Use this type of airway with caution in patients who are receiving anticoagulants, fibrinolytics, or thrombolytics.

39. **Correct Answer: A**
A semi-reclining or upright position will promote upper lobe drainage. Fluid or secretions will collect if the patient is positioned flat.

40. **Correct Answer: B**
If the head is lower than the body intracranial pressure is increased. It is also best to avoid postural drainage in a woman in the last 2–3 months of pregnancy, because the baby will shift toward the lungs and may cause respiratory distress. It is also a good idea to wait an hour after a patient eats before giving an aerosol treatment so as to avoid nausea, vomiting, and possible aspiration.

41. **Correct Answer: D**
Answers A, B, and C are complications of BiPAP. BiPAP must be regulated so as not to cause barotrauma, yet still keep alveoli from collapsing during expiration. The patient may have to be mechanically ventilated at some point if the BiPAP is not effective.

42. **Correct Answer: C**
Virchow's triad consists of venous stasis, hypercoagulability of blood, and injury to vascular endothelium. Beck's triad is indicative of cardiac tamponade.

43. **Correct Answer: A**
Beta$_2$-adrenergic agonists include Brethine, Bronkosol and Proventil. These medications are preferred because they cause fewer cardiovascular effects in patients with respiratory failure. They are selective for respiratory stimulation. Epinephrine and Isuprel are non-respiratory selective. Atrovent is classified as a parasympatholytic.

44. **Correct Answer: B**

The ventilatory pressures caused by excessive force with the BVM can exceed the intrathoracic and intrapleural pressures, causing barotrauma. Such excessive pressures can damage several different organs in the thorax and even organs in the abdomen. The lungs are susceptible to collapse (pneumothorax). Barotrauma may also damage major blood vessels.

45. **Correct Answer: B**

An acute pulmonary embolism can be associated with right heart failure. The patient may have chest pain, dyspnea, tachycardia, hypotension, shock, and possibly coma.

46. **Correct Answer: C**

The patient will have a sudden decrease in the PET CO_2 due to loss of blood flow in the pulmonary vasculature. The decrease in blood flow increases dead space, with a resultant decrease in the PET CO_2.

47. **Correct Answer: A**

In addition, in pulmonary embolism, the EKG may actually be normal, may show right axis deviation, T-wave inversion (leads V_1 and V_4) and ST-segment depression. New-onset atrial fibrillation and RBBB may also occur.

48. **Correct Answer: B**

Severe acute respiratory syndrome (SARS) is a community-acquired pneumonia. Its incubation period is usually 2–14 days, and the pathogen—SARS-associated coronavirus—is spread via droplets. SARS is usually acquired in underdeveloped areas. There is no cure and symptoms are treated as they appear. It is incumbent on the nurse to make certain the patient is placed in a negative-pressure isolation room and that an N-95 respirator mask is used.

49. **Correct Answer: C**

If the D-dimer is elevated it may be caused by multiple other conditions. A normal D-dimer rules out a pulmonary embolism. Hyperventilation will occur subsequent to hypoxemia, so respiratory alkalosis will occur. Heparin does not dissolve existing clots.

50. **Correct Answer: C**

Hamman's sign is a "crunching" sound or a slight clicking sound with each heart sound, auscultated over the apex of the heart.

51. **Correct Answer: B**

If carbon monoxide levels are above 60%, the patient will be comatose and will probably die. Smokers often have CO levels of 5–10%. Normal CO levels in nonsmokers are less than 2%.

52. **Correct Answer: D**

In cases of severe carbon monoxide poisoning, hyperbaric therapy must be utilized to force the CO molecule off the hemoglobin. The CO is then eliminated by the lungs.

53. **Correct Answer: B**

Airway patency is always a priority. Bernard probably inhaled superheated air and toxins. Most of the products found in a home will give off carbon monoxide when burned. These toxins, plus the CO may cause edema of the air passages.

54. **Correct Answer: D**

   Answers A, B, and C decrease lung compliance. Other factors that decrease compliance include atelectasis, fibrotic changes, abdominal distention, pain (causes splinting), and flail chest (pain and loss of structure).

55. **Correct Answer: C**

   The patient must have an absent gag reflex. The laryngeal mask airway (LMA) cannot be inserted by nurses unless they have received specialized training. The LMA does not usually cause hoarseness because it does not pass through the vocal cords. There is a high risk of aspiration with LMA usage.

56. **Correct Answer: C**

   Acetyl-cysteine contains a sulfide group that effectively splits disulfide bonds in mucin molecules, thereby reducing the viscosity of the mucus. Atropine is an anticholinergic. Terbutaline and albuterol are B_2-agonists.

57. **Correct Answer: A**

   Thinning the mucus may promote excessive coughing with resultant bronchospasm. Additional side effects include rhinorrhea, stomatitis, nausea, and vomiting.

58. **Correct Answer: D**

   Beta$_2$-receptor agonists lower cellular calcium levels and relax bronchial smooth muscle. Selective beta$_2$-receptor agonists do not produce cardiac stimulation. The cardiac stimulation can result in tachycardia and reduced cardiac output.

59. **Correct Answer: B**

   Methylzanthines, which also include caffeine and theobromine, are an important class of drugs. They can be found in coffee, tea and cocoa. This class of drugs, when given in low doses, stimulates cortical arousal. In higher doses, they cause insomnia. Methylzanthines can cause tachycardia, increase production of gastric acid and digestive enzymes, and inhibit histamine release.

60. **Correct Answer: B**

   In malignant hyperthermia, the use of anesthetic agents such as halothane cause muscles to contract and the patient to become hypothermic. Caffeine is used diagnostically in such cases because, when given at higher doses, it can contract muscles without the danger of depolarizing cell membranes. The antidote for malignant hyperthermia is dantrolene.

61. **Correct Answer: C**

   Symptoms have a gradual onset. The patient may develop ARDS, but not always. If the pH is > 2.5, very little necrosis will occur. If the pH is < 2.5, there is probability of pulmonary edema, necrosis, bleeding, and atelectasis.

62. **Correct Answer: D**

   Devin has the classic symptoms of Legionnaire's disease. If left untreated, this infection may lead to hypotension, acute kidney injury, shock, respiratory failure, and death.

63. **Correct Answer: B**

   By definition, an open pneumothorax exists because air enters the pleural cavity from the atmosphere. The hole made into the subclavian vein allows for air to pass from the atmosphere to the pleural cavity.

64. **Correct Answer: C**

    Trendelenburg position with left decubitus tilt will minimize the chance of any air migrating through the heart and into the lungs.

65. **Correct Answer: C**

    Pulmonary angiography involves catheterization of the right ventricle, followed by injection of dye into the pulmonary artery. The pulmonary vasculature is easily seen with this study. The location of the embolus is readily identified because the dye trail comes to a sudden end.

66. **Correct Answer: B**

    Neoplasms, obesity, trauma, dysrhythmias, congestive heart failure (CHF), and prolonged immobility are also factors.

67. **Correct Answer: A**

    Other potential causes include central and pulmonary artery catheters, endoscopy, and automatic pressure-driven injectors.

68. **Correct Answer: B**

    The blood gas results show respiratory acidosis with hypoxemia.

69. **Correct Answer: D**

    Fractures, usually long bone fractures, can release free fatty acids, which cause vasculitis. Fat globules float around in the circulation and obstruct the pulmonary vasculature.

70. **Correct Answer: A**

    Prone positioning is the best position to promote drainage and oxygenation. It is often the most difficult position to achieve without proper lifting and safety devices.

71. **Correct Answer: D**

    The fluid volume is kept low. If too much fluid is present, leakage may occur through damaged capillaries into the interstitial space.

72. **Correct Answer: D**

    The strict definition of pulmonary hypertension is that MPAP is greater than 20 mm Hg. One of our students reported that this question was on her PCCN test last year, but we have not heard that it was used on subsequent exams. Perhaps it was tried out as a question to be validated or misunderstood. We added the question here "just in case." This question involves more advanced hemodynamics and should not appear on your exam.

73. **Correct Answer: C**

    The forced vital capacity (FVC) is the total amount of gas exhaled as forcefully and rapidly as possible after taking a maximal inspiration. The result should be above 80%. The forced expiratory volume (FEV) is how much gas is exhaled during the first second of effort. This amount should be 75% or more of the predicted normal value. In individuals with asthma, this value is decreased because of obstruction.

74. **Correct Answer: B**

    When using an auto-transfusion drainage system, make sure to connect the system per the manufacturer's recommendations. Most connections will be color-coded to simplify the connection process. Clamps must remain open to allow for blood collection and to prevent an increase in intrathoracic pressures. Subcutaneous air should be checked by palpation and borders marked for further monitoring. The average adult-size catheter is 28 or 36 Fr. If a one-way valve system and suction is used, water is not required to maintain a seal because the valve performs this function.

75. **Correct Answer: B**
Acidosis, hypercarbia, and hyperthermia will all lead to a right shift in the oxyhemoglobin dissociation curve. Hemoglobin has a decreased affinity for oxygen and enhances tissue uptake of oxygen.

76. **Correct Answer: D**
If a patient has ingested carbonated beverages, the CO_2 production/accumulation within the stomach would lead to inflation of the esophageal detection device (EDD) and a false-positive reading for the ETT placement in the airway. It is best to use auscultation, observation, and improvement in vital signs as primary techniques to confirm endotracheal tube placement and EDD and CO_2 detectors as secondary methods.

77. **Correct Answer: A**
Research into the use of normal saline in tracheal suctioning has proven that normal saline causes anxiety, increases the patient's risk for hospital-acquired pneumonia, and may cause bronchoconstriction. Current recommendations focus on dry suctioning, frequent oral care, balanced hydration, and position changes as means to prevent complications associated with intubation and mechanical ventilation.

78. **Correct Answer: A**
To calculate this value, divide 100 mL by 40 minutes, which equals 2.5. Then multiply by 15 (gtts/mL), which equals 37.5, and finally round up to 38.

79. **Correct Answer: A**
Hypothyroidism, banked blood transfusions, malnutrition, hypophosphatemia, and hexokinase deficiency will all cause a decrease in 2,3-DPG. An increase in 2,3-DPG will be seen with anemia, congenital heart disease, hyperthyroidism, and chronic hypoxemia.

80. **Correct Answer: B**
Usually, central cyanosis is seen when the level of deoxygenated Hgb reaches 5 g/dL. The cyanosis can be seen on the lips and possibly on the mucous membranes. It can be an early sign of hypoxemia in patients with polycythemia. These patients will be cyanotic when 5 g/dL is desaturated. Sometimes these patients are called, "blue bloaters." In anemic patients, this is a late sign and they will not necessarily be cyanotic.

81. **Correct Answer: D**
Succinylcholine combines with acetylcholine to cause smooth muscle relaxation. Prolonged use may cause a change in blocking action and result in potassium-regulated alterations in electrical activity. Other side effects of succinylcholine include malignant hyperthermia and hypertension or hypotension, hyperkalemia, anaphylaxis, and increased intraocular pressure.

82. **Correct Answer: C**
Norcuron is eliminated via the hepatic/biliary system. Use with caution in patients with known or suspected hepatic or biliary compromise, such as cirrhosis or hepatitis and may take up to two times as long to clear patients' systems.

83. **Correct Answer: D**

Uncontrolled asthma symptoms during an attack may lead to prolonged and extensive muscle use to maintain independent respirations. This prolonged effort may result in respiratory failure due to respiratory muscle fatigue. Administration of a neuromuscular blocking agent further inhibits the smooth muscle retractions. Long-term steroid use has been linked to muscle wasting. Ventilatory weaning may be prolonged as respiratory muscles recover from both the disease process and the pharmacologic intervention.

84. **Correct Answer: D**

The nasal cannula is generally considered a low-flow oxygen device unless connected to a high-flow system. If using a flow > 4 L/min, the oxygen should be humidified to prevent drying the mucosal membranes.

85. **Correct Answer: C**

If both exhalation ports have one-way valves, then a flow of near 100% oxygen may be reached. To prevent suffocation in patients where the oxygen is disconnected, non-rebreathing masks now have only one one-way valve to prevent/limit inhalation of room air. This results in decreasing the highest concentration of actual inspired oxygen to 60–80%.

86. **Correct Answer: D**

The accuracy of pulse oximetry is affected by patient motion, low perfusion, venous pulsation, light, poor probe positioning, edema, anemia, and carbon monoxide levels. It is important to compare pulse oximetry values against arterial blood gas results to validate values less than 70%.

87. **Correct Answer: B**

Sepsis may result in lung tissue injury and, consequently, increased pulmonary vascular resistance (PVR). Prostaglandin and oxygen therapies result in pulmonary vasodilatation and decreased PVR.

88. **Correct Answer: A**

Increased metabolic rate would increase the O_2 uptake by tissues, resulting in a lower value as measured by venous blood gases. Answers B, C, and D result in a lower tissue oxygen requirement and, therefore, higher values of oxygen remaining in the bloodstream.

89. **Correct Answer: B**

For women, the average depth for an ETT at the lip is 21 cm when using a 7 to 8 Fr ETT. The average depth for men is 23 cm at the lip when using an 8 to 8.5 Fr ETT. Assessment documentation should always include both of these values, in case the tube becomes dislodged at any time during respiratory support. Please refer to current ACLS guidelines.

90. **Correct Answer: D**

The normal ratio is derived from the lateral diameter, which is one-half the anterior–posterior diameter, so the ratio is 1:2. This information is handy to know because if you measure these distances, you can sometimes note early changes in the thorax, possibly due to emphysema or COPD.

91. **Correct Answer: A**

    Stimulation of the posterior tibial nerve results in plantar flexion of the great toe. Other locations for peripheral nerve stimulation electrode placement include the ulnar nerve and the facial nerve.

92. **Correct Answer: C**

    The progression in which movement of muscles stops is eyes, face, neck, extremities, abdomen, glottis, intercostals, and diaphragm. It is important to recall that muscle movement will return in the reverse order.

93. **Correct Answer: A**

    One to two twitches represents 85–90% blockage. It is important to remember that different muscles may respond differently to neuromuscular blocking agents. As muscles of the face will stop before the diaphragm, one might check twitches on the face and an extremity rather than just on the face. Although the PCCN exam is not supposed to include ventilator-related questions, your patient may have to be intubated emergently and, therefore, may require blockade.

94. **Correct Answer: C**

    These findings indicate compensated metabolic acidosis. The pH is between 7.35 and 7.45, so the value is compensated; because it is closer to 7.35, the value is considered acidotic. To determine whether the acidosis is respiratory or metabolic, find the value that represents acidosis: $HCO_3 < 22$ mEq/L.

95. **Correct Answer: D**

    These findings indicate uncompensated respiratory alkalosis. The pH is greater than 7.45, so the value is uncompensated alkalosis. To determine whether the alkalosis is respiratory or metabolic, find the value that represents alkalosis: $CO_2 < 35$ mm Hg.

96. **Correct Answer: C**

    These findings indicate uncompensated metabolic acidosis. The pH is less than 7.35, so the value is uncompensated acidosis. To determine whether the acidosis is respiratory or metabolic, find the value that represents acidosis: $HCO_3 < 22$ mEq/L.

97. **Correct Answer: A**

    These findings indicate uncompensated (mixed) respiratory/metabolic alkalosis. The pH is greater than 7.45, so the value is uncompensated. To determine whether the acidosis is respiratory or metabolic, find the value that represents alkalosis: $HCO_3 > 26$ mEq/L and $CO_2 < 35$ mm Hg, meaning the cause of the alkalosis is both respiratory and metabolic in nature.

98. **Correct Answer: B**

    The pH is between 7.35 and 7.45; CO_2 (between 35 and 45 mm Hg) and HCO_3 (between 22 and 26 mEq/L) are within normal ranges. This ABG is considered normal.

99. **Correct Answer: D**

    These findings indicate uncompensated respiratory alkalosis. The pH is greater than 7.45, so the value is uncompensated alkalosis. To determine whether the alkalosis is respiratory or metabolic, find the value that represents alkalosis: $CO_2 < 35$ mm Hg.

100. **Correct Answer: B**

These findings indicate compensated respiratory acidosis. The pH is between 7.35 and 7.45, so the value is compensated; because it is closer to 7.35, the value is considered acidotic. To determine whether the acidosis is respiratory or metabolic, find the value that represents acidosis: $CO_2 > 45$ mm Hg.

101. **Correct Answer: A**

These findings indicate uncompensated (mixed) respiratory/metabolic acidosis. The pH is less than 7.35, so the value is uncompensated acidosis. To determine whether the acidosis is respiratory or metabolic, find the value that represents acidosis: $HCO_3 < 22$ mEq/L and $CO_2 > 45$ mm Hg, meaning the cause of the acidosis is both respiratory and metabolic in nature.

102. **Correct Answer: C**

These findings indicate compensated respiratory alkalosis. The pH is between 7.35 and 7.45, so the value is compensated; because it is closer to 7.45, the value is considered alkalotic. To determine whether the alkalosis is respiratory or metabolic, find the value that represents alkalosis: $CO_2 < 35$ mm Hg.

103. **Correct Answer: A**

These findings indicate uncompensated metabolic alkalosis. The pH is greater than 7.45, so the value is uncompensated. To determine whether the alkalosis is respiratory or metabolic, find the value that represents alkalosis: $HCO_3 > 26$ mEq/L.

104. **Correct Answer: B**

These findings indicate uncompensated (mixed) respiratory/metabolic acidosis. The pH is less than 7.35, so the value is uncompensated acidosis. To determine whether the acidosis is respiratory or metabolic, find the value that represents acidosis: $HCO_3 < 22$ mEq/L and $CO_2 > 45$ mm Hg, meaning the cause of the acidosis is both respiratory and metabolic in nature.

105. **Correct Answer: D**

The pH is between 7.35 and 7.45; CO_2 (between 35 and 45 mmHg) and HCO_3 (between 22 and 26 mEq/L) are within normal ranges. This ABG is considered normal.

106. **Correct Answer: D**

These findings indicate uncompensated respiratory acidosis. The pH is less than 7.35, so the value is uncompensated. To determine whether the acidosis is respiratory or metabolic, find the value that represents acidosis: $CO_2 > 45$ mm Hg.

107. **Correct Answer: A**

Answers B, C and D are characteristics of open catheter suctioning. When a closed system is used, its extra weight can increase tension on the catheter or tubing. This may cause the tracheostomy tube to move. Many manufacturers make inline tubing for both endotracheal tubes and tracheostomy tubes, so nurses must make certain they are using the correct tube for suctioning. Another problem with the inline catheters is the extra tubing that hangs out when the catheter is not in use. Patients may easily reach this tubing and extubate themselves or push the catheter down the airway and obstruct air flow.

108. **Correct Answer: D**

Stents can be manufactured in either straight or curved configurations, reflecting the differing nature of individuals' air passages. When the stent rests against the anterior wall of the trachea, it allows for freer passage of air and the patient can breathe spontaneously around the tube.

109. **Correct Answer: C**

The laryngeal mask airway was intended for use as a temporary airway. It requires minimal training to insert, but it cannot be placed by RNs as a matter of course. The patient must be unconscious and/or without gag reflex. The seal around the mask is a low-pressure seal, so it cannot be used on patients with high peak ventilator pressures. The LMA has a significant risk of aspiration as well as laryngospasm.

Advantages with use of this airway are that it is blindly inserted into the hypopharynx, does not require visualization of the vocal cords, and does not traumatize the trachea. Patients will not have hoarseness or lose their voice altogether. At best, patients will complain of a mild sore throat.

110. **Correct Answer: B**

The magnet in the MRI will attract the wires in the tube. Silicone or plastic tubes cannot tolerate repeated cleanings. Use of a one-way speaking valve is contraindicated when using a foam cuff, because the cuff may lie at an angle to the valve due to its orientation in the airway. The cost of such tubes is actually higher to facilities because silicone and plastic tubes are difficult to keep clean and are labor intensive.

111. **Correct Answer: C**

The tracheal tube provides a more stable airway, can be placed in a progressive care setting, and decreases airway resistance. Because the tube is not positioned near the right mainstem bronchus, it will not facilitate intubation of the bronchus. There are a large number of potential complications with the use of a tracheostomy tube—for example, tracheal stenosis, tracheal malacia, aspiration, infection, hemorrhage, subcutaneous emphysema, and pneumothorax.

112. **Correct Answer: D**

Because of the direct connection via the eustachian tube, infection in the ear is possible. If a cervical injury has been stabilized, it is certainly possible for a skilled intubator to place the tube. Additional complications associated with nasal endotracheal tubes include nasal bleeding, sinusitis, accidental esophageal intubation, vocal cord injuries, necrosis, cuff leak or failure, and obstruction.

113. **Correct Answer: A**

Generally, the time it took for the intubator to complete the task is not documented, although if there was an unusual occurrence or a complication, it should be properly documented. The depth of the tube is important to chart because it gives a reference point if any questions arise about tube migration. The size of the tube may be too small or large, so it would have to be adjusted to the next appropriate size. A CXR is done to confirm tube placement; the time it is done should be documented. Any medications given during the procedure should be documented as to reason for administration, patient response, and follow-up such as vital sign measurements or untoward reactions.

114. **Correct Answer: C**

$ETCO_2$ is not a substitute for pulse oximetry. A pulse oximeter measures the availability of sites on the hemoglobin molecule for oxygen transport versus the number of sites occupied. The $ETCO_2$ indicates whether gas exchange is taking place at the cellular level. If CO_2 is being given off, it will react with chemically treated paper in the detector. There is no excuse for not auscultating the patient's lungs to determine correct ETT placement. If the esophagus has been intubated, the $ETCO_2$ may give a false-positive reading if the patient has consumed a carbonated beverage within the past few hours.

115. **Correct Answer: A**

Sinusitis cannot be prevented simply by using a smaller-diameter ET. If anything, it will make the patient's work of breathing more difficult, though it will not necessarily contribute to an infectious process. Orogastric tubes are preferable to nasogastric tubes whenever possible. Good hand washing technique has been shown to be effective in reducing all types of hospital-acquired infections.

116. **Correct Answer: B**

Double effect is a common ethical dilemma. Here an action is justified as long as there is no intent to do further harm. Neither the physician nor the wife wants to hasten the patient's death, but they do want to make him more comfortable. It is the intent behind the use of the narcotic, rather than the use itself, that defines the double effect. At least some good is done with the outcome of the discussion and resolution of the dilemma.

117. **Correct Answer: A**

The N95 respirator is the primary mask to filter for TB particles. It should be test fit prior to use.

118. **Correct Answer: B**

The result will be nullified. False-negative results may occur if the patient has a bacterial infection, a live virus vaccination, renal failure, depleted sensitized T lymphocytes, or immunologic defects.

119. **Correct Answer: B**

The tidal volume is the amount of gas inspired and expired with a normal breath. Think of it as the tide just coming in and going out with no extra effort. It is normally thought to be equivalent to approximately 10 mL per kilogram of body weight.

120. **Correct Answer: B**

The patient's abdominal contents have probably entered the thoracic cavity secondary to a diaphragmatic tear. If air also enters the thoracic cavity, it will increase intrathoracic pressure and help to transmit sound. Usually, the left side of the diaphragm ruptures, and Ian was injured on the left side. (The liver, because it is large, is believed to protect the right side of the diaphragm.) A fractured pelvis usually also results in almost a 50% increased probability of a ruptured diaphragm.

121. **Correct Answer: A**

Diaphragmatic rupture is a medical emergency. Maintenance of the airway and adequate oxygenation are always priorities. The abdominal contents' excursion into the thoracic cavity, along with the increase in intrathoracic pressure, will cause hemodynamic compromise. Preload will be decreased, the patient will become tachycardic and dyspneic, have uneven diaphragmatic movement (on palpation), and may progress to shock. The shoulder pain on the side of the tear may become quite severe, and may further hinder respiratory effort. Complications may include bowel obstruction and/or strangulation. The patient may become so unstable that he must be stabilized before surgery can even be considered.

122. **Correct Answer: C**

A flail chest results when two or more adjacent ribs are broken in two or more places. The chest wall is unstable. Usually during inspiration, the chest wall moves outward with an increase in negative intrathoracic pressure. In cases of flail chest, the opposite movement of the chest wall is seen. This is known as "paradoxical" movement. Eventually the result will be atelectasis and alveolar collapse, with possible development of ARDS.

To adequately stabilize the fracture, neuromuscular blockade is sometimes used. The patient must be given pain medication and sedation. Also, pain management is a priority because the patient's work of breathing (WOB) needs to be reduced. Just think about a time you have had a pain in your side, and how difficult it was to take a full breath.

123. **Correct Answer: C**

Flail chest is a very painful condition that limits respiratory effort because of the pain or from analgesia and sedation that may be required. The CO_2 level will increase, PaO_2 will decrease, and the pH will be below 7.35. The patient will develop respiratory acidosis.

124. **Correct Answer: B**

The pH of the aspirate is very important. If the aspirate is acidic, pulmonary edema develops almost immediately due to the collapse and breakdown of the alveoli, capillaries, and their interface. Atelectasis, possible intra-alveolar hemorrhage, and some interstitial edema lead to hypoxia. Alkalotic aspirate destroys surfactant, which causes alveolar collapse, leading to hypoxia. Other factors to identify are the type of material aspirated and the amount. Syrup of ipecac is used for ingestions. ABG results would be considered more of a diagnostic tool.

125. **Correct Answer: C**

To evacuate fluids, the tube is placed low in the thoracic cavity and gravity is used to help clear the fluid. If a hemothorax is not completely removed, an infection may potentially occur, which can lead to empyema. When assessing a patient, it is a good idea to ask (if possible) about the origin of small scars on the thoracic area. It may take years to cause a problem.

126. **Correct Answer: B**

In this type of respiratory failure, $PaCO_2$ may be either decreased or normal. A ventilation/ perfusion mismatch (pneumonia, atelectasis) may occur as a result of an intrapulmonary shunt. Alternatively, there may be increased alveolar dead space (shock, pulmonary embolism). Pulmonary fibrosis may reduce diffusion capacity (COPD, ARDS).

127. **Correct Answer: C**

Cor pulmonale also results from right ventricular failure or dilation secondary to pulmonary hypertension caused by lung disease. The important distinction here is that the condition is not caused by any problem with the left ventricle. Acute cor pulmonale is usually the result of a massive pulmonary embolism that raises the PVR and causes increased preload and strain on the right heart.

128. Correct Answer: D

If a pulmonary embolism decreases oxygen availability, the work of breathing increases, as does the respiratory rate. The thoracic respiratory muscles and the diaphragm will increase their oxygen demand, and respiratory muscle fatigue may result. Oxygen may be diverted to these muscles and deplete the oxygen and nutrient supplies necessary for other vital organs. These organs may become ischemic and develop multiple organ dysfunction. Answers A, B, and C may all contribute to the formation of a pulmonary embolus.

129. Correct Answer: A

Traditionally, nurses were taught to assess Homan's sign: dorsiflexion of the ankle while bending the knee. If that action elicited pain, the patient had a problem with circulation and possibly DVT. Moses' sign is elicited by pressing the calf toward the tibia, which may also elicit pain. These results are not exclusive to DVT, but may complement a diagnosis.

130. Correct Answer: C

The most likely diagnosis is COPD. No information was given about a possible fever or lung sounds.

131. Correct Answer: D

The airway is always the priority. After placing the mask and notifying the charge nurse, you have other options. If the patient is stable, you can notify the attending physician and see if he wants to reintubate the patient or leave on the mask, change to another form of O_2 delivery and/or FiO_2, draw ABGs, or do nothing. If the patient's condition deteriorates, you may have the option of asking the ED physician to intubate the patient. The wife may have innocently believed she was doing good, but she may be a facilitator for her husband's drinking and behavior. She would certainly bear close watching if she is allowed to stay on the unit. This question is multi-faceted and allows for different interpretations and requires application of critical thinking skills.

132. Correct Answer: D

Dairy products may actually increase bronchospasm and may cause an increase in phlegm. Fluid intake should be increased to approximately 3 L/day. Serevent is a long-lasting inhaler and can take up to an hour to work.

133. Correct Answer: C

Answers A, B, and D are to be avoided: They will diminish the respiratory drive and may cause bronchoconstriction. You would expect to use steroids, mucolytics, and bronchodilators.

134. Correct Answer: B

In the bifurcation of the internal and external carotid arteries, carotid bodies, and aortic bodies (in the carotid arch) are chemoreceptors. When the supply of oxygen decreases, stimulation of the aortic and/or carotid bodies occurs and, in turn, stimulates cortical activity. The result is adrenal gland secretions (epinephrine, norepinephrine), tachycardia, tachypnea, increased respiratory rate, and increased blood pressure.

135. Correct Answer: B

The formula for functional residual capacity is FRC = ERV (expired residual volume) + RV (residual volume). The normal FRC in healthy lungs is approximately 2,000–3,000 mL.

136. **Correct Answer: C**
Subcutaneous emphysema usually occurs in the thorax as a result of a pulmonary air leak. This air leak may be secondary to the patient receiving positive-pressure ventilation or from alveolar rupture from a pneumothorax. The air travels along under the skin, where it may be easily palpated and feel like a crackling sensation. Patients who have chest tubes often have at least a small amount of subcutaneous emphysema at the tube insertion site. Sometimes the patient will feel pain when palpation is performed because the air tears the tissue. The free air must be reabsorbed, a process that may take several days.

137. **Correct Answer: A**
Bilirubin is not within the color spectrum that will interfere with pulse oximetry results. Dark nail polish, especially black, brown, blue, and green, will interfere with light transmission and cause an artificial lowering of the SpO_2. Patients who have bruising under the nails may also have SpO_2 values that are artificially decreased.

138. **Correct Answer: B**
During resuscitation, blood pressure and blood flow may vary. The pharmacologic effects of medications used during resuscitation (such as vasoactive drugs) will compromise SpO_2 values.

139. **Correct Answer: B**
SpO_2 values are not the same as PaO_2 values. A slight drop in SpO_2 is reflective of a major change in PaO_2 values. That is why the alarm limits should never exceed 5% of the acceptable baseline. Also, heart rate alarms can be set in accordance with any EKG limits.

140. **Correct Answer: B**
Pulse oximetry values do not directly correlate to PaO_2. You must use ABGs to determine PaO_2, the amount of oxygen available to the tissues. By comparison, SpO_2 measures the number of hemoglobin binding sites that are occupied compared to the number of hemoglobin binding sites available. The columns listed below show the correlation.

Values of Pulse Oximetry	Probable PaO_2
97	100
95	80
94	70
90	60
85	50
75	40
57	30
32	20
10	10

141. **Correct Answer: B**
With the Vollman Prone Positioner, one person is positioned on either side of the bed, and the third person at the head of the bed. The person at the head of the bed is responsible for maintaining cervical stability, the stability and positioning of the endotracheal tube, ventilator tubing, intravenous lines, and any monitoring cables.

142. **Correct Answer: D**
If the abdomen is open, the area may be covered with synthetic material and an abdominal binder used to help secure the abdomen. Additional contraindications would include an unstable spine, an unstable chest wall, an open chest, a bifurcated endotracheal tube, and blood pressures < 90 mm Hg in a patient who is receiving vasoactive medications.

143. **Correct Answer: C**
Adding a capnography device will help assure appropriate positioning of the endotracheal tube while turning the patient and when the patient is in the prone position. All EKG leads should be removed from the anterior chest wall and all wound dressings should be changed prior to placing the patient prone. All colostomy and ileostomy bags should be emptied because the patient's weight may cause the bags to rupture.

144. **Correct Answer: C**
Maintaining suction at levels higher than –40 cm H_2O may cause reexpansion pulmonary edema, pleural air leaks, and lung tissue entrapment. The lung may not be able to expand properly.

145. **Correct Answer: D**
If a mediastinal chest tube is in place, bubbling in the water seal chamber may indicate a communication between the mediastinal space and the pleural space. The physician should be notified immediately. However, some sporadic bubbling will occur when suction is first turned on because fluid must displace air in the collection chamber. Chest tube tubing that is dependent or coiled will allow for the accumulation of drainage, and this obstruction may increase pressure in the lung.

146. **Correct Answer: A**
This patient is exhibiting the classic symptoms of a tension pneumothorax. Air has leaked into the pleural space and, because the thorax is closed, increasing pressure has caused the lung to collapse. Tension pneumothorax is a medical emergency.

147. **Correct Answer: A**
The needle is actually placed just above the third rib at the midclavicular line on the affected side. This placement, using the edge of the bone to guide the needle, should lessen the possibility of damaging the artery, vein, and nerve that are located just below each rib. Additional complications could include cellulitis, localized hematoma, pleural infection, and pneumothorax if the patient did not have a tension pneumothorax.

148. **Correct Answer: D**
A high pleural fluid to serum protein ratio will cause a fluid shift and result in an effusion. This is a reason for performing a thoracentesis. Contraindications for performing a thoracentesis include coagulation disorders or patients receiving anticoagulants, abnormal anatomy (normal landmarks cannot be clearly identified), and splenomegaly. In patients with a pneumonectomy, a thoracentesis may damage the remaining lung or drastically change intrapleural pressure, possible collapse of the lung.

149. **Correct Answer: C**
Physiologic PEEP is the amount of positive pressure that remains in the alveoli after exhalation and keeps the alveoli from totally collapsing. Auto-PEEP occurs when the patient is mechanically ventilated and an amount of PEEP remains in the alveoli.

Auto-PEEP is in addition to physiologic PEEP. Causes of auto-PEEP include use of a small-diameter endotracheal tube, bronchospasm, water in the ventilator tubing, high minute ventilation, and high respiratory rates. Patients actually have increased work of breathing because, to initiate a breath on the ventilator, they have to overcome the set sensitivity and the amount of Auto-PEEP. Corrective measures include use of a large-diameter endotracheal tube, slower respiratory rates, emptying the water from the ventilatory tubing, use of sedatives and/or narcotics, and adjustment of the ventilator to shorten inspiratory time and lengthen exhalation time.

150. **Correct Answer: B**
Compliance is the ability of the lung and the chest wall to freely move (distensibility)—that is, the ability of the lung and chest wall to stretch. Emphysema patients often exhibit a barrel-shaped chest. ARDS, atelectasis, obesity, pulmonary fibrosis, pulmonary edema, kyphoscoliosis, and pneumonia are conditions that inhibit lung and chest wall movement (compliance).

151. **Correct Answer: D**
Albuterol administration would decrease lung resistance because resistance means how easy it is to move gases through airways. Albuterol is a bronchodilator, so it increases the size of the lumen, facilitating ventilation through the bronchi. Conditions that decrease the size of the bronchi lumen increase resistance.

152. **Correct Answer: D**
A buildup of ketones results from impaired glucose utilization. Additional causes of metabolic acidosis include diarrhea, renal failure, methanol poisoning, aspirin overdose, and lactic acidosis. Nasogastric suction removes chloride and causes metabolic alkalosis.

153. **Correct Answer: C**
Emphysema causes air to become trapped in the lungs. Also, it results in less consolidation (density), so sound travels more readily through this area. Percussion is performed to determine whether an area is filled with fluid, air, or solids. The liver would give off a dull sound because it is solid. A total thoracotomy or pneumonia would produce a flat sound because of consolidation.

154. **Correct Answer: A**
Generally, the patient will be hypoxic and demonstrate right heart failure, rather than left heart failure. Pulmonary hypertension leads to right heart failure. Chronic hypoxia also causes an increase in red blood cells (polycythemia). The clubbing of the fingers has no known etiology, but occurs with chronic COPD.

155. **Correct Answer: B**
Smoking remains the number one cause of COPD. Smoking generates carbon monoxide and those molecules cause a hypoxic state by occupying receptor sites on the hemoglobin molecule. Oxygen has a lower affinity for these sites. Smoking causes vasoconstriction and increases afterload. Smoking will also cause bronchoconstriction and decrease the efficiency of cilia and macrophages. Sputum production is increased. Pollution is now a major cause of COPD, and there has been a documented increase in all types of allergens. An individual's occupation may certainly be a factor with COPD, but that alone will rarely cause the condition.

156. **Correct Answer: D**
Headaches may be caused by multiple factors, but are not a cardinal sign of respiratory failure. Patients will exhibit tachypnea, diaphoresis, and restlessness as the body attempts to compensate for the respiratory distress and then exhibit signs of oxygen deprivation and starvation.

157. **Correct Answer: C**
Surya's anxiety probably resulted in hyperventilation. Carbon dioxide would be blown off and the pH would fall and he would become alkalotic. Flail chest is very painful, and this pain may have contributed to the patient's increased respiratory rate. If Surya was medicated, it might also hinder his respiratory efforts. It is a delicate balance.

158. **Correct Answer: C**
As many as 20% of patients treated with ACE inhibitors will develop a dry cough, though this cough may take one week to six months to occur after starting therapy. Sometimes, it will take weeks for the cough to disappear.

159. **Correct Answer: D**
Tachycardia is a direct result of carbon dioxide retention, as is restlessness. Cyanosis is a late sign of respiratory failure. Recognition of these signs is important, because early treatments such as O_2, aerosols, suctioning, and even repositioning can prevent or mitigate respiratory failure.

160. **Correct Answer: B**
Normally, the colloid osmotic pressure is 10–25 mm Hg higher than the pulmonary capillary wedge pressure (PAOP). Colloid osmotic pressure from proteins and albumin keeps fluid in the intravascular space. If this pressure decreases, fluid leaks from the pulmonary capillaries. This fluid will also leak if the wedge pressure increases.

161. **Correct Answer: A**
Carbon anhydrase is an enzyme that helps convert water and carbon dioxide to bicarbonate. This form of CO_2 comprises about 70% of the total circulating CO_2. Approximately 10% of carbon dioxide is dissolved and becomes arterial $PaCO_2$. The remaining 20% exists as carbaminohemoglobin in hemoglobin.

162. **Correct Answer: B**
When a chest tube is correctly placed in the pleural space, it can drain air or fluid. A tube could be in the mediastinal space, but it is referred to as a mediastinal tube, not a chest tube.

163. **Correct Answer: C**
Prednisone decreases the effectiveness of isoniazid.

164. **Correct Answer: D**
Neupogen stimulates granulocyte and macrophage proliferation and differentiation as well as some end-cell functions.

165. **Correct Answer: A**
Neupogen stimulates the bone marrow to increase production of macrophages and granulocytes. Bone pain and muscle aches are common.

166. **Correct Answer: D**

The pH indicates partial compensation, CO_2 is compensated, and HCO_3 is low (metabolic).

167. **Correct Answer: D**

Even with the FiO_2 at 30%, the patient can only maintain her oxygenation. There has been an increase of dead air space secondary to her pulmonary embolus.

168. **Correct Answer: B**

These symptoms are classic for a pneumothorax. Remember that the air must be expelled, usually via a thoracentesis, and chest tubes will be placed. Be alert for hemodynamic compromise. Pain management will be necessary, although be aware of the possibility of respiratory depression.

169. **Correct Answer: B**

The most common size is 40 mcg. This size will greatly reduce the dangers of microembolization.

170. **Correct Answer: C**

Old blood sometimes collects in the pleural cavity, and a change in position may cause it to flow into the tube. If there is any question as to the origin, check the patient's blood pressure and do a thorough assessment.

171. **Correct Answer: B**

Venturi mask systems allow for high-flow oxygen at predetermined concentrations with specific adapters. This method is advantageous for patients who need greater flow or inspiratory pressure without the high oxygen concentration.

BIBLIOGRAPHY

Adhikari, N., Burns, K. E. A., & Meade, M. O. (2004). Pharmacologic therapies for adults with acute lung injury and acute respiratory distress syndrome. *Cochrane Database of Systematic Reviews, 4,* Art No CD004477, pub 2, DOI: 10.1002/14651858.

Agbaht, K., Lisboa, T., Pobo, A., Rodriguez, A., Sandiumenge, A., Diaz, E., et al. (2007). Management of ventilator-associated pneumonia in a multidisciplinary intensive care unit: Does trauma make a difference? *Intensive Care Medicine, 33*(8), 1387–1395.

Ahrens, T., & Sona, C. (2003). Capnography application in acute and critical care. *AACN Clinical Issues, 14,* 123–132.

Ahrens, T. (2006). *Critical care nursing certification.* Columbus, OH: McGraw-Hill.

American Association of Critical-Care Nurses. (2004). *Ventilator associated pneumonia (VAP). Practice alert series.* Aliso Viejo, CA: Author.

American Association of Critical-Care Nurses. (2006). *Core curriculum for critical care nursing* (6th ed.). Philadelphia: Saunders.

American Association of Critical-Care Nurses. (2007). *AACN certification and core review for high acuity and critical care* (6th ed.). Philadelphia: Saunders.

American Heart Association. (2005). *Guidelines 2005 for cardiopulmonary resuscitation and emergency cardiovascular care.* Retrieved July 18, 2008, from http://circ.ahajournals.org/content/vol112/24_suppl/

American Heart Association. (2007). *Guidelines 2005 for cardiopulmonary resuscitation and emergency cardiovascular care: Update.* Retrieved July 18, 2008, from http://circ.ahajournals.org/content/vol112/24_suppl/

American Lung Association. (2005). Lung transplants: Treatments and support. Retrieved February 2, 2005, from http://www.lungusa.org/site/c.dvLUK9O0E/b.23012/k.A039/Lung_Transplants.htm

American Thoracic Society. (2005). Consensus statement: Guidelines for the management of adults with hospital-acquired, ventilatory-associated, and healthcare-associated pneumonia. *American Journal of Respiratory Critical Care Medicine, 171,* 388–416.

Andenaes, R., Kalfoss, M. H., & Wahl, A. (2004). Psychological distress and quality of life in hospitalized patients with chronic obstructive pulmonary disease. *Journal of Advanced Nursing, 46*(5), 523–530.

Arora, S., Lang, I., Nayyar, V., Stachowski, E., & Ross, D. L. (2007). Atrial fibrillation in a tertiary care multidisciplinary intensive care unit: Incidence and risk factors. *Anesthesia and Intensive Care, 35*(5), 707–713.

Association of Operating Room Nurses. (2007). AORN guideline for prevention of venous stasis. *AORN Journal, 85*(3), 607–624.

Azu, M. C., McCormack, J. E., Huang, E. C., Lee, T. K., & Shapiro, M. J. (2007). Venous thromboembolic events in hospitalized trauma patients. *American Surgeon, 73*(12), 1228–1231.

Bailey, P. H., Colella, T., & Mossey, S. (2004). COPD-intuition or template: Nurses' stories of acute exacerbations of chronic obstructive pulmonary disease. *Journal of Clinical Nursing, 13*(6), 756–764.

Barnes, P. J., & Adcock, I. M. (2003). How do corticoid steroids work in asthma? *Annals of Internal Medicine, 139*(5, pt 1), 359–370.

Berkowitz, D. S., & Coyne, N. C. (2003). Understanding primary pulmonary hypertension. *Critical Care Nursing Quarterly, 26*(1), 28–34.

Bialk, J. L. (2004). Ethical guidelines for assisting patients with end-of-life decision making. *Medsurg Nursing, 13*(2), 87–90.

Bigatello, L. M., Davidson, K. R., & Stelfox, H. T. (2005). Respiratory mechanics and ventilatory waveforms in the patient with acute lung injury. *Respiratory Care, 50,* 235–245.

Booker, R. (2004). The effective assessment of acute breathlessness in a patient. *Nursing Times, 100*(24), 61–63.

Booker, R. (2005). Chronic obstructive pulmonary disease: Non-pharmacological approaches. *British Journal of Nursing, 14*(1), 14–18 (review).

Borges, J. B., Okamoto, V. N., Matos, G. F. J., Caramez, M. P., Arantes, P. R., Barros, F., et al. (2006). Reversibility of lung collapse and hypoxemia in early acute respiratory distress syndrome. *American Journal of Respiratory and Critical Care Medicine, 174*(3), 268–278.

Boron, W. F., & Boulpaep, E. L. (2004). *Medical physiology*. Philadelphia: Saunders.

Boyle, A. H., & Locke, D. L. (2004). Update on chronic obstructive pulmonary disease. *Medsurg Nursing, 13*(1), 42–48.

Burgess, A. W. (2005). Death by catheterization? Sudden, unexpected deaths of older adults are often not questioned. *American Journal of Nursing, 105*(4), 56–59.

Burns, D. M. (2003). Tobacco-related diseases. *Seminars in Oncology Nursing, 19*(4), 244–249.

Burns, S. M. (2003). Working with respiratory waveforms: How to use bedside graphics. *AACN Clinical Issues, 14,* 133–144.

Burns, S. M. (2004). The science of weaning: When and how? *Critical Care Nursing Clinics of North America, 16*(3), 379–386, ix.

Burns, S. M. (Ed.). (2007). *American Association of Critical-Care Nurses (AACN): AACN protocols for practice: Healing environments* (2nd ed.). Sudbury, MA: Jones and Bartlett.

Celli, B. R., MacNee, W., & ATS/ERS Task Force. (2004). Standards for the diagnosis and treatment of patients with COPD: A summary of the ATS/ERS position paper. *European Respiratory Journal, 23,* 932–946.

Chasen, E. R., & Umlauf, M. G. (2003). Nocturia: A problem that disrupts sleep and predicts obstructive sleep apnea. *Geriatric Nursing, 24*(2), 76–81.

Chojnowski, D. (2003). "GOLD" standards for acute exacerbation in COPD. *Nursing Practice, 28*(5), 26–35.

Conner, B., & Meng, A. (2003). Pulmonary function testing in asthma: Nursing applications. *Critical Care Nursing Clinics of North America, 38*(4), 571–583.

Conover, M. B. (2003). *Understanding electrocardiography* (8th ed.). St. Louis, MO: Mosby/Elsevier.

Cooper, S. J. (2004). Methods to prevent ventilator-associated lung injury: A summary. *Critical Care Nurse, 20*(6), 358–365.

Copstead, L., & Banasik, J. L. (2000). *Pathophysiology: Biological and behavioral perspectives.* (2nd ed.). Philadelphia: Saunders/Elsevier.

Corbridge, S. J., & Corbridge, T. C. (2004). Severe exacerbations in asthma. *Critical Care Nursing Quarterly, 27,* 207–228.

Costello, J., & Hogg, C. T. (2003). CT pulmonary angiogram compared with ventilation–perfusion scan for the diagnosis of pulmonary embolism in patients with cardiorespiratory disease. *Emergency Medicine Journal, 20,* 547–548.

Criner, G. J., Scharf, S. M., Falk, J. A., Gaughan, J. P., Sternberg, A. L., Patel, N. B., et al. (2007). Effect of lung volume reduction surgery on resting pulmonary hemodynamics in severe emphysema. *American Journal of Respiratory and Critical Care Medicine, 176*(3), 253–260.

Curley, M. A. Q. (1998). Patient–nurse synergy: Optimizing patients' outcomes. *American Journal of Critical Care, 7,* 64–72.

de Perrot, M., Granton, J., & Fadel, E. (2006). Pulmonary hypertension after pulmonary emboli: An underrecognized condition. *Canadian Medical Association Journal, 174*(12), 1706–1707.

Dells, P. L. (2004). Advances in prostacyclin therapy for pulmonary arterial hypertension. *Critical Care Nurse, 24,* 42–54.

Dossey, B. M., Keegan, L., & Guzzetta, C. (2003). *Holistic nursing: A handbook for practice* (3rd ed.). Sudbury, MA: Jones and Bartlett.

Dueker, C. W. (2004). Immersion in fresh water and survival. *Chest, 126*(6), 2027–2028.

Durbin, C. G. (2005). Applied respiratory physiology: Uses of ventilator waveforms and mechanics in the management of critically ill patients. *Respiratory Care, 50,* 287–293.

Ecklund, M. M., & Kurluk, S. A. (2004). Caring for the bariatric patient with obstructive sleep apnea. *Critical Care Nursing Clinics of North America, 16*(3), 311–317.

Edwards, D. F. (1999). The Synergy Model: Linking patient needs to nurse competencies. *Critical Care Nurse, 19*(1), 88–98.

Eli-Masri, M. M., Williamson, K. M., & Fox-Wasylyshyn, S. M. (2004). Severe acute respiratory syndrome: Another challenge for critical care nurses. *AACN Clinical Issues, 15*(1), 150–159.

Ellstrom, K. (2006). *The pulmonary system: Core curriculum for critical care nursing* (6th ed.). St. Louis, MO: Saunders.

Emergency Nurses Association & Newberry, L. (2003). *Sheehy's emergency nursing: Principles and practice* (5th ed.). St. Louis, MO: Mosby/Elsevier.

Estabrooks, C. A., Midodzi, W. K., Cummings, G. G., Ricker, K. L., & Giovannetti, P. (2005). The impact of hospital nursing characteristics on 30-day mortality. *Nursing Research, 54*(2), 74–84.

Fedullo, P. F., & Tapson, V. F. (2003). Clinical practice: The evaluation of suspected pulmonary embolism. *New England Journal of Medicine, 349*, 1247–1256.

Fehrenbach, C. (2005). Initiatives to improve outcomes for chronic obstructive pulmonary disease. *Journal of Professional Nursing, 20*(6), 43–45.

Fenstermacher, D., & Hong, D. (2004). Mechanical ventilation: What have we learned? *Critical Care Nursing Quarterly, 27*, 258–294.

Finesilver, C. (2003). Pulmonary assessment: What you need to know. *Progress in Cardiovascular Nursing, 18*, 83.

Finkelmeier, B. A. (2000). *Cardiothoracic surgical nursing* (2nd ed.). Philadelphia: Lippincott, Williams & Wilkins.

Fost, S. D., Brotman, D. J., & Michota, F. A. (2003). Rational use of D-dimer measurements to exclude acute venous thromboembolic disease. *Mayo Clinic Proceedings, 78*, 1385–1391.

Frazier, S. C. (2005). Implications of the GOLD report for chronic obstructive pulmonary disease for the home care clinician. *Home Health Nurse, 23*(2), 109–114.

Giulliano, K. K., & Higgins, T. L. (2005). New generation pulse oximetry in the care of critically ill patients. *American Journal of Critical Care, 14*, 26–39.

Goldrick, B. A. (2005). Infection in the older adult: Long-term care poses particular risk. *American Journal of Nursing, 105*(6), 31–34.

Gronkiewicz, C., & Borkgen-Okonek, M. (2004). Acute exacerbation of COPD: Nursing application of evidence-based guidelines. *Critical Care Nursing Quarterly, 27*(4), 336–352.

Guyton, A. C., & Hall, J. E. (2005). *Textbook of medical physiology* (11th ed.). Philadelphia: Saunders.

Hanneman, S. (2004). Weaning from short-term mechanical ventilation. *Critical Care Nurse, 24*(1), 70.

Hardie, J. A., Vollmer, W. M., Buist, A. S., Ellingsen, I., & Mørkve, O. (2004). Reference values for arterial blood gases in the elderly. *Chest, 125*, 2053.

Hardin, S. R., & Kaplow, R. (Eds.). (2004). *Synergy for clinical excellence: The AACN Synergy Model for Patient Care.* Sudbury, MA: Jones and Bartlett.

Heinzer, M. M., Bish, C., & Detwiler, R. (2003). Acute dyspnea as perceived by patients with chronic obstructive pulmonary disease. *Clinical Nursing Research, 12*(1), 85–101.

Hickey, J. V. (2002). *The clinical practice of neurological and neurosurgical nursing* (5th ed.). Philadelphia: Lippincott, Williams & Wilkins.

Hogg, J. C., Chu, F., Utokaparch, S., Woods, R., Elliott, W. M., Buzatu, L., et al. (2004). The nature of small-airway obstruction in chronic obstructive pulmonary disease. *New England Journal of Medicine, 350*, 2645–2653.

Hughes, J. M. B. (2007). Review series: Lung function made easy: Assessing gas exchange. *Chronic Respiratory Disease, 4*(4), 205–214.

Jesurum, J. (2004). SvO_2 monitoring. *Critical Care Nurse, 24*, 73–76.

Jones, P. W. (2003). Ultrasound-guided thoracentesis: Is it a safer method? *Chest, 123*, 418.

Kaczorowski, D. J., & Zuckerbraun, B. S. (2007). Carbon monoxide: Medicinal chemistry and biological effects. *Current Medicinal Chemistry, 14*(25), 2720–2725.

Kallet, R. H., & Katz, J. A. (2003). Respiratory system mechanics in acute respiratory distress syndrome. *Respiratory Care Clinics of North America, 9,* 297.

Kane, C., & Galanes, S. (2004). Adult respiratory distress syndrome. *Critical Care Nursing Quarterly, 27*(4), 325–335.

Kanervisto, M., Paavilainen, E., & Astedt-Kurki, P. (2003). Impact of chronic obstructive pulmonary disease on family functioning. *Heart and Lung, 32*(6), 360–367.

Katis, P. G. (2005). Atraumatic hemopericardium in a patient receiving warfarin therapy for a pulmonary embolus. *Journal of the Canadian Association of Emergency Physicians, 7*(3), 168–170.

Keenan, S. P., Sinuff, T., Cook, D. J., & Hill, N. S. (2004). Does noninvasive positive pressure ventilation improve outcome in acute hypoxemic respiratory failure: A systematic review. *Critical Care Medicine, 32,* 2516–2523.

King, J. E. (2003). Could my patient have deep vein thrombosis? *Nursing, 33*(9), 24.

Kollef, M. H. (2004). Prevention of hospital-associated pneumonia and ventilatory-associated pneumonia. *Critical Care Medicine, 6,* 1396.

Koschel, M. J. (2004). Pulmonary embolism: Quick diagnosis can save a patient's life. *American Journal of Nursing, 140*(6), 46–50.

Kreamer, K. M. (2003). Getting the lowdown on lung cancer. *Nursing, 33*(11), 36–42.

Kress, T., & Krueger, D. (2004). Identifying carbon monoxide poisoning. *Nursing, 34*(11), 68–69.

Kumar, D., Farrell, T., & Tierney, E. (2007). A frightening complication of general anesthesia for pediatric dental extractions. *Pediatric Surgery International, 23*(6), 613–616.

Lindgren, V. A., & Ames, N. J. (2005). Caring for patients on mechanical ventilation: What research indicates is best practice. *American Journal of Nursing, 105*(5), 50–60.

Lipson, J. G., Dibble, S. L., & Minarik, P. A. (Eds.). (1996). *Culture and nursing care: A pocket guide.* San Francisco, CA: UCSF Nursing Press.

Lomborg, K., Bjorn, A., Dahl, R., & Kirkevold, M. (2005). Body care experienced by people hospitalized with severe respiratory disease. *Journal of Advanced Nursing, 50*(3), 262–271.

Lynes, D., & Kelly, C. (2003). The psychological needs of patients with chronic respiratory disease. *Nursing Times, 99*(33), 44–45.

MacIntyre, N. R. (2004). Evidence-based ventilator weaning and discontinuation. *Respiratory Care, 49*(7), 830–836.

Majer, S., & Graber, P. (2007). Postpartum pneumomediastinum (Hamman's syndrome). *Canadian Medical Association Journal, 177*(1), 32.

Markou, N. K., Myrianthefs, P. M., & Batopoulos, G. J. (2004). Respiratory failure: An overview. *Critical Care Nursing Quarterly, 27*(4), 353–379.

McQuillan, D. P., Duncan, R. A., & Craven, D. E. (2005). Ventilator-associated pneumonia: Emerging principles of management. *Infections in Medicine, 22*(3), 104–118.

McQuillan, K. A., Von Rueden, K. T., Hartsock, R. L., Flynn, M. B., & Whalen, E. (Eds.). (2002). *Trauma nursing: From resuscitation through rehabilitation* (3rd ed.). Philadelphia: Saunders/Elsevier.

Medina, J., & Puntillo, K. (2006). *AACN protocols for practice: Palliative care and end-of-life issues in critical care.* Sudbury, MA: Jones and Bartlett.

Merrel, P., & Mayo, D. (2004). Inhalation injury in the burn patient. *Critical Care Nursing Clinics of North America, 16*(1), 27–38.

Merritt, S. L., & Berger, B. E. (2004). Obstructive sleep apnea–hypopnea syndrome. *American Journal of Nursing, 104*(7), 49–52.

Mullan, B., Snyder, M., Lindgren, B., Finkelstein, S. M., & Hertz, M. I. (2003). Home monitoring for lung transplant candidates. *Progress in Transplantation, 13*(3), 176–182.

Muno, N. (2003). Cardiac bypass without the pump. *RN, 66*(10), 28–32.

Musto, P. K. (2003). General principles of asthma management: Education. *Nursing Clinics of North America, 38*(4), 621–633.

Nilsestuen, J. O., & Hargett, K. D. (2005). Using ventilator graphics to identify patient–ventilator asynchrony. *Respiratory Care, 50,* 202–234.

O'Shea Forbes, M. (2007). Prolonged ventilator dependence: Perspective of the chronic obstructive pulmonary disease patient. *Clinical Nursing Research, 16*(3), 231.

Pagana, K. D., & Pagana, J. (2005). *Mosby's manual of diagnostic and laboratory tests* (3rd ed.). St. Louis, MO: Mosby/Elsevier.

Petty, M. (2003). Lung and heart–lung transplantation: Implications for nursing care when hospitalized outside the transplant center. *Medsurg Nursing, 12*(4), 250–259.

Poulose, B. K., Griffin, M. R., Zhu, Y., Smalley, W., Richards, W. O., Wright, J. K., et al. (2005). National analysis of adverse patient safety events in bariatric surgery. *American Surgeon, 71*(5), 406–413.

Powers, J., & Daniels, D. (2004). Turning points: Implementing kinetic therapy in the ICU. *Nursing Management, 35*(5 suppl), 1–7.

Pruitt, B., & Jacobs, M. (2005). Caring for a patient with asthma. *Nursing, 35*(2), 48–51.

Ramirez, E. G. (2003). Management of asthma emergencies. *Nursing Clinics of North America, 38*(4), 713–724.

Rance, M. (2005). Kinetic therapy positively influences oxygenation in patients with ALI/ARDS. *Nursing Critical Care, 10*(1), 35–41.

Roberts, J. (2003). The new asthma guidelines: A patient-centered approach to asthma. *Journal of Professional Nursing, 18*(7), 379–382.

Roch, A., Blayac, D., Ramiara, P., Chetaille, B., Marin, V., Michelet, P., et al. (2007). Comparison of lung injury after normal or small volume optimized resuscitation in a model of hemorrhagic shock. *Intensive Care Medicine, 33*(9), 1645–1654.

Rowe, C. (2004). Development of clinical guidelines for prone positioning in critically ill adults. *Nursing Critical Care, 9*(2), 50–57.

Salomez, F., & Vincent, J. L. (2004). Drowning: A review of epidemiology, pathophysiology, treatment and prevention. *Resuscitation, 63*(3), 261–268.

Seidel, H. M. (2003). *Mosby's guide to physical examination* (3rd ed.). St. Louis, MO: Mosby.

Sevransky, J. E., Levy, M. M., & Marini, J. J. (2004). Mechanical ventilation in sepsis-induced acute lung-injury/acute respiratory distress syndrome: An evidence-based review. *Critical Care Medicine, 32,* S548–S553.

Simmons, P., & Simmons, M. (2004). Informed nursing practice: The administration of oxygen to patients with COPD. *Medsurg Nursing, 13*(2), 82–85.

Sims, J. M. (2003). Guidelines for treating asthma. *Dimensions of Critical Care Nursing, 22*(6), 247–250.

Skidmore-Roth, L. (2004). *Mosby's 2004 nursing drug reference.* St. Louis, MO: Mosby/Elsevier.

Smeltzer, S., & Bare, B. G. (2003). *Brunner and Suddarth's textbook of medical–surgical nursing* (10th ed.). Philadelphia: Lippincott, Williams & Wilkins.

Sole, M. L., Hartshorn, J., & Lamborne, M. L. (2001). *Introduction to critical care nursing* (3rd ed.). Philadelphia: Saunders/Elsevier.

Spector, N., & Connoly, M. (2003). *Dyspnea. Protocols for Practice Series.* Aliso Viejo, CA: American Association of Critical Care.

Squara, P. (2004). Matching total body oxygen consumption and delivery: A crucial objective? *Intensive Care Medicine, 30,* 2170–2179.

St. John, R. E. (2003). End-tidal CO_2 monitoring. *Critical Care Nurse, 23,* 83–88.

St. John, R. E. (2004). Airway management. *Critical Care Nurse, 4*(2), 93–96.

Tablan, O. C., Anderson, L. J., Besser, R., Bridges, C., Hajjeh, R., CDC, et al. (2004). Guidelines for preventing health care–associated pneumonia, 2003: Recommendations of CDC and the Healthcare Infection Control Practices Advisory Committee. *MMWR Recommendations and Reports, 53,* 1–36.

Tillie-Leblond, I., Gosset, P., & Tonnel, A. B. (2005). Inflammatory events in severe acute asthma. *Allergy, 60*(1), 23.

Tsangaris, I., Galiatsou, E., Kostanti, E., & Nakos, G. (2007). The effect of exogenous surfactant in patients with lung contusions and acute lung injury. *Intensive Care Medicine, 33*(5), 851–855.

Turpie, A. G. G., Chin, B. S. P., & Lip, G. L. H. (2002). Venous thromboembolism: Pathophysiology, clinical features, and prevention. *British Medical Journal, 325,* 887–890.

United Network for Organ Sharing. (2005). Information for transplant professionals about the lung allocation score system. Retrieved February 20, 2005, from http://www.unos.org/SharedContentDocuments/Lung_pro.pdf

Urden, L. D., Stacy, K. M., & Lough, M. E. (2007). *Thelan's critical care nursing: Diagnosis and management* (5th ed.). St. Louis, MO: Mosby.

U.S. Organ Procurement and Transplantation Network (OPTN). (2005). Scientific Registry of Transplant Recipients (SRTR): OPTN/SRTR annual report. Retrieved February 20, 2005 from http://www.ustransplant.org/annual_Reports/archives/2005/default.htm

Vahid, B., & Marik, P. E. (2007). Severe emphysema associated with cocaine smoking. *Journal of Respiratory Diseases, 28*(11), 485.

Vecchiarino, P., Bohannon, R. W., Ferullo, J., Maljanian, R. (2004). Short-term outcomes and their predictors for patients hospitalized with community-acquired pneumonia. *Heart and Lung, 33,* 301–307.

Veronesi, J. F. (2004). Trauma nursing: Blunt chest injuries. *RN, 67*(3), 47–54.

Vollman, K. M. (2004). Prone positioning in the patient who has acute respiratory distress syndrome: The art and science. *Critical Care Nurse Clinics of North America, 16*(3), 431–443.

Walker, S. (2003). Updates in small cell lung cancer treatment. *Clinical Journal of Oncology Nursing, 7*(5), 562–568.

Weir, P. (2004). Quick asthma assessment: A stepwise approach to treatment. *Advanced Nursing Practice, 12*(1), 53–56.

Wiegand, D. J. L., & Carlson, K. K. (Eds.). (2005). *AACN procedure manual for critical care* (5th ed.). Philadelphia: Elsevier.

Wilkins, R. L., Stoller, J. K., & Scanlan, C. L. (2003). *Egan's fundamentals of respiratory care* (8th ed.). St. Louis, MO: Mosby.

Williams, T. A., & Leslie, G. D. (2004). A review of the nursing care of enteral feeding tubes in critically ill adults: Part I. *Intensive and Critical Care Nursing, 20*(6), 330–343.

Williams, T. A., & Leslie, G. D. (2004). A review of the nursing care of enteral feeding tubes in critically ill adults: Part II. *Intensive and Critical Care Nursing, 21*(5), 5–15.

Williamson, J. P., Illing, R., Gertler, P., & Braude, S. (2004). Near-drowning treated with therapeutic hypothermia. *Medical Journal of Australia, 181*(9), 500–501.

Wisniewski, A. (2003). Chronic bronchitis and emphysema: Clearing the air. *Nursing, 33*(5), 46–49.

Woods, S., Sivarajan Froelicher, E. S., & Motzer, S. U. (2000). *Cardiac nursing* (4th ed.). Philadelphia: Lippincott, Williams & Wilkins.

Wynne, R., & Botti, M. (2004). Postoperative pulmonary dysfunction in adults after cardiac surgery with cardiopulmonary bypass: Clinical significance and implications for practice. *American Journal of Critical Care, 13,* 384–393.

Yang, J. C. (2005). Prevention and treatment of deep vein thrombosis and pulmonary embolism in critically ill patients. *Critical Care Nursing Quarterly, 28*(1), 72–79.

Yoneyama, T., Yoshida, M., Ohrui, T., Mukaiyama, H., Okamoto, H., Hoshiba, K., et al. (2003). Oral care reduces pneumonia in older patients in nursing homes. *Journal of the American Geriatrics Society, 51,* 1018–1022.

Yusen, R. D., Lefrak, S. S., & Gierada, D. S. (2003). A prospective evaluation of lung volume reduction surgery in 200 consecutive patients. *Chest, 123,* 1026–1037.

QUESTIONS

1. Sandra M., a 31-year-old female, is admitted to the progressive care unit after a cholecystectomy due to her morbid obesity. She has a recent history of gastric bypass surgery for weight loss. You find her confused with slurred speech and diaphoretic. Her BP is 90/40, pulse 120, and her blood sugar is 28. Your first action should be to
   A. Notify the physician and recheck the blood sugar.
   B. Open the intravenous fluid and give the patient orange juice with sugar.
   C. Give one amp of D_{50} per hospital policy, notify the physician, and recheck the blood sugar in 30 minutes.
   D. Recheck the blood sugar with the hospital lab.

2. What is the pathophysiology of acute hypoglycemia?
   A. Oral antihyperglycemic agents will cause the disease.
   B. Glucose consumption exceeds glucose production.
   C. Insulinoma is the primary cause.
   D. Alcoholism reduces the number of cells that produce glycogen.

3. Which of the following therapies would be appropriate to use in the treatment of acute hypoglycemia (blood sugar less than 50 mg/dL)?
   A. Small, frequent meals, increased carbohydrate consumption
   B. Intravenous D_{50} administration, oral glucose, treat the cause
   C. Increased carbohydrate diet, intravenous glucose
   D. Treat the cause, increased carbohydrate consumption

4. What is the most common precipitating factor in the development of diabetic ketoacidosis (DKA)?
   A. Hypoglycemia only
   B. Hypoglycemia with obesity and family history
   C. Hyperglycemia only
   D. Hyperglycemia with concurrent illness or injury

5. Which of the following are some of the signs and symptoms associated with diabetic ketoacidosis (DKA)?
   A. Polyuria, polydipsia, polyphagia, dilute urine
   B. Polyuria, polydipsia, polyphagia, fruity breath, dehydration, marked fatigue
   C. Hyperactivity, confusion, nausea, vomiting
   D. Kussmaul's respirations, dilute urine

6. Sid has been admitted to the progressive care unit with DKA. His insulin drip is at 5 units per hour. His current blood sugar is 290, and his anion gap is 28. Which changes in his care should you anticipate?

   A. Change intravenous fluid to D_5W and continue the insulin drip
   B. Change intravenous fluids to D_5NS and continue insulin drip
   C. Discontinue insulin drip, start blood sugars every 4 hours
   D. No changes in therapy

7. Which of the following diabetic patients are most likely to develop DKA?

   A. Type I, well controlled on 70/30 insulin
   B. Type I, noncompliant, with cellulitis of his left leg
   C. Type II, with $HgbA_{1c}$ of 6.5 and minor surgery
   D. Type II, noncompliant, with a mild upper respiratory tract infection

8. Arthur is a 50-year-old patient with a history of DKA. He currently has a blood glucose of 460 mg/dL and a potassium level of 6.2. You have started an insulin drip. You know that the insulin drip will

   A. Draw more potassium from the intracellular space.
   B. Draw more potassium from the extracellular space.
   C. Not change potassium levels.
   D. Move potassium back into the intracellular space.

9. Kayexalate is often given for hyperkalemia. What is the mechanism of action of this drug?

   A. Kayexalate causes diarrhea, thereby removing potassium from the gastrointestinal tract.
   B. Kayexalate preserves the sodium pump.
   C. Kayexalate exchanges sodium ions for potassium ions.
   D. Kayexalate moves potassium into the intracellular space.

10. Nathan is a 42-year-old who has a crush injury to his right thigh. Why does this put Nathan at risk for hyperkalemia?

    A. There is actually a greater risk for hypokalemia.
    B. He is not at risk for hyperkalemia.
    C. Cellular destruction leads to increased circulating potassium levels.
    D. Wound infection decreases potassium levels.

11. Which EKG changes are seen with hyperkalemia?

    A. Narrow QRS, peaked T waves and U waves
    B. Widening QRS, peaked T waves, loss of P waves
    C. Wide QRS, normal T waves, U waves
    D. Narrow QRS, normal T waves, rapid rate

12. How does hyperglycemic, hyperosmolar, nonketotic syndrome (HHNS) differ from diabetic ketoacidosis (DKA)?

    A. HHNS has the same onset, higher blood sugars, and more dehydration compared to DKA.
    B. HHNS has a slower onset, lower blood sugars, and less dehydration compared to DKA.
    C. HHNS has a slower onset, much higher blood sugars, and more profound dehydration than DKA.
    D. HHNS has the same onset, lower blood sugars, and no dehydration than DKA.

13. **Which lab results would you anticipate for a patient with hyperglycemic, hyperosmolar, nonketotic syndrome (HHNS)?**
    A. Glucose 550, positive ketones, serum osmolality 280 mOsm/L
    B. Glucose 1,258, negative ketones, serum osmolality 375 mOsm/L
    C. Glucose 700, negative ketones, serum osmolality 270 mOsm/L
    D. Glucose 600, positive ketones, serum osmolality 240 mOsm/L

14. **Bernie is an 87-year-old man found unconscious in his board and care room. He was admitted to your progressive care unit an hour ago. His blood sugar is 1,525, he has negative serum ketones, and his serum osmolality is 348. What do you anticipate for medical treatment of this condition?**
    A. D_5 ½NS intravenous fluids 300 mL/h and an insulin drip with sliding-scale coverage
    B. Normal saline at 200 mL/h, subcutaneous insulin with sliding-scale coverage every 4 hours and monitor potassium
    C. Intravenous fluids with normal saline in high volumes, insulin drip with sliding-scale coverage, monitor electrolyte levels
    D. Normal saline intravenously, bicarbonate drip, monitor electrolytes

15. **What is the difference between the Somoygi effect and the dawn phenomenon?**
    A. They are essentially the same process.
    B. The dawn phenomenon is nocturnal hypoglycemia, and the Somoygi effect is greatly increased blood sugars in the early morning.
    C. The Somoygi effect is nocturnal hypoglycemia with rebound hyperglycemia, and the dawn phenomenon is increased morning glucose without nocturnal hypoglycemia.
    D. The dawn phenomenon is morning hypoglycemia, and the Somoygi effect is nocturnal hyperglycemia.

16. **Your 20-year-old patient has been diagnosed with Cushing syndrome. Which diagnostic tests do you anticipate?**
    A. Computerized tomography of the brain, chest, and abdomen; 24-hour urine cortisol levels; ACTH serum concentrations
    B. Computerized tomography of the brain, chest, and abdomen; thyroid levels; basic metabolic panel
    C. Serum and urine cortisol levels; thyroid panels; beta-naturetic peptide levels
    D. Urine ACTH concentrations; thyroid panel; C-reactive protein level

17. **Which physical symptoms do you expect with Cushing syndrome?**
    A. Moon facies, edema, weight loss
    B. Moon facies, acne, weight loss
    C. Moon facies, purple striae on trunk, buffalo hump
    D. Moon facies, easy bruising, weight loss

18. **Functions of the thyroid gland, adrenal gland, and male and female reproductive glands are regulated by the**
    A. Pineal gland of the brain.
    B. Thyroid gland.
    C. Pineal–pituitary axis.
    D. Hypothalamic–pituitary axis.

19. **Where is the pituitary gland located?**
    A. Inferior to the hypothalamus and sits in the sella turcica of the skull
    B. Superior to the hypothalamus gland, near the optic chiasm
    C. Between the thalamus and hypothalamus in the midbrain
    D. Superior to the pons and brain stem

20. **Which of the following hormones are produced by the anterior pituitary gland?**
    A. GRF, TSH, Substance P
    B. ADH, TSH, FSH
    C. FSH, LH, TSH, ACTH
    D. Vasopressin and oxytocin

21. **Your patient's thyroid-stimulating hormone (TSH) level is 0.001. Which condition does this value indicate?**
    A. Hypoactive anterior pituitary function
    B. Hyperactive anterior pituitary function
    C. Hypothyroidism
    D. Hyperthyroidism

22. **Where is the thyroid gland located?**
    A. Just below the hyoid bone
    B. In the throat on either side of the trachea
    C. Above the larynx
    D. On top of the thymus gland

23. **What is an important teaching point for a patient with hypothyroidism?**
    A. Take thyroid medication at the same time every day; there is no need to fast.
    B. Take thyroid medication at the same time every day, 30 minutes before breakfast.
    C. Take thyroid medication each evening before bed.
    D. Take thyroid medication daily with food.

24. **John had a thyroidectomy yesterday for thyroid cancer. Today he is delirious, vomiting, hyperthermic, and tachycardic. It is imperative to notify the physician stat because**
    A. John has a postoperative infection.
    B. John may have had a cerebrovascular accident.
    C. John may be having a thyrotoxic crisis.
    D. John is hypoxic and needs a tracheostomy.

25. **Treatment for a thyrotoxic crisis includes**
    A. Administration of PTH and symptomatic care.
    B. Symptomatic care and wait for symptoms to subside.
    C. Synthroid administration and supportive care.
    D. No need for treatment, the crisis will resolve spontaneously.

26. **Which feature is unique to the pancreas?**
    A. The pancreas does not have any unique features.
    B. The pancreas is both an endocrine and an exocrine gland.
    C. The pancreas is the largest gland in the body.
    D. The location and size make the pancreas unique.

27. **Where are the parathyroid glands located?**
    A. Anterior to the thyroid gland
    B. Posterior to the thyroid gland
    C. On top of the thyroid gland
    D. Below the thyroid gland

28. **Janet was admitted to your progressive care unit with an anaphylactic reaction to a bee sting. Multiple labs are drawn, and her calcium level is 11.9 mg/dL. This value may indicate which of the following conditions?**
    A. Hypoparathyroidism
    B. Excessive calcium intake
    C. Hyperparathyroidism
    D. Recent fracture of a long bone

29. **Which precipitating condition might cause hypoparathyroidism?**
    A. Trauma
    B. Hypercalcemia
    C. Hypophosphatemia
    D. Thyroid or neck surgery

30. **Where is the pancreas located in the abdomen?**
    A. Right lower quadrant of the abdomen
    B. Right upper quadrant of the abdomen
    C. Left upper quadrant of the abdomen
    D. Left lower quadrant of the abdomen

31. **What is the purpose of testing HgbA$_{1c}$ in diabetes mellitus?**
    A. It is of little help in managing diabetes mellitus.
    B. It measures blood sugars over a 6-month period.
    C. It measures the effectiveness of diabetes mellitus.
    D. It measures red blood cell activity in diabetes mellitus.

32. **Erin is a 20-year-old female who was admitted to your progressive care unit for new-onset diabetic ketoacidosis. You are teaching her about diabetes mellitus and HgbA$_{1c}$. Which of the following HgbA$_{1c}$ values should be Erin's goal for good control of her diabetes mellitus?**
    A. 7–8%
    B. 4–5%
    C. 8–9%
    D. 6–7%

33. **Why are hyperglycemia and hyperlipidemia seen concurrently in diabetes mellitus?**
    A. Very-low-density lipoprotein (VLDL) production increases in response to increased insulin production.
    B. Insulin resistance promotes VLDL production.
    C. Lipid breakdown is hindered by hyperinsulinemia.
    D. Glucose increases cause the liver to increase lipid production.

34. **Which of the following are considered risk factors in the development of diabetes mellitus?**
    A. Obesity (BMI of 42), blood pressure 160/95, HDL 28, brother with diabetes mellitus
    B. Obesity (BMI of 27), blood pressure 120/70, HDL 42, no family history of diabetes mellitus
    C. Obesity (BMI of 26), Caucasian ancestry, blood pressure 190/100, family history of diabetes mellitus
    D. Obesity (BMI of 40), blood pressure 100/50, HDL 50, no family history of diabetes mellitus

35. **Which hormones are secreted by the islets of Langerhans?**
    A. Insulin and amylase
    B. Glucagon and amylase
    C. Glucagon and insulin
    D. Insulin and lipase

36. **How is insulin secretion regulated?**
    A. Hormonal, insulin, and neuronal controls
    B. Chemical, hormonal, and neuronal controls
    C. Chemical, glucagon, and insulin controls
    D. Hormonal, exocrine gland secretion, and glucose controls

37. **What is the role of glucagon?**
    A. It acts on the liver to decrease blood sugar.
    B. It acts on the liver to increase blood sugar.
    C. It acts on the pancreas to decrease blood sugar.
    D. It acts on the pancreas to increase blood sugar.

38. **John, who has Type I diabetes, asks you why he is so thirsty when his blood sugars rise. Which of the following explanations might be appropriate to help explain his condition?**
    A. Polyuria is increased urine output due to high blood sugars.
    B. Polyphagia is seen with increased glucose secondary to extracellular dehydration.
    C. Polydipsia is seen with increased glucose due to intracellular dehydration.
    D. Polyphagia is seen with increased appetite, which in turn leads to excess thirst.

39. **Which level of beta cell function must be lost before hyperglycemia occurs?**
    A. 60–70%
    B. 25–45%
    C. 50–60%
    D. 80–90%

40. **What is non-alcohol steatohepatitis (NASH)?**
    A. Fatty liver infiltrates seen as a precursor to diabetes mellitus Type II
    B. Fatty liver from hepatitis B infection
    C. Fatty liver from poor diet
    D. Fatty liver from obesity and excess consumption of dietary fats

41. **Glenda, a 49-year-old female with Type II diabetes, is admitted to the progressive care unit with acute coronary syndrome (ACS). She is NPO for angiography. She calls you to her room and tells you she feels "funny." You note that Glenda is pale, diaphoretic, anxious, and restless. What is your next step in evaluating this patient?**
    A. Check vital signs and temperature
    B. Check vital signs, repeat cardiac enzymes, and obtain a stat EKG
    C. Check vital signs and blood sugar
    D. Check vital signs and obtain a pulse oximetry reading

42. **Continuing with the scenario from Question 41, Glenda's blood sugar is 37. What is your next action?**
    A. Do nothing; the intravenous fluid will correct the blood sugar
    B. Notify the physician and give Glenda a glass of orange juice with 3 packets of sugar
    C. Notify the physician and increase the intravenous fluids
    D. Give one amp of D_{50} intravenously per your hospital protocol and notify the physician

43. **Gastroparesis is usually associated with**
    A. Alcohol abuse.
    B. Long-term diabetes mellitus, either type.
    C. Acute pancreatitis.
    D. Acute cholecystitis.

44. **What are the three major problems associated with macrovascular disease along with diabetes mellitus?**
    A. Retinopathy, coronary artery disease, cerebral vascular accident
    B. Peripheral neuropathy, coronary artery disease, cerebral vascular accident
    C. Coronary artery disease, cerebral vascular accident, peripheral vascular disease
    D. Diabetic peripheral neuropathy, peripheral vascular disease, cerebral vascular accident

45. **What is the pathophysiology of microvascular disease in diabetes mellitus?**
    A. Increased atherosclerotic plaques on the intima
    B. Changes in the capillary basement membrane causing hypoxia on the cellular level
    C. Vasoconstriction from hyperglycemia
    D. Repeated hypoglycemic events

46. **Floyd was admitted to your unit with a diagnosis of acute kidney injury. He has a history of diabetes mellitus. What is the first sign of renal damage in a patient with diabetes mellitus?**
    A. Proteinuria
    B. Elevated blood urea nitrogen and creatinine levels
    C. Oliguria
    D. Hematuria

47. **Where is renin stored?**
    A. Renal tubules
    B. Loop of Henle
    C. Juxtoglomerular cells of the nephron
    D. Adrenal cortex

48. Which of the following conditions or medications can trigger the renin–angiotensin mechanism?
    A. Aldosterone, diuretics
    B. Diuretics, decreased renal blood flow
    C. Diuretics, adrenergic blockers
    D. Increased renal blood flow, diuretics

49. What is the correct order of the renin–angiotensin mechanism when there is a decrease in blood flow to the kidneys?
    A. Renin, ACTH, angiotensin I
    B. Increased ADH, renin, angiotensin I, angiotensin II
    C. Renin, angiotensinogen, angiotensin I, angiotensin I converting enzyme, angiotensin II, aldosterone
    D. Renin, aldosterone, angiotensin I, angiotensin I converting enzyme, angiotensin II

50. Where are the catecholamines produced?
    A. Liver
    B. Kidneys
    C. Adrenal cortex
    D. Adrenal medulla

51. Frank is admitted to the progressive care unit for treatment of diabetic ketoacidosis. As his nurse, you know his insulin drip will be titrated by sliding scale and based on his anion gap. What does the anion gap measure?
    A. It estimates cations and anions.
    B. An estimate of unmeasured anions
    C. An estimate of anions in the blood
    D. It estimates the correction of the acid/base balance.

52. Continuing with the scenario from Question 51, Frank has arterial blood gases drawn. Which of the following results would you expect to see with diabetic ketoacidosis?
    A. pH 7.55; CO_2 22 mm Hg; HCO_3 26 mEq/L
    B. pH 7.36; CO_2 54 mm Hg; HCO_3 33 mEq/L
    C. pH 7.15; CO_2 24 mm Hg; HCO_3 12 mEq/L
    D. pH 7.40; CO_2 41 mm Hg; HCO_3 25 mEq/L

53. Your new patient with diabetic ketoacidosis is slowly improving. What do the following arterial blood gases represent for this patient: pH 7.32; CO_2 50 mm Hg; HCO_3 20 mEq/L.
    A. Fully compensated respiratory acidosis
    B. Fully compensated metabolic alkalosis
    C. Partially compensated metabolic acidosis
    D. Partially compensated respiratory acidosis

54. A new graduate nurse admits a patient with diabetic ketoacidosis who has a HCO_3 level of 10 mEq/L. In addition to an insulin drip, you should anticipate which of following treatments or actions?

A. Sodium bicarbonate drip with frequent HCO_3 levels

B. Sodium bicarbonate bolus and repeat every 4–6 hours

C. Increase the insulin drip to hasten the resolution of the metabolic acidosis

D. Decrease the insulin drip, because the acidosis is resolving

55. Fred is a 60-year-old male admitted to the progressive care unit for an acute myocardial infarction. He has a schizoaffective disorder for which he has taken lithium for 15 years. You note he has a very high urine output—approximately 800 cc/h—and an SpG of 1.001. What is wrong?

A. Fred is experiencing the diuretic effect of a low-sodium diet.

B. Fred has diabetes insipidus from long-term lithium use.

C. Fred has excessive oral fluid intake.

D. Fred has neurogenic diabetes insipidus.

56. Mrs. Z. is admitted to the progressive care unit with myxedema coma. She is receiving intravenous thyroid replacement therapy when she suddenly develops hypotension, hypoglycemia, nausea, and vomiting. What has probably happened?

A. An allergic response to the thyroid medication

B. She needs an increased dose of thyroid medication.

C. She needs a lower dose of thyroid medication.

D. The patient is experiencing Addisonian crisis.

57. Gina has end-stage renal disease (ESRD) stage IV and is on hemodialysis every Monday, Wednesday, and Friday. Her calcium is 6.3 mg/dL and her PTH is 70 mg/mL. What is happening to this patient?

A. Hypoparathyroidism

B. Secondary hypoparathyroidism

C. Secondary hyperthyroidism

D. Hypothyroidism

58. The anterior pituitary gland controls which of the following glands?

A. Parathyroid, adrenal medulla, gonads

B. Thyroid, adrenal medulla, gonads

C. Parathyroid, thyroid, gonads

D. Thyroid, adrenal cortex, gonads

59. What is the function of antidiuretic hormone (ADH)?

A. Water balance

B. Sodium balance

C. Aldosterone production

D. Potassium balance

60. What inhibits antidiuretic hormone (ADH) production?

A. Pituitary tumors

B. Water intoxication

C. Increased serum osmolality

D. Increased potassium levels

61. **Which symptoms are seen with diabetes insipidus?**
    A. Low urine output, hypertension, bradycardia
    B. Excessive urine output, hypertension, tachycardia
    C. Excessive urine output, hypotension, tachycardia
    D. Low urine output, hypotension, tachycardia

62. **Why is diabetes insipidus (DI) common in patients with basilar skull fractures?**
    A. Cerebral edema
    B. Hematomas, especially epidural hematomas
    C. DI is not common in basilar skull fractures
    D. Damage to the sella turcica and, therefore, to the pituitary gland

63. **What is the most common presentation of a patient with syndrome of inappropriate antidiuretic hormone (SIADH)?**
    A. Excessive, dilute urine output
    B. Hypotension
    C. Seizures
    D. Tetany

64. **Paul has been diagnosed with diabetes insipidus. Which of the following lab results could probably be seen with this condition?**
    A. Serum osmolality 275, sodium 137, urine specific gravity 1.020
    B. Serum osmolality 315, sodium 165, urine specific gravity 1.003
    C. Serum osmolality 283, sodium 119, urine specific gravity 1.015
    D. Serum osmolality 265, sodium 150, urine specific gravity 1.001

65. **Which of the following is responsible for the symptoms of hypothyroidism?**
    A. Low levels of T_4 (thyroxine)
    B. Low levels of T_3 (triiodothyronine)
    C. Decreased thyrocalcitonin
    D. Increased thyrocalcitonin

66. **Which of the following conditions must be present for calcium to be utilized by the body?**
    A. Increased oral calcium
    B. Increased phosphorus
    C. A euthyroid state
    D. Adequate vitamin D levels

67. **Trousseau's sign is seen with which condition?**
    A. Increased serum calcium
    B. Decreased serum calcium
    C. Decreased serum phosphorus
    D. Hypothyroidism

68. **Which of the following signs may be seen with hypocalcemia?**
    A. Short QT interval
    B. Hyperparathyroidism
    C. Chvostek's sign
    D. Cullen's sign

69. **Which glands regulate thyroid function?**
    A. Posterior pituitary and hypothalamus
    B. Anterior pituitary and thalamus
    C. Anterior pituitary and hypothalamus
    D. Posterior pituitary and thalamus

70. **Which of the following can cause a thyroid storm in a patient with hyperthyroidism?**
    A. Overdose of propylthyrouricil (PTU)
    B. Increased iodine intake
    C. Trauma or infection
    D. Decreased iodine intake

71. **Which symptoms are to be expected with thyrotoxic crisis?**
    A. Hypotension, bradycardia
    B. Hyperthermia, bradycardia
    C. Flushing, hypoventilation
    D. Hypertension, hyperthermia

72. **Your patient is in thyrotoxic crisis. Which medication would you give to reduce her symptoms?**
    A. Propranolol
    B. Levophed
    C. Adenosine
    D. Digoxin

73. **Mr. Y. is admitted to the progressive care unit in hypertensive crisis. You notice large fluctuations in his blood pressure even though you have not changed his nitroprusside drip. The physician orders a plasma catecholamine level. His fractional epinephrine level is very high. What does this indicate?**
    A. Cocaine use
    B. Pheochromocytoma
    C. Adrenal cortex tumor
    D. Hyperthyroidism

74. **Continuing with the scenario from Question 73, part of your patient education for Mr. Y. includes dietary restrictions. Which of the following foods should he avoid?**
    A. Cream cheese
    B. Red meat
    C. Aged cheddar cheese
    D. Chocolate

75. **What is the treatment of choice once a diagnosis of pheochromocytoma is made?**
    A. Dietary changes
    B. Antihypertensive medications
    C. Surgical removal of the tumor
    D. Diuretics

This concludes the Endocrine Questions section.

ANSWERS

1. **Correct Answer: C**
   The most important issue is to increase the blood sugar and notify the physician. Orange juice and sugar should not be given to a new postoperative patient. Her gastric bypass and NPO status increase her risk for hypoglycemia. Other causes of acute hypoglycemia include alcohol abuse, insulinoma, medications, and adrenal insufficiency.

2. **Correct Answer: B**
   Lack of food or inability of the liver to provide glucogenesis causes a drop in blood glucose to less than 50 mg/dL. The other answers are risk factors for hypoglycemia.

3. **Correct Answer: B**
   D_{50}, oral glucose, and treating the cause are the most effective ways to manage acute hypoglycemia. The other answers include increased carbohydrate consumption which would be prohibited. The optimal diet would consist of small, frequent meals and reduced carbohydrates.

4. **Correct Answer: D**
   DKA is seen with illness or injury such as infection, surgery, trauma, or UTI. It is defined as a fasting blood sugar greater than 250 mg/d to approximately 1,000 mg/dL.

5. **Correct Answer: B**
   Polyuria, polydipsia, and polyphagia are known as the "three P's." The fruity breath is from ketone production when fatty acids are broken down. Dehydration is due to osmotic diuresis. Fatigue is due to potassium shifting from inside the cells to the intravascular space.

6. **Correct Answer: B**
   Once the blood glucose is less than 300 mg/dL, D_5WNS should be added to slow the drop in glucose. Hourly blood glucose levels should be continued. The anion gap should slowly be lowered to less than 20.

7. **Correct Answer: B**
   DKA is more common in insulin-dependent diabetics, especially those with an illness or infection such as cellulitis. However, 20–30% of patients with DKA have no identified precipitating factors. A person with well-controlled diabetes is at low risk for DKA. Individuals with Type II diabetes are more likely to develop HHNS.

8. **Correct Answer: D**
   Potassium is pulled from the intracellular space due to metabolic acidosis. The insulin drip will help correct the metabolic acidosis allowing the potassium to return to normal levels.

9. **Correct Answer: C**
   Kayexalate permanently exchanges 1 g of medication for 1 mEq of potassium. Other therapies include IV insulin, $D_{50}W$, and sodium bicarbonate; these therapies allow quick, effective, short-term correction of the potassium level. Hemodialysis and Kayexalate are the only two methods that permanently remove excess potassium.

10. **Correct Answer: C**

    Crush injuries cause a massive release of potassium into the bloodstream. Each cell contains approximately 135–145 mEq of potassium.

11. **Correct Answer: B**

    Hyperkalemia slows conduction, leading to a widened QRS, peaked T waves, and loss of P waves. If the condition becomes severe, the patient can develop asystole.

12. **Correct Answer: C**

    HHNS develops slowly in the setting of Type II diabetes. It most often occurs in elderly patients or those with undiagnosed diabetes mellitus. The blood sugars are generally more than 600 mg/dL and can exceed 1,500 mg/dL. The other differentiation between HHNS and DKA is the lack of ketones seen with HHNS.

13. **Correct Answer: B**

    Blood sugars over 600 mg/dL with negative serum ketones and a serum osmolality greater than 310 mOsm/L are typical of hyperglycemic, hyperosmolar, nonketotic syndrome (HHNS). The pH is usually greater than 7.3 and the blood urea nitrogen (BUN) may be elevated. Osmolality is the best predictor of survivability than blood sugar levels.

14. **Correct Answer: C**

    Normal saline is given in large volumes until the depletion is corrected, then D_5NS is administered once blood glucose is in the 250–300 mg/dL range. An insulin drip at about 15 units per hour with hourly glucose monitoring and frequent electrolyte monitoring would also be implemented. If the patient is given D_5 ½NS too early in the treatment, it could lead to cerebral edema.

15. **Correct Answer: C**

    The Somoygi effect is nocturnal hypoglycemia with rebound hyperglycemia. It is more common in patients with Type I diabetes, especially children. The dawn phenomenon is morning hyperglycemia without nocturnal hypoglycemia; it is caused by growth hormone secretion in the early-morning hours.

16. **Correct Answer: A**

    Cushing syndrome is usually seen with Cushing's disease. It is important to rule out tumors of the pituitary gland, tumors of the chest area (small-cell cancer of the lung), adrenal tumors, and pheochromocytomas. These tumors cause excessive ACTH production, leading to the physical changes seen with Cushing syndrome, such as moon facies, buffalo hump, truncal obesity, and purple striae on the abdomen.

17. **Correct Answer: C**

    Numerous physical changes occur with Cushing syndrome or Cushing's disease: thinning hair, acne, moon facies, increased body hair, buffalo hump on the upper back, purple striae on the trunk, truncal obesity with thin extremities, and easy bruising.

18. **Correct Answer: D**

    The hypothalamic–pituitary axis releases a number of hormones that inhibit or release several other hormones that affect body functions.

19. **Correct Answer: A**

The pituitary gland is inferior to the hypothalamus and sits in the sella turcica of the sphenoid bone. The correct order is the thalamus, hypothalamus, infidibulum, and pituitary gland.

20. **Correct Answer: C**

The anterior pituitary gland produces numerous hormones: TSH, LH, FSH, ACTH, melanocyte-stimulating hormone. Substance P is a hormone released by the hypothalamus. Vasopressin and oxytocin are released by the posterior pituitary gland.

21. **Correct Answer: D**

This lab value indicates hyperthyroidism or thyrotoxicosis. Causes can include goiter, Graves disease, thyroid carcinoma, and TSH-secreting pituitary adenoma. Hyperthyroidism without toxicosis is most often related to excessive intake of thyroid hormones.

22. **Correct Answer: B**

The thyroid gland is located below the larynx, on either side of the trachea.

23. **Correct Answer: B**

Thyroid medications should be taken on an empty stomach 30 minutes before breakfast. Other teaching points include the need for regular follow-up labs to monitor TSH and T_4, symptoms of myxedema, and symptoms of hyperthyroidism. Taking thyroid medication in the evening can lead to insomnia.

24. **Correct Answer: C**

Thyrotoxic crisis is a rare but serious problem in post-thyroidectomy patients, patients with under-treated hyperthyroidism, patients with cardiopulmonary disease, and patients undergoing hemodialysis.

25. **Correct Answer: A**

Treatment of thyrotoxic crisis includes PTH to decrease levels of thyroid-stimulating hormone and thyroid hormones, plus symptomatic care.

26. **Correct Answer: B**

The pancreas is both an endocrine gland (it secretes glucagon and insulin) and an exocrine gland (it secretes amylase and lipase).

27. **Correct Answer: B**

The parathyroid glands are located posterior to the thyroid gland and may consist of four to six small glands. The parathyroid glands produce parathyroid hormone (PTH), which regulates serum calcium, magnesium, and phosphorus levels. PTH also stimulates the kidneys to produce bioavailable vitamin D.

28. **Correct Answer: C**

Hyperparathyroidism can be either primary or secondary in nature. Primary hyperparathyroidism is the excess secretion of parathyroid hormone (PTH) and may be related to a breakdown of the feedback system to the glands or overgrowth of the gland. Secondary hyperparathyroidism is generally related to a chronic disorder such as chronic renal failure or a malabsorption state.

29. **Correct Answer: D**

Hypoparathyroidism is usually caused by damage to the parathyroid gland. This damage leads to increased phosphatemia and lowered calcium levels.

30. **Correct Answer: C**

    The pancreas is located in the left upper quadrant of the abdomen and sits behind the stomach near the spleen and duodenum.

31. **Correct Answer: C**

    $HgbA_{1c}$ measures the effectiveness of diabetes mellitus therapy. Hemoglobin and glucose have an affinity for each other joining together to form a glycolated hemoglobin. The $HgbA_{1c}$ level rises and falls in direct correlation with blood sugars. The American College of Endocrinologists recommends an $HgbA_{1c}$ level of less than 6.5%, whereas the American Diabetes Association recommends an $HgbA_{1c}$ level of less than 7%. Patients with $HgbA_{1c}$ values of less than 6% are considered nondiabetic.

32. **Correct Answer: D**

    An $HgbA_{1c}$ of 6–7% means that Erin's glucose was in the range of 100–150 mg/dL over a 3-month period. A value of 4–5% is considered normal, and values of 7–8%, 8–9%, or more are indicative of poorly controlled diabetes mellitus.

33. **Correct Answer: B**

    Insulin resistance predisposes the patient to elevated blood glucose and increased insulin production. Very-low-density lipoprotein (VLDL) production increases with hyperinsulinemia.

34. **Correct Answer: A**

    Risk factors for the development of diabetes mellitus include blood pressure greater than 140/90, first-degree relative with diabetes mellitus, nonwhite ancestry, obesity (BMI greater than 30), and high-density lipoprotein (HDL) less than 35.

35. **Correct Answer: C**

    Beta cells of the islets of Langerhans secrete glucagon and insulin. Amylase and lipase are enzymes that are produced by the exocrine pancreas along with trypsin, chymotrypsin, and carboxypeptidase.

36. **Correct Answer: B**

    Insulin secretion is controlled by chemicals such as glucose and amino acids; hormones such as GI hormones, prostaglandin, and neuronal control such as the sympathetic response to increased glucose levels.

37. **Correct Answer: B**

    Glucagon is produced by the alpha cells of the pancreas.

38. **Correct Answer: A**

    Polyuria (excessive urinary output) is caused by changes in the osmotic pressure as the body attempts to correct hemoconcentration. This dehydration leads to stimulation of the thirst center by the hypothalamus.

39. **Correct Answer: D**

    Approximately 80–90% of the beta cell function of the islets of Langerhans is lost before hyperglycemia occurs.

40. **Correct Answer: A**

    Non-alcohol steatohepatitis (NASH) is characterized by fatty liver infiltrates and is often seen with insulin resistance, obesity, and increased triglycerides. NASH may progress to cirrhosis if the patient does not make any lifestyle changes.

41. **Correct Answer: C**

   Glenda is most likely experiencing a hypoglycemic event due to her NPO status. The other options are not wrong, but the question asks about a diabetic that is NPO.

42. **Correct Answer: D**

   The most important action is to raise Glenda's blood sugar safely using D_{50} intravenously. It would also be prudent to recheck her blood sugar in one hour. The physician must be notified. To do nothing for a patient with hypoglycemia is negligence.

43. **Correct Answer: B**

   Gastroparesis is a visceral neuropathy that occurs with long-term or uncontrolled diabetes mellitus. The hallmark of this condition is decreased gastric motility. Other visceral neuropathies include cranial nerve pain, Bell's palsy, urinary retention, sexual dysfunction, decreased cardiac reflexes, orthostatic hypotension, and radiculopathies.

44. **Correct Answer: C**

   Coronary artery disease, cerebral vascular accident, and peripheral vascular disease are the three major problems associated with macrovascular disease and are seen in Type II diabetes mellitus. Mortality or morbidity in these patients is due to macrovascular changes. Diabetes leads to early atherosclerosis and atherosclerotic heart disease. The other problems listed (retinopathy, peripheral neuropathy, and diabetic nephropathy) are microvascular diseases.

45. **Correct Answer: B**

   Prolonged hyperglycemia thickens the capillary basement membrane. This thickening leads to decreased blood flow, hypoxia, and a lack of nutrients at the cellular level. The eyes and kidneys are the organs most susceptible to this process.

46. **Correct Answer: A**

   Proteinuria is the first sign of renal dysfunction. It is a reliable symptom, especially when the proteinuria is prolonged. Continued proteinuria is usually associated with a life expectancy of less than 10 years. The exact pathophysiology is not fully understood, but glomerular destruction allows proteins to leak into the filtrate.

47. **Correct Answer: C**

   Renin is stored in a crystalline form in the juxtaglomerular cells of the kidneys. When the kidneys perceive a decreased blood flow, the sympathetic response triggers the release of renin which converts angiotensinogen to angiotensin I, a mild vasoconstrictor. If the problem is not resolved, the lungs release angiotensin I converting enzyme to create angiotensin II, a powerful vasoconstrictor. Angiotensin II triggers the release of aldosterone from the adrenal glands, which causes sodium and water retention, thereby increasing blood pressure.

48. **Correct Answer: B**

   Anything that causes a perceived drop in renal blood flow triggers the renin–angiotensin mechanism. Renin release can also be triggered by sodium and volume depletion, such as seen with diuretic use.

49. **Correct Answer: C**

   The kidneys perceive a drop in blood flow leading to the release of renin from the juxtaglomerular cells of the nephron. This stimulates the release of angiotensinogen, which stimulates the release of angiotensin I. If the blood pressure is not corrected, the lungs release angiotensin I converting enzyme, which in turn causes the secretion of angiotensin II. Angiotensin II causes the release of aldosterone from the adrenal glands causing the retention of sodium and water retention and increasing blood pressure.

50. **Correct Answer: D**
The adrenal medulla produces 75–85% of epinephrine (a catecholamine) and 25% of norepinephrine from phenylalanine.

51. **Correct Answer: B**
The anion gap measures anions not generally measured in routine labs; it is an estimate of the degree of lactic acidosis. The formula for figuring the anion gap is Na – (HCO_3 + Cl). A normal level is 10–20 mEq/L. With diabetic ketoacidosis, the anion gap is greater than 30 mEq/L.

52. **Correct Answer: C**
This blood gas shows uncompensated metabolic acidosis. The body has depleted its HCO_3 while trying to correct the acidosis. The ABG is uncompensated because the pH is low and the CO_2 is elevated. Answer A indicates acute respiratory alkalosis; answer B indicates respiratory acidosis with metabolic alkalosis; and answer D is a normal ABG. Normal values for ABG results are pH 7.35–7.45; CO_2 35–45 mm Hg; and HCO_3 22–27 mEq/L.

53. **Correct Answer: C**
With the pH near normal (7.35 –7.45), the increased CO_2, and near-normal HCO_3 means the body has tried to correct the acidosis. As the condition resolves, the ABG's should continue to improve.

54. **Correct Answer: A**
A sodium bicarbonate drip should be anticipated to replace the HCO_3. This will help resolve the metabolic acidosis. Boluses would be given only if the pH was very low. The insulin drip will not directly correct the HCO_3.

55. **Correct Answer: B**
This patient has nephrogenic diabetes related to lithium use. The lithium causes insensitivity to vasopressin in the renal tubule making the tubule incapable of absorbing water. Treatment involves administration of hydrochlorothiazide or indomethicin.

56. **Correct Answer: D**
Subclinical adrenal insufficiency may co-exist with myxedema. The treatment of choice is intravenous hydrocortisone therapy.

57. **Correct Answer: B**
This patient has secondary hyperparathyroidism. In ESRD, vitamin D synthesis is decreased thus causing hypocalcemia. The calcium is also bound to phosphorus, further reducing the calcium levels. This decrease stimulates the parathyroid glands to secrete parathyroid hormone in an attempt to correct the calcium levels.

58. **Correct Answer: D**
The anterior pituitary or adenohypophysis controls the function of the thyroid gland with thyroid-stimulating hormone (TSH), the adrenal cortex with antidiuretic hormone (ADH), and the gonads with luteinizing hormone (LH) or interstitial cell-stimulating hormone (ICSH).

59. **Correct Answer: A**

    Antidiuretic hormone (ADH) helps regulate thirst and water balance. This hormone is produced by the posterior pituitary gland. When the plasma becomes concentrated or there is a reduced blood volume, the posterior pituitary gland releases ADH, causing water retention and concentration of urine. ADH production is regulated by a feedback mechanism in the pituitary gland.

60. **Correct Answer: C**

    Antidiuretic hormone (ADH) production is controlled by a negative feedback system. Production is decreased when the osmoreceptors of the hypothalamus recognize hemodilution or hemoconcentration and adjust ADH production accordingly.

61. **Correct Answer: C**

    Diabetes insipidus is caused by low antidiuretic hormone levels and water absorption is greatly reduced. The hypotension and tachycardia are due to volume depletion.

62. **Correct Answer: D**

    The pituitary gland sits in the sella turcica at the base of skull and can be easily damaged with any head trauma. An anterior basilar skull fracture is the most common fracture leading to diabetes insipidus.

63. **Correct Answer: C**

    Seizures are among the most common presenting symptoms of syndrome of inappropriate antidiuretic hormone (SIADH). SIADH causes hemodilution and a relative decrease in serum sodium levels. Once the sodium falls below 120, the patient is at great risk for seizures. Excessive urine output and hypotension are symptoms of diabetes insipidus.

64. **Correct Answer: B**

    The volume is lost through hemoconcentration with excess fluid loss. The kidneys are unable to concentrate urine.

65. **Correct Answer: A**

    The decreased T_4 leads to hypothyroid symptoms of cold, dry skin, hair loss, periorbital edema, and possible thyroid enlargement.

66. **Correct Answer: D**

    Calcium cannot be utilized by the body without adequate vitamin D levels. Fifteen minutes of daylight on the skin without use of sunblock allows the body to create its own vitamin D. An increased phosphorus level would bind the calcium, making it unavailable.

67. **Correct Answer: B**

    Trousseau's sign, also known as carpal–pedal spasm, is seen with decreased calcium levels. Hypocalcemia can occur with end-stage renal disease (increased phosphorus) and decreased vitamin D levels. It is also seen in patients who receive 3 or more units of red blood cells that are treated with calcium citrate.

68. **Correct Answer: C**

    Chvostek's sign is seen with hypocalcemia. It is elicited by tapping the cheek over the zygomatic arch and causes facial twitching. The QT interval would be prolonged with hypocalcemia. Cullen's sign is ecchymosis around the umbilicus and is often seen with pancreatitis.

69. **Correct Answer: C**
   The anterior pituitary gland secretes thyroid-stimulating hormone (TSH). The hypothalamus regulates the anterior pituitary gland with thyrotropin-releasing hormone (TRH).

70. **Correct Answer: C**
   Injury or infection, as well as manipulation of the thyroid gland, can trigger a thyroid storm and thyrotoxicosis.

71. **Correct Answer: D**
   Thyrotoxic crisis symptoms include hypertension, hyperthermia, flushing, tachycardia (especially atrial tachyarrhythmia), high-output heart failure, nausea and vomiting, psychosis, and delirium. Treatment includes supportive care and medications to block catecholamine effects.

72. **Correct Answer: A**
   Propranolol (Inderal) would be used for this patient. It is a beta blocker and would decrease the effects of the sympathetic stimulation of thyrotoxic crisis. It controls heart rate, hypertension, and oxygen consumption.

73. **Correct Answer: B**
   Pheochromocytoma is a tumor of the adrenal medulla. These tumors are rarely malignant. They cause release of large amounts of catecholamines such as dopamine, epinephrine, and norepinephrine. Hypertension with pheochromocytoma can be triggered by consumption of foods such as cheese, alcohol, yogurt, and caffeine.

74. **Correct Answer: C**
   Hypertension with pheochromocytoma can be triggered by foods such as cheese, alcohol, yogurt, and caffeine. It is important to give the patient a list of foods to avoid. Crises often occur after stressful life events where these foods might be consumed.

75. **Correct Answer: C**
   The best treatment option for pheochromocytoma is surgical removal of the tumor. Alpha-adrenergic blockers or beta-adrenergic blockers may be used to treat hypertension until surgery can be performed.

BIBLIOGRAPHY

Ahrens, T. (2006). *Critical care nursing certification*. Columbus, OH: McGraw-Hill.

American Association of Critical-Care Nurses. (2006). *Core curriculum for critical care nursing* (6th ed.). Philadelphia: Saunders.

American Association of Critical-Care Nurses. (2007). *AACN certification and core review for high acuity and critical care* (6th ed.). Philadelphia: Saunders.

American Heart Association. (2007). *Guidelines 2005 for cardiopulmonary resuscitation and emergency cardiovascular care: Update*. Retrieved July 21, 2008 from http://circ.ahajournals.org/content/vol112/24_suppl

Boyle, P. J. (2007). Diabetes mellitus and macrovascular disease: Mechanisms and mediators. *American Journal of Medicine: Optimizing Cardiovascular Outcomes in Diabetes Mellitus, 120*(9B), S12.

Brimioulle, S., Orellana-Jimenez, C., Aminian, A., & Vincent, J. L. (2008). Hyponatremia in neurological patients: Cerebral salt wasting versus inappropriate antidiuretic hormone secretion. *Intensive Care Medicine, 34*(1), 125–131.

Burns, S. M. (Ed.). (2007). *American Association of Critical-Care Nurses (AACN): AACN protocols for practice: Healing environments* (2nd ed.). Sudbury, MA: Jones and Bartlett.

Conover, M. B. (2003). *Understanding electrocardiography* (8th ed.). St. Louis, MO: Mosby/Elsevier.

Copstead, L., & Banasik, J. L. (2000). *Pathophysiology: Biological and behavioral perspectives* (2nd ed.). Philadelphia: Saunders/Elsevier.

Curley, M. A. Q. (1998). Patient–nurse synergy: Optimizing patients' outcomes. *American Journal of Critical Care, 7*, 64–72.

Dossey, B. M., Keegan, L., & Guzzetta, C. (2003). *Holistic nursing: A handbook for practice*. (3rd ed.). Sudbury, MA: Jones and Bartlett.

Dunn, J. P., & Jagasia, S. M. (2007). Case study: Management of Type 2 diabetes after bariatric surgery. *Clinical Diabetes, 25*(3), 112–114.

Edwards, D. F. (1999). The Synergy Model: Linking patient needs to nurse competencies. *Critical Care Nurse, 19*(1), 88–98.

Eldin, W. S., Ragheb, A., Klassen, J., & Shoker, A. (2008). Evidence for increased risk of prediabetes in the uremic patient. *Nephron, 108*(1), c47–c55.

Emergency Nurses Association & Newberry, L. (2003). *Sheehy's emergency nursing: Principles and practice* (5th ed.). St. Louis, MO: Mosby/Elsevier.

Feldman, B. J., Rosenthal, S. M., Vargas, G. A., & Gitelman, S. E. (2005). Nephrogenic syndrome of inappropriate antidiuresis (NSIAD): A paradigm for activating mutations causing endocrine dysfunction. *New England Journal of Medicine, 352*(18), 1884–1890.

Finkelmeier, B. A. (2000). *Cardiothoracic surgical nursing* (2nd ed.). Philadelphia: Lippincott, Williams & Wilkins.

Gaines, K. K. (2004). Desmopressin (DDAVP) for enuresis, diabetes insipidus. *Urologic Nursing, 24*(6), 520–523.

Gale, S. C., Sicoutris, C., Reilly, P. M., Schwab, C. W., & Gracias, V. H. (2007). Poor glycemic control is associated with increased mortality in critically ill trauma patients. *American Surgeon, 73*(5), 454–460.

Hardin, S. R., & Kaplow, R. (Eds.). (2004). *Synergy for clinical excellence: The AACN Synergy Model for Patient Care*. Sudbury, MA: Jones and Bartlett.

Haskal, R. (2007). Current issues for nurse practitioners: Hyponatremia. *Journal of the American Academy of Nurse Practitioners, 19*(11), 563–579.

Hickey, J. V. (2002). *The clinical practice of neurological and neurosurgical nursing* (5th ed.). Philadelphia: Lippincott, Williams & Wilkins.

Inoue, T., & Node, K. (2007). Statin therapy for vascular failure. *Cardiovascular Drugs and Therapy, 21*(4), 281–295.

Jane, J. A., Edward, M. L., & Laws, R. (2006). Neurogenic diabetes insipidus. *Pituitary, 9*(4), 327–329.

Johnson, A. L., & Criddle, L. M. (2004). Pass the salt: Indications for and implications of using hypertonic saline. *Critical Care Nurse, 24*(5), 36–38, 40–44, 46 passim.

Lath, R. (2005). Hyponatremia in neurological diseases in ICU. *Indian Journal of Critical Care Medicine, 9*(1), 47–51.

Lipson, J. G., Dibble, S. L., & Minarik, P. A. (Eds.). (1996). *Culture and nursing care: A pocket guide.* San Francisco, CA: UCSF Nursing Press.

Livingstone, C., & Rampes, H. (2006). Lithium: A review of its metabolic adverse effects. *Journal of Psychopharmacology, 20*(3), 347–355.

McQuillan, K. A., Von Rueden, K. T., Hartsock, R. L., Flynn, M. B., & Whalen, E. (Eds.). (2002). *Trauma nursing: From resuscitation through rehabilitation* (3rd ed.). Philadelphia: Saunders/Elsevier.

Medina, J., & Puntillo, K. (2006). *AACN protocols for practice: Palliative care and end-of-life issues in critical care.* Sudbury, MA: Jones and Bartlett.

Musch, W., Hedeshi, A., & Decaux, G. (2004). Low sodium excretion in SIADH patients with low diuresis. *Nephron, 96*(1), p11–p18.

Oksanen, T., Skrifvars, M. B., Varpula, T., Kuitunen, A., Pettilä, V., Nurmi, J., et al. (2007). Strict versus moderate glucose control after resuscitation from ventricular fibrillation. *Intensive Care Medicine, 33*(12), 2093–2100.

Pagana, K. D., & Pagana, J. (2005). *Mosby's manual of diagnostic and laboratory tests* (3rd ed.). St. Louis, MO: Mosby/Elsevier.

Paydas, S., Araz, F., & Balal, M. (2008). SIADH induced by amiodarone in a patient with heart failure. *International Journal of Clinical Practice, 62*(2), 337.

Sata, A., Hizuka, N., Kawamata, T., Hori, T., & Takano, K. (2006). Hyponatremia after transsphenoidal surgery for hypothalamo-pituitary tumors. *Neuroendocrinology, 83*(2), 117–122.

Skidmore-Roth, L. (2004). *Mosby's 2004 nursing drug reference.* St. Louis, MO: Mosby/Elsevier.

Smeltzer, S., & Bare, B. G. (2003). *Brunner and Suddarth's textbook of medical–surgical nursing* (10th ed.). Philadelphia: Lippincott, Williams & Wilkins.

Sobel, B. E. (2007). Optimizing cardiovascular outcomes in diabetes mellitus. *American Journal of Medicine: Optimizing Cardiovascular Outcomes in Diabetes Mellitus, 120*(9B), S3.

Sole, M. L., Hartshorn, J., & Lamborne, M. L. (2001). *Introduction to critical care nursing* (3rd ed.). Philadelphia: Saunders/Elsevier.

Sommerfield, A. J., Wilkinson, I. B., Webb, D. J., & Frier, B. M. (2007). Vessel wall stiffness in Type I diabetes and the central hemodynamic effects of acute hypoglycemia. *American Journal of Physiology: Endocrinology and Metabolism, 293*(5), E1274.

Su, H., Sun, X., Ma, H., Zhang, H. F., Yu, Q. J., Huang, C., et al. (2007). Acute hyperglycemia exacerbates myocardial ischemia/reperfusion injury and blunts cardioprotective effect of GIK. *American Journal of Physiology: Endocrinology and Metabolism, 293*(3), E629.

Sugimoto, A. K. (2007). No elevation of blood urea level in a dehydrated patient with central diabetes insipidus. *QJM, 100*(12), 800.

Thomas, G., Rojas, M. C., Epstein, S. K., Balk, E. M., Liangos, O., & Jaber, B. L. (2007). Insulin therapy and acute kidney injury in critically ill patients: A systematic review. *Nephrology, Dialysis, Transplantation, 22*(10), 2849–2855.

Toprak, O., Cirit, M., Ersoy, R., Uzüm, A., Ozümer, O., Çobanoğlu, A., et al. (2005). New-onset type II diabetes mellitus, hyperosmolar non-ketotic coma, rhabdomyolysis and acute renal failure in a patient treated with sulpiride. *Nephrology, Dialysis, Transplantation, 20*(3), 662–663.

Urden, L. D., Stacy, K. M., & Lough, M. E. (2007). *Thelan's critical care nursing: Diagnosis and management.* (5th ed.). St. Louis, MO: Mosby.

Venkataraman, S., Munoz, R., Candido, C., & Feldman-Witchel, S. (2007). The hypothalamic–pituitary–adrenal axis in critical illness. *Reviews in Endocrine & Metabolic Disorders, 8*(4), 365–373.

Wiegand, D. J. L., & Carlson, K. K. (Eds.). (2005). *AACN procedure manual for critical care* (5th ed.). Philadelphia, PA: Elsevier.

Woods, S., Sivarajan Froelicher, E. S., & Motzer, S. U. (2000). *Cardiac nursing* (4th ed.). Philadelphia: Lippincott, Williams & Wilkins.

Yeates, K. E., & Morton, A. R. (2006). Vasopressin antagonists: Role in the management of hyponatremia. *American Journal of Nephrology, 26*(4), 348–355.

Hematology/Immunology

QUESTIONS

1. You are working in the capacity of a charge nurse in the telemetry unit. Your patient population is comprised of recent surgical patients and two patients waiting for lung transplants. As a progressive care nurse, you are aware that the chain of infection includes which of the following components?
   A. Understaffing
   B. Having all transplant patients in strict isolation
   C. Use of non-alcohol-based hand washes
   D. Availability of bag-valve masks in each patient room

2. Cyclosporine has significant adverse effects that include
   A. Hypotension.
   B. Hepatotoxicity.
   C. Acute pancreatitis.
   D. Hypokalemia.

3. An antirejection drug that is classified as an antimetabolite is
   A. Cyclosporine.
   B. Terralimus.
   C. Prednisolone.
   D. Imuran.

4. Martha is a 45-year-old patient admitted for observation following placement of a coronary stent. You note that the patient received Reo Pro during the procedure. As a nurse, you know this patient must be monitored for
   A. Increased bleeding for 48 hours, because Aggrastat is used with Reo Pro.
   B. Aggrastat toxicity.
   C. HITS and bleeding at the sheath insertion site.
   D. Coagulopathies.

5. A patient can be presensitized and is more likely to undergo organ rejection if there is a history of
   A. Multiple pregnancies.
   B. Small or reduced lumens in the bile ducts.
   C. Destruction of small airways.
   D. Cytomegalovirus (CMV) infection.

6. **An absolute contraindication for a single-lung, double-lung, or heart–lung transplant would be**
   A. Previous cardiothoracic surgery.
   B. Kidney disease.
   C. Liver disease.
   D. Psychiatric illness.

7. **The most common cause of DIC is**
   A. Carcinoma.
   B. Surgery.
   C. Sepsis.
   D. Vasculitis.

8. **Mrs. C. was a direct admission to your unit from her physician's office following sudden epistaxis with severe headache. She is now obtunded. During your initial assessment, you note gingival bleeding, generalized ecchymosis, and petechial hemorrhages on both legs. You suspect Mrs. C. may have**
   A. DIC.
   B. Pulmonary emboli.
   C. A fat embolism.
   D. ITP.

9. **Patients who undergo renal transplants often have electrolyte imbalances. Which of the following values would likely occur?**
   A. Serum K^+ 6.9 mEq/L
   B. Sodium bicarbonate 12 mEq/L
   C. Serum Na 156 mEq/L
   D. Serum Ca 7.3 mEq/L

10. **A 38-year-old posttransplant patient was admitted to your unit five days after the surgery. He was stable for the entire time he was in the ICU. About an hour after transfer to your unit, he suddenly exhibits sinus bradycardia. You anticipate administration of**
    A. Atropine.
    B. Digoxin.
    C. Indocin.
    D. Epinephrine.

11. **Factor VIII deficiency is also known as**
    A. Hemophilia B.
    B. Sickle cell anemia.
    C. Aplastic anemia.
    D. Von Willebrand's disease.

12. Your patient has received platelet transfusions. It is important to closely monitor the patient and perform a one or two hour post-transfusion platelet count. You must also carefully assess the patient for
    A. Hematuria.
    B. Fever.
    C. Petechiae.
    D. Ecchymosis.

13. The blood component that contains factor VIII is
    A. FFP.
    B. PRBCs.
    C. Salt-poor albumin.
    D. Cryoprecipitate.

14. A fluid that causes decreased platelet aggregation and possibly an allergic reaction is
    A. Dextran.
    B. Hetastarch.
    C. Lactated Ringer's.
    D. D_5/Isolyte M.

15. What medication is specific for cryptococcal meningitis?
    A. Amphotericin B
    B. Rifampin
    C. Famvir
    D. Acyclovir

16. When patients receive multiple transfusions, they are susceptible to increased
    A. Potassium levels.
    B. BUN and creatinine levels.
    C. Bilirubin and amylase levels.
    D. Sodium and magnesium levels.

17. Adam was injured at work and has been fairly sedentary since his accident. He has now developed DVT. He has been on a heparin drip for three days. Which lab value would indicate that Adam is maintaining a therapeutic level of heparin?
    A. Negative Cullen's sign
    B. The platelet count has returned to 100,000 mm^3.
    C. Activated partial thromboplastin time of 45 seconds
    D. Resolution of oozing around IV insertion sites

18. Your patient has been diagnosed with immune thrombocytopenic purpura (ITP). Which of the following laboratory values would be expected for this patient?
    A. Elevated PT and PTT
    B. 0.5 capillary fragility test
    C. Platelet count of 11,000
    D. Positive anti-RH immunosuppression

19. **Your patient has been diagnosed with hemolytic anemia. She has been in the progressive care unit for three days. You believe her condition was caused by**
    A. An inappropriate TPN solution.
    B. Reduced folate deficiency.
    C. Bone marrow aspiration.
    D. Intra-aortic balloon counterpulsation (IABP).

20. **A medication that may cause hemolytic anemia is**
    A. Phenobarbital.
    B. Quinidine.
    C. Furosemide.
    D. Captopril.

21. **As a progressive care nurse, you know that Mrs. N.'s abrupt-onset DIC may be due to a previously undiagnosed cause. This cause could include**
    A. Viral infection.
    B. Abdominal aneurysm and hepatic cirrhosis.
    C. Influenza.
    D. Trauma.

22. **The blood component that carries factor VIII, factor XIII, and fibrinogen is**
    A. FFP.
    B. PRBC.
    C. Salt-poor albumin.
    D. Cryoprecipitate.

23. **In the progressive care setting, patients with DIC are at a high risk of developing**
    A. Deficiencies in vitamin K and folate.
    B. Increased fibrinogen levels.
    C. A decreased D-dimer (less than 300).
    D. Dependency on heparin to maintain hemostasis.

24. **A possible cause of thrombocytopenia is**
    A. Portal hypertension.
    B. MI.
    C. Latex.
    D. Low protein diet.

25. **Patients with Type II HIT are at great risk for developing**
    A. Generalized bleeding.
    B. Thrombosis.
    C. Pericarditis.
    D. Limb amputation.

26. **Nursing interventions by the progressive care nurse should include which of the following to minimize risk to a patient with HIT?**
    A. Avoid the use of heparin flushes
    B. Assess the need for manual blood pressure measurements
    C. Monitor platelet counts
    D. Observe for petechiae

27. **What is the most common cause of a fatal transfusion reaction?**
    A. Immunocompromised recipient
    B. Mismatched blood
    C. Volume overload
    D. Severe hyperkalemia

28. **Rejection of a transplanted organ usually occurs as a result of**
    A. Cellular immunity.
    B. Humoral immunity.
    C. Delayed hypersensitivity reaction.
    D. Complement cascade.

29. **Harry is a 34-year-old patient who was envenomated by a rattlesnake on his left forearm this afternoon while gardening. His entire left arm is ecchymotic. The best course of treatment would be**
    A. Clotting factors and antivenin.
    B. Clotting factors and heparin.
    C. IV at 150 mL/h and antivenin.
    D. IV at 150 mL/h and heparin.

30. **Adin is a 30-year-old who was thrown from a horse onto a fence and suffered abdominal trauma with a splenic rupture. While awaiting surgery in the telemetry unit, because the operating rooms were full, he received 12 units of PRBCs. As a telemetry nurse, you know that Adin should also receive**
    A. Potassium.
    B. Whole blood.
    C. Platelets.
    D. Heparin.

31. **Organ rejection that occurs 3–5 days post transplant, is antibody mediated, with fever and oliguria is known as**
    A. Chronic rejection.
    B. Acute rejection.
    C. Accelerated acute rejection.
    D. Hyperacute rejection.

32. **A snake bite will result in activation of the**
    A. Fibrinolytic system.
    B. Anti-thrombin system.
    C. Intrinsic cascade.
    D. Extrinsic cascade.

33. **Quincy had a renal transplant about one year ago. He was admitted to your unit for severe flu-like symptoms. Which sign or symptom would lead you to suspect that Quincy is having an acute rejection episode?**
    A. Pelvic pain
    B. Hypotension
    C. Increased urine output
    D. Decreased urine osmolality

34. An anti-rejection agent that is used for induction therapy for patients who undergo lung transplants and lowers the number of circulating T cells is
    A. Daclizumab.
    B. Muromonab.
    C. A polyclonal antibody.
    D. Paroxetine.

35. Back pain or abdominal pain with itching can be indicators of acute rejection in what organ?
    A. Pancreas
    B. Lung
    C. Kidney
    D. Liver

36. Following heart–lung transplants, prostaglandin (PGE_1) is used to
    A. Provide inotropic support.
    B. Augment the heart rate.
    C. Promote pulmonary vasodilation.
    D. Promote wound healing.

37. Chris ingested shellfish and is having an anaphylactic reaction. He had been on a regular diet in the hospital when his family brought him dinner from an outside restaurant. To treat the anaphylaxis, Chris received epinephrine via Epi-pen and intravenously. He is now intubated because he had severe airway obstruction due to swelling and will be transferred to the MICU. Epinephrine is given in anaphylaxis because it
    A. Prevents localized edema.
    B. Promotes temporary changes in ST segments.
    C. Prevents third space fluid loss.
    D. Promotes bronchodilation and inhibits additional mediator release.

38. Why is DIC usually fatal if untreated?
    A. Exsanguination
    B. Intracranial hemorrhage
    C. Myocardial infarction
    D. Cerebral thrombosis

39. Oat-cell carcinomas are primarily found in the
    A. Central airways.
    B. Genital area.
    C. Bronchial wall.
    D. Pancreas.

40. Hemoglobin is phagocytized primarily in the
    A. Liver.
    B. Spleen.
    C. Kidneys.
    D. Lungs.

41. **Acute post-hemorrhagic anemia develops after**
    A. Rapid loss of erythrocytes.
    B. The spleen is damaged.
    C. Iron levels decrease by more than 15%.
    D. Bone marrow is damaged.

42. **The most prevalent type of anemia is**
    A. Chronic.
    B. Acute.
    C. Pernicious.
    D. Iron-deficiency.

43. **Patient teaching for a patient with thalassemia would include**
    A. Keeping the limbs flat to help avoid a stasis ulcer.
    B. Avoiding oral stimulants (i.e., smoking).
    C. Eating fewer, larger high-protein meals.
    D. Using warm water to cleanse the skin.

44. **A decrease in the available number of erythrocytes caused by bone marrow production failure is called**
    A. Chronic anemia.
    B. Aplastic anemia.
    C. Hemolytic anemia.
    D. Pernicious anemia.

45. **High blood viscosity and low oxygen tension are the cause of which of the following types of anemia?**
    A. Pernicious anemia
    B. Aplastic anemia
    C. Sickle cell anemia
    D. Hemolytic anemia

46. **Samantha was admitted for low H and H, epistaxis, and bleeding into the diaphragm. She is bleeding from her gums, even with only the lightest stimulus. Petechiae are noted on her chest and arms. Her platelet count is < 100,000. Samantha's probable diagnosis is**
    A. Aplastic anemia.
    B. ITP.
    C. Hemolytic anemia.
    D. Pernicious anemia.

47. **How does low–molecular-weight heparin (LMWH) differ from unfractionated heparin?**
    A. LMWH is more difficult to administer.
    B. There are more side effects with LMWH.
    C. LMWH is more stable.
    D. Unfractionated heparin is easier to administer.

48. **Clopidogrel may interfere with the metabolism of which of the following drugs?**
    A. Phenobarbitol
    B. Phenytoin
    C. Cimetidine
    D. Estrogen

49. **Ethacrynic acid works on the body by**
    A. Inhibiting the aldosterone mechanism.
    B. Blocking carbonic anhydrase.
    C. Increasing osmotic pressure.
    D. Inhibiting reabsorption of Na and Cl.

50. **A diuretic that is classified as a carbonic anhydrase inhibitor is**
    A. Methazolamide.
    B. Mannitol.
    C. Urea.
    D. Metolazone.

51. **Potential complications of loop diuretics include**
    A. Hypercalcemia.
    B. Increased BUN.
    C. Hypokalemia.
    D. Hypertension.

52. **Mannitol would be classified as which type of diuretic?**
    A. Loop
    B. Thiazide
    C. Osmotic
    D. Potassium-sparing

53. **Effects of nesiritide include**
    A. Vasoconstriction.
    B. Decreased left heart pressure.
    C. Anemia.
    D. Decreased cardiac output.

54. **Adverse effects of Epogen include**
    A. Hypertension.
    B. Increased iron.
    C. Decreased thrombosis.
    D. Decreased BUN.

55. **Your patient with a renal condition needs to undergo a radiologic procedure that requires contrast dye. He has no allergies. Which of the following medications administered prior to the test would be effective in this patient?**

    A. Bicarbonate

    B. NSAIDs

    C. BNP

    D. Mucomyst

56. A normal value for intracellular potassium (K$^+$) is

    A. 4.5 mEq/L.

    B. 140 mEq/L.

    C. 45 mEq/L.

    D. 104 mEq/L.

57. A normal value for bicarbonate (HCO$_3$) in the intravascular space is

    A. 11 mEq/L.

    B. 45 mEq/L.

    C. 24 mEq/L.

    D. 80 mEq/L.

58. Which hormone would be released if your patient's CVP suddenly rose from 6 to 17?

    A. BNP

    B. Aldosterone

    C. ANP

    D. ADH

59. Which of the following solutions would be used to expand the intravascular volume?

    A. Hypertonic saline

    B. D$_5$W

    C. 0.45% NS

    D. 0.9% NS

60. If your patient has a decreased extracellular fluid volume, which of the following hemodynamic profiles would be indicative of this condition?

    A. Decreased CO and increased CVP

    B. Increased CVP and CO

    C. Decreased CVP and increased CO

    D. Decreased CVP and CO

61. Sam was aggressively treated with 0.3% hypertonic saline for profound hyponatremia. Now, Sam is having tremors, LOC changes, and paresthesias. Sam is probably developing

    A. A paranoid psychosis.

    B. Hyponatremia veridans.

    C. Osmotic demyelinization syndrome.

    D. Red cell sequestration.

62. Matthew is a 17-year-old who has not been eating correctly for about two weeks because he is stressed out about asking a girl to the prom. He eats a diet of cereals, pastas, and high-calorie, high-sugar foods. Matthew collapsed at work today after becoming dyspneic. His EKG shows sinus tachycardia without ectopy, he is pale, somewhat irritable, and he complains of a headache. His initial diagnosis is folic acid deficiency. Tomorrow Matthew is scheduled for more tests to determine whether an underlying disease process is present. You suspect that he simply has a dietary deficiency and prepare to instruct him about foods that contain high amounts of folic acid. These foods would include
    A. Green beans.
    B. Fish.
    C. Oranges.
    D. Peanut butter.

63. Which of the following types of cell would be considered a nongranular leukocyte?
    A. Eosinophil
    B. Neutrophil
    C. Basophil
    D. Monocyte

64. Cellular humoral immunity is mediated by
    A. T lymphocytes.
    B. Eosinophils.
    C. B lymphocytes.
    D. Killer cells.

65. All the clotting factors in blood are synthesized in the liver except
    A. VIII and XIII.
    B. V and IX.
    C. IX and III.
    D. IIa and IXa.

66. Which of the following drugs is useful in the treatment of DIC to inhibit fibrinolysis?
    A. Heparin
    B. Cryoprecipitate
    C. Amicar
    D. Prednisone

67. Teresa is 40 years old and has a history of hemolytic anemia. She was admitted today for chest pain, fever, and heart failure. These symptoms would indicate Teresa is probably suffering from
    A. A myocardial infarction.
    B. Pulmonary edema.
    C. DIC.
    D. Hemolytic crisis.

68. **Immune-mediated HITT usually begins about _____ after the initiation of heparin therapy.**
    A. 48 hours
    B. 72 hours
    C. 4 days
    D. 5–7 days

69. **The diagnosis of immune thrombocytopenic purpura may be made based on**
    A. Thrombin time.
    B. Platelet antibody screening.
    C. PTT.
    D. PT.

70. **Your patient has immune thrombocytopenic purpura that has worsened and become refractory to treatments, including plasmapheresis and injections of gamma globulin and glucocorticoid therapy. The patient will be undergoing a splenectomy. One preoperative treatment to expect with this patient is**
    A. Interferon.
    B. Anti-Rh immunoglobulin.
    C. *Haemophilus influenzae* type B vaccination.
    D. Colchicine.

71. **Blood component replacement therapy for DIC may include all of the following except**
    A. FFP.
    B. Cryoprecipitate.
    C. Amicar.
    D. Platelets.

72. **A transfusion reaction that usually occurs within 5–30 minutes of the start of the transfusion is known as**
    A. An acute intravascular hemolytic reaction.
    B. A febrile reaction.
    C. An allergic reaction.
    D. An acute extravascular hemolytic reaction.

73. **Henry is a 76-year-old gentleman who was admitted for end-stage mesothelioma. Which of the following occupations would lend itself to a diagnosis of mesothelioma?**
    A. Bricklayer
    B. Gardener
    C. Office manager
    D. Shipbuilder

74. **Pernicious anemia results from a lack of**
    A. Vitamin B_6.
    B. Vitamin A.
    C. Vitamin B_{12}.
    D. Vitamin E.

75. You are asked to draw a CBC on a patient. You should collect the sample in a
_____-topped tube.
    A. gray
    B. purple
    C. green
    D. red

76. Your employer asks that you be immunized for hepatitis B. You should expect
    A. One dose, with a booster every 10 years.
    B. Two doses, with the second dose at 4–8 weeks.
    C. Three doses, with the second dose at 1–2 months and the third dose at 4–6 months.
    D. One dose every 4 years.

77. The normal range for a hematocrit in an adult female is
    A. 20–40%.
    B. 28–35%.
    C. 37–47%.
    D. 42–55%.

This concludes the Hematology/Immunology Questions section.

ANSWERS

1. **Correct Answer: A**
   When areas are understaffed, the risk of nosocomial infection is increased. Standards of care, such as suctioning, turning patients, and use of aseptic technique are frequently not met.

2. **Correct Answer: B**
   Other adverse effects include nephrotoxicity, hypertension, hyperkalemia, leg cramps, headache, seizures, and development of neoplasms.

3. **Correct Answer: D**
   Antimetabolites interfere with RNA and DNA synthesis and inhibit T- and B-lymphocyte proliferation.

4. **Correct Answer: C**
   Reo Pro may affect platelet function for as long as 48 hours. It places the patient at risk for HITS because Reo Pro is frequently used with heparin and aspirin. Aggrastat and Integrilin are also inhibitors, but usually affect platelet function up to only eight hours.

5. **Correct Answer: A**
   Other possible causes include transfusions, previous organ transplants, and blood-type incompatibilities. Answers B, C, and D are the results of organ rejection, not causes.

6. **Correct Answer: D**
   Patients with a history of psychiatric illness may be unable to comprehend or follow through with a complicated postoperative medication regimen.

7. **Correct Answer: C**
   Sepsis is the most common cause of DIC. In sepsis, endotoxins stimulate production of tissue factor and the extrinsic pathway is activated. If this process continues, thrombi in capillaries can lead to hypoperfusion and metabolic acidosis, causing free radical formation and damage to tissues. Tissue factor is released, resulting in DIC. Answers A, B, and D are also causes of DIC.

8. **Correct Answer: A**
   Disseminated intravascular coagulation is an overstimulation of the clotting cascade. Both the intrinsic and extrinsic pathways are activated at the same time, which accelerates the clotting process. When the clots lyse, the fibrin split products are anticoagulants. Eventually, all the clotting factors are used up and no further clots can form. Heparin is sometimes used to interrupt the clotting cycle.

9. **Correct Answer: B**
   Potassium, sodium, and bicarbonate levels are decreased due to diuresis post transplant.

10. **Correct Answer: D**
    A transplanted heart is denervated and does not respond to atropine. Epinephrine or isoproterenol may be of use in this situation.

11. **Correct Answer: D**
    Hemophilia A and B are factor IX deficiencies.

12. **Correct Answer: B**
    Fever usually causes increased destruction of platelets. Answers A, C, and D are signs and symptoms, not causes.

13. **Correct Answer: D**
    Cryoprecipitate is quick frozen and contains large amounts of factor VIII. Cryoprecipitate does have disadvantages: (1) It is expensive; (2) newer recombinant factor VIII products are available; and (3) it carries the risk of transmission of hepatitis A, hepatitis C, hepatitis G, and HIV.

14. **Correct Answer: A**
    Sometimes Dextran causes acute tubular necrosis because it is made of polymers of high-molecular weight polysaccharides.

15. **Correct Answer: A**
    This form of meningitis is caused by a fungus, and amphotericin B is an antifungal. Rifampin is an antibacterial, Famvir and acyclovir are antivirals.

16. **Correct Answer: A**
    When blood is transfused, sometimes the cells lyse and the intracellular potassium is released. This can also occur when the cells strike the floating ball in the infusion chamber. It is sound practice to monitor electrolytes after each two units of blood given. Remember to monitor the patient for dysrhythmias.

17. **Correct Answer: C**
    The activated partial thromboplastin time of 45 seconds is correct because therapeutic results are standardized at 2–2½ times the normal time for the patient's blood to clot (20–30 seconds).

18. **Correct Answer: C**
    ITP usually occurs after a viral infection. The first symptoms may be purpura and petechiae on the distal extremities. The PT and PTT results will be normal because they test for nonplatelet parts of the coagulation pathway. The result of the capillary fragility test will be greater than 1. The Anti-RH immunoglobulin is a treatment for the disease. The patient should be continually monitored for signs and symptoms of intracranial hemorrhage.

19. **Correct Answer D**
    Usually at about the third day following admission, patients develop anemias. A reduced folate level would lead to megaloblastic anemia. Bone marrow aspiration is a diagnostic procedure, and TPN solutions would not lead to anemia. The IABP could, indeed, cause cells to lyse, as could prosthetic heart valves, heart–lung bypass, and bacterial endotoxins.

20. **Correct Answer B**
    Phenobarbital may cause aplastic anemia, furosemide may cause a generalized anemia, and captopril causes pancytopenia. In addition, quinidine, procainamide, and acetaminophen may cause hemolytic anemia.

21. **Correct Answer: B**
    Additional causes include progressive gram-negative bacterial infections and malignancies such as prostate cancer. Trauma may result in a bacterial infection.

22. **Correct Answer: D**

Cryoprecipitate does carry factor VIII, factor XIII, and fibrinogen. It is also associated with a risk of disease transmission and transfusion reactions.

23. **Correct Answer: A**

DIC often leads to malnutrition and nutritional deficits.

24. **Correct Answer: A**

Other potential causes include sepsis, viral infection, burns, and radiation therapy. Medications such as thiazides, furosemide, penicillins, sulfonamides, ranitidine, and heparin may cause thrombocytopenia. Chemotherapy is another cause.

25. **Correct Answer: B**

HIT is sometimes called "white clot syndrome." Thrombi are primarily venous in origin and can lead to DVT, pulmonary emboli, thrombotic stroke, limb ischemia, and myocardial infarction.

26. **Correct Answer: A**

HIT stands for "heparin-induced thrombocytopenia."

27. **Correct Answer: B**

Mismatched blood causes a hemolytic reaction resulting in systemic cellular lysis. The overwhelming destruction of cells cannot be corrected rapidly enough by the bone marrow.

28. **Correct Answer: A**

The function of T cells is to provide cellular immunity. These cells recognize the transplanted organ cells as foreign resulting in a mounted attack that could potentially lead to organ rejection. Immunosuppressive drugs suppress this normal response.

29. **Correct Answer: A**

Rattlesnakes envenomate with an enzyme called hyaluronidase, which breaks down the hyaluronic acid barriers on cells. As a consequence, the cells lyse and exudative products enter the bloodstream. Treatment is very similar to a patient with DIC, because fibrin split products (anticoagulants) are released. The patient may need to receive multiple vials of antivenin.

30. **Correct Answer: C**

PRBCs contain no platelets, and platelets must be given to aid in hemostasis.

31. **Correct Answer: C**

Answer C is the standard definition of this type of rejection.

32. **Correct Answer: D**

Damage to the tissues and vessels initiates the extrinsic cascade. Thromboplastin and factor VII are released and are activated in the presence of calcium.

33. **Correct Answer: A**

The transplanted kidney is placed in the pelvic area, so pelvic pain is an ominous sign. Patients who have undergone kidney transplants should be educated to notify their physicians immediately if they experience pelvic pain, as it is a symptom of rejection.

34. **Correct Answer: C**

Polyclonal antibodies are also used for episodes of acute rejections. Answers A and B are monoclonal antibodies. They can also be used for induction therapy; they alter T cells so the cells cannot recognize antigens. Paroxetine (Paxil) is an antidepressant.

35. **Correct Answer: D**

Additional indicators would include elevated liver enzymes, elevated bilirubin, jaundice, and elevated ammonia levels (a late sign). The itching results from the presence of bilirubin deposits in the skin.

36. **Correct Answer: C**

Prostaglandin relaxes the smooth muscles within the pulmonary airways and causes vasodilation within arteries. Inotropic support is usually accomplished with epinephrine. Heart rate is usually augmented with isoproterenol. Wound healing is promoted with a small single dose of methylprednisolone.

37. **Correct Answer: D**

Epinephrine counteracts the bronchoconstrictive and vasodilator actions of histamine by stimulating alpha, $beta_1$, and $beta_2$ receptors. Epinephrine is also useful in treating hayfever and urticaria.

38. **Correct Answer: B**

DIC is characterized by the depletion of clotting factors, and the patient becomes thrombocytopenic.

39. **Correct Answer: C**

Oat-cell carcinoma is a small-cell carcinoma. On CXR, a central mass will be seen. This type of carcinoma easily spreads to the brain, bone, liver, and adrenal glands and has a very poor prognosis.

40. **Correct Answer: A**

Hemoglobin consists of two parts: (1) "heme," which causes the reddish color and contains iron and porphyrin, and (2) globin, a protein. Hemoglobin combines with oxygen to form oxyhemoglobin. Hemoglobin also binds with CO_2 and carries it to alveoli to be expired. When the hemoglobin is phagocytized, it breaks down into heme and globin components. The iron in the hemoglobin is processed and reused to manufacture new hemoglobin. The porphyrin converts to bilirubin and is excreted in urine and feces.

41. **Correct Answer: A**

Acute post-hemorrhagic anemia may result from hemorrhage, a cancerous lesion, an ulcerative lesion that erodes an arterial wall, trauma to a major vessel, or rupture of an aneurysm. After hemorrhage, plasma is lost and vasoconstriction takes place. The concentration of erythrocytes increases because the fluid volume is low. In other words, the cells are not diluted in the usual amount of fluid, so the count is artificially high. It can take about six weeks for hemoglobin levels to return to normal.

42. **Correct Answer: D**

Iron-deficiency anemia is the most frequently occurring anemia seen around the world. It can be caused by an iron-poor diet or an excessive loss of iron. Trauma is a primary cause of acute loss and can result from bleeding. Blood donations, menses, GI bleeding, malabsorption syndromes, pica, and excessive diarrhea are all potential causes of this type of anemia. If you could view the erythrocytes in iron-deficiency anemia, they look kind of "puny": They are pale from lack of hemoglobin and tend to be smaller.

43. **Correct Answer: B**

In thalassemia, the erythrocytes (known as "target cells") are very thin and fragile. The serum bilirubin is very elevated, so you should caution the patient against scratching. Cool water and lotion may be used for skin care. Oral stimulants could lead to vaso-constriction. The integrity of the skin is weakened, so careful positioning is paramount. The patient may require ongoing transfusions. Multiple transfusions may actually lead to too much iron that might have to be chelated out.

44. **Correct Answer: B**

Approximately 50% of all cases of aplastic anemia are caused by toxins. The other 50% have an unknown cause. Some of the causes are radiation (x-rays, radioactive isotopes, radium), benzene, streptomycin, carbon tetrachloride, DDT, chloramphenicol, and sulfonamides. Many types of pesticides other than DDT are thought to contribute to aplastic anemia.

45. **Correct Answer: C**

Sickle cell anemia occurs primarily in the African-American population. Affected individuals are homozygous for HgS and have more HgS than HgA. This causes some cells to form a "sickle" shape—curved with rough edges. A crisis can occur when the low oxygen tension (postulated) causes a proliferation of these cells. The sharp edges of these cells travel through the microcirculation and damage capillaries. Even a simple thing like cold weather can precipitate massive sickling. Other identified risk factors include dehydration, vomiting, diarrhea, high altitude, excessive exercise, and stress. When the cells break apart, they occlude the microcirculation and lower oxygen tension, which initiates even more sickling. A crisis is a very painful time for the patient and oxygen, pain management, and fluids are very important.

46. **Correct Answer: B**

Idiopathic thrombocytopenia purpura (ITP) is the result of a low platelet count. Sometimes platelets are destroyed early and systematically. The cause is thought to be an autoimmune response. Hemorrhages may occur in the brain, which may lead to stroke and an increased intracranial pressure.

47. **Correct Answer: C**

LMWH (Lovenox) is so stable and predictable that PTT's are not required. This type of heparin is also easy to administer at home.

48. **Correct Answer: B**

Plavix will interfere with the activity of phenytoin, tamoxifen, tolbutamide, fluvastin, toresemide, and warfarin. It also may affect the effectiveness of nonsteroidal anti-inflammatories. Plavix does not seem to affect the effectiveness of estrogen, cimetidine, or phenobarbitol.

49. **Correct Answer: D**

Ethacrynic acid is a loop diuretic that prevents reabsorption of Na and Cl at the ascending loop of Henle (in the medulla of the kidney). Loop diuretics include furosemide, torsemide, bumetanide, and ethacrynic acid. As a group, they have vasodilatory effects on the renal vasculature.

50. **Correct Answer: A**
    Additional carbonic anhydrase inhibitors include dichlorphenamide and acetazo-lamide sodium. This type of diuretic blocks carbonic anhydrase and promotes excre-tion of water, Na^+, K^+, and bicarbonate. Potential complications include hypokalemia and hyperchloremic acidosis.

51. **Correct Answer: C**
    Because of the high volume of urine excreted, additional complications include hypocalcemia, dilutional hyponatremia, hyperglycemia, and hypochloremic acidosis.

52. **Correct Answer: C**
    Mannitol and urea are osmotic diuretics. They increase the osmotic pressure of the fil-trate, which attracts water and electrolytes and prevents reabsorption. The problem is that they can cause a rebound volume expansion, hyponatremia, and hyperkalemia. Mannitol may be used in lieu of sodium bicarbonate to manage hemoglobinuria and myoglobinuria secondary to rhabdomyolysis or severe crush injury. If large volumes of fluid are also used, this may reduce or prevent renal tubular obstruction.

53. **Correct Answer: B**
    Nesiritide is a synthetic brain naturetic peptide (BNP) that is used in the management of heart failure associated with prerenal azotemia. The BNP causes vasodilation, decreased systemic resistance (SVR), decreased left heart pressures, increased cardiac output (or cardiac index), diuresis, and decreased renin–angiotensin activity.

54. **Correct Answer: A**
    Epogen and Procrit are recombinant erythropoietin and they are used to correct the anemia that can occur with chronic renal failure. Adverse effects include clotting at the site of vascular access, depletion of iron, and may cause increases of potassium, creatinine, and BUN.

55. **Correct Answer: D**
    Mucomyst N-acetylcysteine or (NAC) is used to help reduce renal failure or worsening of symptoms caused by contrast media. The contrast media can cause contrast-induced neuropathy. Mucomyst has antioxidant properties that may counteract the reactive oxygen species that occur when the contrast media causes tubular epithelial cell toxicity.

56. **Correct Answer: B**
    Intracellular fluid contains high concentrations of potassium, magnesium, proteins, phosphates, and sulfates.

57. **Correct Answer: C**
    Bicarbonate in the interstitial spaces contains about three mEq/L more than the con-centration of bicarbonate in the intravascular space, which averages 24 mEq/L.

58. **Correct Answer: C**
    Atrial naturetic peptide (ANP) is released by the atria as a response to fluid overload. It increases excretion of sodium and water from the kidneys, which in turn lowers the blood pressure. The excretion of sodium and water decreases the release of antidiuretic hormone (ADH) and aldosterone.

59. **Correct Answer: A**

    D_5W will be distributed equally between the intravascular and extravascular spaces. The hypertonic saline will expand the intravascular volume only. Other solutions used for volume replacement include Dextran (hetastarch) and Hextend, both of which are synthetic colloidal solutions.

60. **Correct Answer: D**

    If all the fluid is present in the ECF, the systemic vascular resistance is increased. The fluid in the intravascular space is therefore low, and all the other parameters are decreased.

61. **Correct Answer: C**

    Treatment should have occurred at a slower pace to prevent shrinkage and lysis of brain cells. If this condition is discovered early enough, fluid and electrolyte replacement can be slowed. If permanent damage is done, the patient may develop quadriparesis, flaccidity, and other neurological deficits. Seizure precautions should be in place.

62. **Correct Answer: D**

    Additional foods that are high in folic acid include red beans, broccoli, asparagus, liver, and beef.

63. **Correct Answer: D**

    Monocytes and lymphocytes are classified as agranulocytes. The monocyte is the largest leukocyte, but accounts for a small amount of the total cell count for WBCs. When the monocytes mature, they become tissue macrophages and work as phagocytes. When a phagocyte is found in the liver, it is called a Kupffer cell. When it is found in the lungs, it is called an alveolar macrophage. When it is found in the connective tissues, it is called a histiocyte.

    Macrophages contain lysosomal enzymes and chemicals that can destroy bacteria. If the macrophage is activated by an antigen, it will secrete monokines, which control communication between all the cells involved in an immune response.

64. **Correct Answer: C**

    B lymphocytes originate and mature in bone marrow. They form antibodies (immunoglobulins) that formulate a response to a specific antigen that bound itself to the B cell's receptor sites. The B cell then forms a specific antibody for that particular antigen. Five types of immunoglobulins are available: IgG, IgA, IgM, IgE, and IgD. After the antibodies are synthesized, the specific antibody can attach to its antigen and set off the reaction to allow for phagocytosis. The cells retain a "memory" for the specific antigen so that if another exposure occurs, the subsequent response will be quicker and stronger.

65. **Correct Answer: A**

    All factors except VIII and XII are synthesized in the liver, which is why liver injuries can bleed so much and are so dangerous. While we were researching and confirming this question, we found out that the factors in the clotting cascades were numbered by order of discovery, not in the order of use. Just FYI!

66. **Correct Answer: C**

    Aminocaproic acid (Amicar) interferes with plasmin and inhibits fibrinolysis. Synthetic antithrombin III inhibits thrombin and can be very useful in treating DIC.

67. **Correct Answer: D**

   Patients who have hemolytic anemia may remain healthy until they are exposed to a major stressor such as infection, trauma, surgery, or a psychological stressor such as divorce. The patient may be overwhelmed and hemolysis accelerates and may cause tissue hypoxia and ischemia, which then progress to necrosis and infarction. Treatment is supportive and targeted to presenting symptoms.

68. **Correct Answer: D**

   If a severe reaction develops, the patient will have chest pain due to cardiac ischemia, neurologic impairment and LOC changes, and paresthesias because of cerebral ischemia. The patient may develop pulmonary emboli, dyspnea, extremity pain and pallor due to thrombosis, and possibly arterial thrombosis. This reaction usually takes 5–7 days to manifest, but can occur in a much shorter time.

69. **Correct Answer: B**

   The PT, PTT, and thrombin time are normal with ITP because these tests measure only nonplatelet factors in the coagulation cascade. The platelet antibody screen measures the presence of IgG and IgM antiplatelet antibodies.

70. **Correct Answer: C**

   Interferon is not applicable. Answers B and D are treatments for ITP that have probably been tried prior to the decision to perform a splenectomy. The patient may also be vaccinated for pneumococcal and meningococcal organisms to lower the risk of postoperative infection.

71. **Correct Answer: C**

   Amicar inhibits fibrinolysis. It is used in the treatment of DIC, but it may also change a simple bleeding issue into DIC. This medication must be used in combination with heparin. DIC is usually treated with FFP, cryoprecipitate, and platelets. Cryoprecipitate contains more than 5–10 times more fibrinogen than FFP. A good rule of thumb is to give 10 units of cryoprecipitate for each 3 units of FFP. If the patient is actively bleeding, platelets are commonly used as part of treatment.

72. **Correct Answer: A**

   The patient may experience chills, fever, tachycardia, hypotension, hematuria, back pain, and may exhibit additional signs of shock. The extravascular hemolytic reaction may manifest as fever, low H and H even after transfusion, and elevated bilirubin.

73. **Correct Answer: D**

   Mesothelioma is a cancer of the mesothelium. Most cases of this relatively rare cancer begin in the pleura or peritoneum. Approximately 2,000 new cases of mesothelioma are diagnosed in the United States each year. The disease occurs more often in men than in women and the risk increases with age. Symptoms of mesothelioma may not appear until 30–50 years after the initial exposure to asbestos. An increased risk of developing mesothelioma has been found among shipyard workers, people who work in asbestos mines and mills, producers of asbestos products, workers in the heating and construction industries, and other tradespeople. Symptoms include dyspnea, pleural effusion, weight loss, and abdominal pain and swelling due to an excess of fluid in the abdomen. Other potential symptoms of peritoneal mesothelioma include bowel obstruction, clotting disorders, anemia, and fever. Symptoms with metastases may include pain, dysphagia, or swelling of the neck or face.

Asbestos has been widely used in many industrial products, including cement, duct linings, sound insulation, brake linings, roof shingles, flooring products, textiles, and thermal insulation. If tiny asbestos particles float in the air, especially during the manufacturing process, they may be inhaled or swallowed, and can cause serious health problems. In addition to mesothelioma, exposure to asbestos increases the risk of lung cancer, asbestosis, and cancers of the trachea, larynx, and kidney. Smoking does not appear to increase the risk of mesothelioma, but the combination of smoking and exposure increases a person's risk of developing bronchial cancer.

While we were researching this topic, we discovered a sobering piece of information: More than 110,000 schools in the U.S. still contain some form of asbestos.

74. Correct Answer: C

Pernicious anemia results from a lack of protein intrinsic factor in the stomach that helps the body absorb vitamin B_{12}. The stress placed on the heart from the resultant hypoxia can cause heart murmurs, tachycardias, arrhythmias, hypertrophy, and heart failure. A lack of vitamin B_{12} raises the homocysteine level, and high levels of homocysteine add to the buildup of fatty deposits. A lack of vitamin B_{12} can damage nerve cells, causing problems such as paresthesias in the hands and feet and problems with ambulation and balance. Memory loss, visual disturbances, and confusion may develop. This condition was named "pernicious" because it was often fatal before the cause was discovered to be a lack of vitamin B_{12}.

75. Correct Answer: B

The purple-topped tubes are standardized within the U.S. hematology system as containing the additives EDTA K2 and EDTA K3. These additives bind with calcium in the serum to prevent coagulation. EDTA K2 tubes are also used to determine viral load for patients with HIV.

Gray-topped tubes are used for testing of glucose, blood alcohol, lactate, and bicarbonate levels. Potassium oxalate and sodium fluoride, sodium fluoride/Na2 EDTA, and sodium fluoride are the additives. Oxalate and EDTA prevent coagulation. The additives prevent glucose uptake by the cells when there may be a delay in processing.

Green-topped tubes are used for clinical chemistry tests. The heparin based additives produce a whole blood specimen and do not allow coagulation.

Red-topped tubes are used for immunohematology and serology testing. There are no additives, and clotting of the specimen is expected.

76. Correct Answer: C

Hepatitis B vaccine is given in three doses. The initial dose is given then the second dose is given at 1–2 months, followed by the third dose at 4–6 months. Blood titers can be drawn to determine the level of protection and the need for a booster shot.

77. Correct Answer: C

Normal adult female hematocrit levels are 37–47%.

BIBLIOGRAPHY

Aberg, F., Koivusalo, A. M., Hockerstedt, K., & Isoniemi, H. (2007). Renal dysfunction in liver transplant patients: Comparing patients transplanted for liver tumor or acute or chronic disease. *Transplant International, 20*(7), 591–599.

Ahrens, T. (2006). *Critical care nursing certification.* Columbus, OH: McGraw-Hill.

American Association of Critical-Care Nurses. (2006). *Core curriculum for critical care nursing* (6th ed.). Philadelphia: Saunders.

American Association of Critical-Care Nurses. (2007). *AACN certification and core review for high acuity and critical care* (6th ed.). Philadelphia: Saunders.

American Heart Association. (2007). *Guidelines 2005 for cardiopulmonary resuscitation and emergency cardiovascular care: Update.* Retrieved July 21, 2008, from http://circ.ahajournals.org/content/vol112/24_suppl

Aster, R. H., & Bougie, D. W. (2007). Drug-induced immune thrombocytopenia: Current concepts. *New England Journal of Medicine, 357*(6), 580–587.

Barroso, J., Wells Pence, B., Salahuddin, N., Harmon, J. L., & Leserman, J. (2008). Physiological correlates of HIV-related fatigue. *Clinical Nursing Research, 17*(1), 5.

Bhullar, I. S., Braman, R., & Block, E. F. J. (2007). Recombinant factor VII as an adjunct to control of hemorrhage from chest trauma in a Jehovah's Witness. *American Surgeon, 73*(8), 818–819.

Biagini, E., Spirito, P., Leone, O., Picchio, F. M., Coccolo, F., Ragni, L., et al. (2008). Heart transplantation in hypertrophic cardiomyopathy. *American Journal of Cardiology, 101*(3), 387.

Bonatti, H., Dougerty, M., Martin, K., Hinder, R. A., Nguyen, J. H., & Haddad, M. A. (2007). Whipple procedure for chronic pancreatitis in a Jehovah's Witness. *American Surgeon, 73*(9), 935–936.

Burns, S. M. (Ed.). (2007). *American Association of Critical-Care Nurses (AACN): AACN protocols for practice: Healing environments* (2nd ed.). Sudbury, MA: Jones and Bartlett.

Caliskan, M., Erdogan, D., Gullu, H., Tok, D., Bilgi, M., & Muderrisoglu, H. (2007). Original paper: Low serum bilirubin concentrations are associated with impaired aortic elastic properties, but not impaired left ventricular diastolic function. *International Journal of Clinical Practice, 61*(2), 218–224.

Campbell, M. S., Constantinescu, S., Furth, E. E., Reddy, K. R., & Bloom, R. D. (2007). Effects of hepatitis C–induced liver fibrosis on survival in kidney transplant candidates. *Digestive Diseases and Sciences, 52*(10), 2501–2507.

Chierakul, W., Tientadakul, P., Suputtamongkol, Y., Wuthiekanun, V., Phimda, K., Limpaiboon, R., et al. (2008). Activation of the coagulation cascade in patients with leptospirosis. *Clinical Infectious Diseases, 46*(2), 254.

Clark, N., Witt, D., Delate, T., Trapp, M., Garcia, D., Ageno, W., et al. (2008). The clinical consequence of subtherapeutic anticoagulation: The Low INR Study (LINeRS). *Journal of Thrombosis and Thrombolysis, 25*(1), 127–128.

Cohney, S. J., Walker, R. G., Haeusler, M. N., Francis, D. M., & Hogan, C. J. (2007). Blood group incompatibility in kidney transplantation: Definitely time to re-examine! *Medical Journal of Australia, 187*(5), 306–308.

Conover, M. B. (2003). *Understanding electrocardiography* (8th ed.). St. Louis, MO: Mosby/Elsevier.

Copstead, L., & Banasik, J. L. (2000). *Pathophysiology: Biological and behavioral perspectives* (2nd ed.). Philadelphia: Saunders/Elsevier.

Curley, M. A. Q. (1998). Patient–nurse synergy: Optimizing patients' outcomes. *American Journal of Critical Care, 7*, 64–72.

Danes, A. F., Cuenca, L. G., Rodriguez Bueno, S., Mendarte Barrenechea, L., & Montoro Ronsano, J. B. (2008). Efficacy and tolerability of human fibrinogen concentrate administration to patients with acquired fibrinogen deficiency and active or in high-risk severe bleeding. *Vox Sanguinis, 94*(3), 221–226.

Delclaux, C., Zerah-Lancner, F., Bachir, D., Habibi, A., Monin, J. L., Godeau, B., et al. (2005). Factors associated with dyspnea in adult patients with sickle cell disease. *Chest, 128*(5), 3336–3344.

Dhaliwal, G., Cornett, P. A., & Tierney, L. M. (2004). Hemolytic anemia. *American Family Physician, 69*(11), 2599–2606.

Domen, R. E., & Hoeltge, G. A. (2003). Allergic transfusion reactions: An evaluation of 273 consecutive reactions. *Archives of Pathology & Laboratory Medicine, 127*(3), 316–320.

Dossey, B. M., Keegan, L., & Guzzetta, C. (2003). *Holistic nursing: A handbook for practice* (3rd ed.). Sudbury, MA: Jones and Bartlett.

Douketis, J. D., Gu, S. Z., Schulman, S., Ghirarduzzi, A., Pengo, V., & Prandoni, P. (2007). The risk for fatal pulmonary embolism after discontinuing anticoagulant therapy for venous thromboembolism. *Annals of Internal Medicine, 147*(11), 766–774.

Drent, G., De Geest, S., & Haagsma, E. B. (2006). Prednisolone noncompliance and outcome in liver transplant recipients. *Transplant International, 19*(4), 342–343.

Dvorak, C. C., & Cowan, M. J. (2008). Hematopoietic stem cell transplantation for primary immunodeficiency disease. *Bone Marrow Transplantation, 41*(2), 119–126.

Dwyer, J. (2008). Developing the duty to treat: HIV, SARS, and the next epidemic. *Journal of Medical Ethics, 34*(1), 7.

Eby, C. S., Harris, J. K., Gage, B. F., Ridker, P. M., Goldhaber, S. Z., & Birman-Deych, E. (2008). Pharmacogenetic factors affecting INR control during warfarin initiation. *Journal of Thrombosis and Thrombolysis, 25*(1), 98.

Edwards, D. F. (1999). The Synergy Model: Linking patient needs to nurse competencies. *Critical Care Nurse, 19*(1), 88–98.

El-Husseini, A., Sabry, A., Zahran, A., & Shoker, A. (2007). Can donor implantation renal biopsy predict long-term renal allograft outcome? *American Journal of Nephrology, 27*(2), 144–151.

Emergency Nurses Association & Newberry, L. (2003). *Sheehy's emergency nursing: Principles and practice* (5th ed.). St. Louis, MO: Mosby/Elsevier.

Ezidiegwu, C. N., Lauenstein, K. J., Rosales, L. G., Kelly, K. C., & Henry, J. B. (2004). Febrile nonhemolytic transfusion reactions: Management by premedication and cost implications in adult patients. *Archives of Pathology & Laboratory Medicine, 128*(9), 991–995.

Finkelmeier, B. A. (2000). *Cardiothoracic surgical nursing* (2nd ed.). Philadelphia: Lippincott, Williams & Wilkins.

Goldstein, G., Toren, A., & Nagler, A. (2007). Transplantation and other uses of human umbilical cord blood and stem cells. *Current Pharmaceutical Design, 13*(13), 1363–1373.

Gurm, H. S., & Eagle, K. A. (2008). Use of anticoagulants in ST-segment elevation myocardial infarction patients: A focus on low-molecular-weight heparin. *Cardiovascular Drugs and Therapy, 22*(1), 59–69.

Halkes, P., & Algra, A. (2007). Anticoagulants, aspirin and dipyridamole in the secondary prevention of cerebral ischaemia: Which is the best for which patient? *Cerebrovascular Diseases: S1, 24*, 107–111.

Hardin, S. R., & Kaplow, R. (Eds.). (2004). *Synergy for clinical excellence: The AACN Synergy Model for Patient Care.* Sudbury, MA: Jones and Bartlett.

Hedner, U., & Brun, N. C. (2007). Recombinant factor VIIa (rFVIIa): Its potential role as a hemostatic agent. *Neuroradiology, 49*(10), 789–793.

Heparin-induced thrombocytopenia: A quick review of recent studies. (2007). *Journal of Respiratory Diseases, 28*(9), 396.

Hickey, J. V. (2002). *The clinical practice of neurological and neurosurgical nursing* (5th ed.). Philadelphia: Lippincott, Williams & Wilkins.

Hirohata, A., Nakamura, M., Waseda, K., Honda, Y., Lee, D. P., Vagelos, R. H., et al. (2007). Changes in coronary anatomy and physiology after heart transplantation. *American Journal of Cardiology, 99*(11), 1603.

Ishibashi, H., Takashi, O., Hosaka, M., Sugimoto, I., Takahashi, M., Nihei, T., et al. (2005). Heparin-induced thrombocytopenia complicated with massive thrombosis of the inferior vena cava after filter placement. *International Angiology, 24*(4), 387–390.

James, A. H. (2007). Prevention and management of venous thromboembolism in pregnancy. *American Journal of Medicine: Management of Venous Thromboembolism, 120*(10B), S26.

Kamoun, M., & Grossman, R. A. (2008). Kidney-transplant rejection and anti-MICA antibodies. *New England Journal of Medicine, 358*(2), 196; author reply, 196.

Khan, B. A., Deel, C., & Hellman, R. N. (2006). Tumor lysis syndrome associated with reduced immunosuppression in a lung transplant recipient. *Mayo Clinic Proceedings, 81*(10), 1397–1399.

Krentz, A. J., & Wheeler, D. C. (2005). New-onset diabetes after transplantation: A threat to graft and patient survival. *Lancet, 365*(9460), 640–642.

Krishnamoorthy, P., Alyaarubi, S., Abish, S., Gale, M., Albuquerque, P., & Jabado, N. (2006). Primary hyperparathyroidism mimicking vaso-occlusive crises in sickle cell disease. *Pediatrics, 118*(2), 786–787.

Kuznetsov, A. V., Schneeberger, S., Seiler, R., Brandacher, G., Mark, W., Steurer, W., et al. (2004). Mitochondrial defects and heterogeneous cytochrome c release after cardiac cold ischemia and reperfusion. *American Journal of Physiology: Heart and Circulatory Physiology, 286*(5), H1633–H1641.

Labbé, E., Herbert, D., & Haynes, J. (2005). Physicians' attitude and practices in sickle cell disease pain management. *Journal of Palliative Care, 21*(4), 246–251.

Leichtman, A. B. (2007). Balancing efficacy and toxicity in kidney-transplant immunosuppression. *New England Journal of Medicine, 357*(25), 2625–2627.

Levi, M., & Cate, H. T. (1999). Disseminated intravascular coagulation. *New England Journal of Medicine, 341*(8), 586–592.

Lipson, J. G., Dibble, S. L., & Minarik, P. A. (Eds.). (1996). *Culture and nursing care: A pocket guide.* San Francisco, CA: UCSF Nursing Press.

Lisman, T., & Leebeek, F. W. G. (2007). Hemostatic alterations in liver disease: A review on pathophysiology, clinical consequences, and treatment. *Digestive Surgery, 24*(4), 250–258.

Marik, P. E. (2006). Adrenal-exhaustion syndrome in patients with liver disease. *Intensive Care Medicine, 32*(2), 275–280.

McNally, P. (2001). *GI/liver secrets* (2nd ed.). Philadelphia: Hanley & Belfus/Elsevier.

McQuillan, K. A., Von Rueden, K. T., Hartsock, R. L., Flynn, M. B., & Whalen, E. (Eds.). (2002). *Trauma nursing: from resuscitation through rehabilitation* (3rd ed.). Philadelphia: Saunders/Elsevier.

Medina, J., & Puntillo, K. (2006). *AACN protocols for practice: Palliative care and end-of-life issues in critical care.* Sudbury, MA: Jones and Bartlett.

Mitka, M. (2007). Dual antithrombotic therapy's increased risks not always offset by benefit. *Journal of the American Medical Association, 298*(13), 1504.

Mongardon, N., Bruneel, F., Henry-Lagarrigue, M., Legriel, S., Revault d'Allonnes, L., Guezennec, P., et al. (2007). Shock during heparin-induced thrombocytopenia: Look for adrenal insufficiency! *Intensive Care Medicine, 33*(3), 547–548.

Neff, G. W., Kemmer, N., Kaiser, T. E., Zacharias, V. C., Alonzo, M., Thomas, M., et al. (2007). Combination therapy in liver transplant recipients with hepatitis B virus without hepatitis B immune globulin. *Digestive Diseases and Sciences, 52*(10), 2497–2500.

Norris, W. E. (2004). Acute hepatic sequestration in sickle cell disease. *Journal of the National Medical Association, 96*(9), 1235–1239.

Olson, J. D., Brandt, J. T., Chandler, W. L., Van Cott, E. M., Cunningham, M. T., Hayes, T. E., et al. (2007). Laboratory reporting of the international normalized ratio: Progress and problems. *Archives of Pathology & Laboratory Medicine, 131*(11), 1641–1647.

Orens, J. B. (2007). Lung transplantation for pulmonary hypertension. *International Journal of Clinical Practice, 61*(s158), 4–9.

Pagana, K. D., & Pagana, J. (2005). *Mosby's manual of diagnostic and laboratory tests* (3rd ed.). St. Louis, MO: Mosby/Elsevier.

Prasad, V. K., & Kurtzberg, J. (2008). Emerging trends in transplantation of inherited metabolic diseases. *Bone Marrow Transplantation, 41*(2), 99–108.

Ratnovsky, A., Elad, D., Izbicki, G., & Kramer, M. R. (2006). Mechanics of respiratory muscles in single-lung transplant recipients. *Respiration, 73*(5), 642–650.

Rizzi, E. B., Schininá, V., Rovighi, L., Cristofaro, M., Bordi, E., Narciso, P., et al. (2008). HIV-related pneumococcal lung disease: Does highly active antiretroviral therapy or bacteremia modify radiologic appearance? Review of. *AIDS Patient Care & STDs, 22*(2), 105.

Shorr, A. K., Helman, D. L., Davies, D. B., & Nathan, S. D. (2004). Sarcoidosis, race, and short-term outcomes following lung transplantation. *Chest, 125*(3), 990–996.

Silverborn, M., Ambring, A., Nilsson, F., Friberg, P., & Jeppsson, A. (2006). Vascular resistance and endothelial function in cyclosporine-treated lung transplant recipients. *Transplant International, 19*(12), 974–981.

Skidmore-Roth, L. (2004). *Mosby's 2004 nursing drug reference.* St. Louis, MO: Mosby/Elsevier.

Smeltzer, S., & Bare, B. G. (2003). *Brunner and Suddarth's textbook of medical–surgical nursing* (10th ed.). Philadelphia: Lippincott, Williams & Wilkins.

Smith, W. R., Penberthy, L. T., Bovbjerg, V. E., McClish, D. K., Roberts, J. D., Dahman, B., et al. (2008). Daily assessment of pain in adults with sickle cell disease. *Annals of Internal Medicine, 148*(2), 94–101.

Sole, M. L., Hartshorn, J., & Lamborne, M. L. (2001). *Introduction to critical care nursing* (3rd ed.). Philadelphia: Saunders/Elsevier.

Stewart, S. (2007). Pulmonary infections in transplantation pathology. *Archives of Pathology & Laboratory Medicine, 131*(8), 1219–1231.

Swanson, K., Dwyre, D. M., Krochmal, J., & Raife, T. J. (2006). Transfusion-related acute lung injury (TRALI): Current clinical and pathophysiologic considerations. *Lung, 184*(3), 177–185.

Tien, H., Nascimento, B., Callum, J., & Rizoli, S. (2007). An approach to transfusion and hemorrhage in trauma: Current perspectives on restrictive transfusion strategies. *Canadian Journal of Surgery, 50*(3), 202–209.

Toso, C., Al-Qahtani, M., Alsaif, F. A., Bigam, D. L., Meeberg, G. A., James Shapiro, A. M., et al. (2007). ABO-incompatible liver transplantation for critically ill adult patients. *Transplant International, 20*(8), 675–681.

Unkle, D. W. (2007). Heparin-induced thrombocytopenia. *Orthopaedic Nursing, 26*(6), 383–387.

Urden, L. D., Stacy, K. M., & Lough, M. E. (2007). *Thelan's critical care nursing: Diagnosis and management* (5th ed.). St. Louis, MO: Mosby.

Villar, E., Boissonnat, P., Sebbag, L., Hendawy, A., Cahen, R., Trolliet, P., et al. (2007). Poor prognosis of heart transplant patients with end-stage renal failure. *Nephrology, Dialysis, Transplantation, 22*(5), 1383–1389.

Wiegand, D. J. L., & Carlson, K. K. (Eds.). (2005). *AACN procedure manual for critical care* (5th ed.). Philadelphia: Elsevier.

Williams, S., Wynn, G., Cozza, K., & Sandson, N. B. (2007). Cardiovascular medications. *Psychosomatics, 48*(6), 537–547.

Woods, S., Sivarajan Froelicher, E. S., & Motzer, S. U. (2000). *Cardiac nursing* (4th ed.). Philadelphia: Lippincott, Williams & Wilkins.

Yasunaga, H. (2007). Risk of authoritarianism: Fibrinogen-transmitted hepatitis C in Japan. *Lancet, 370*(9604), 2063–2067.

Yip, N. H., Lederer, D. J., Kawut, S. M., Wilt, J. S., D'Ovidio, F., Wang, Y., et al. (2006). Immunoglobulin G levels before and after lung transplantation. *American Journal of Respiratory and Critical Care Medicine, 173*(8), 917–921.

Zhang, D., Zhang, F., Zhang, Y., Gao, X., Li, C., Ma, W., et al. (2007). Erythropoietin enhances the angiogenic potency of autologous bone marrow stromal cells in a rat model of myocardial infarction. *Cardiology, 108*(4), 228–236.

Neurology

QUESTIONS

1. **Your response to a stressful situation, such as resuscitation of a patient, causes a sympathetic nervous system response. A sympathetic response to a stimuli results in**
   A. Heightened awareness, increased blood pressure, bronchial constriction, and increased glucogenesis.
   B. Dilated pupils, bronchial relaxation, increased gastric motility, and normal urine output.
   C. Vasodilatation, increased blood pressure, decreased gastric secretions, and pupils at 3 mm.
   D. Increased respiratory depth, increased heart rate, decreased gastric motility, and sphincter dilation.

2. **Nursing care for a patient with glaucoma would not include**
   A. Applying cool compresses to the patient's forehead.
   B. Darkening the environment.
   C. Providing a quiet and private space.
   D. Encouraging the patient to cough.

3. **Meniere's disease is characterized by**
   A. Headache, nausea, macular degeneration, and central vision loss.
   B. Pain in the left lower quadrant, diarrhea, food allergies, and nausea.
   C. Vertigo, tinnitus, sweating, and nausea.
   D. Headache, tinnitus, and vision loss.

4. **The type of shock that might be caused by spinal anesthesia or severe pain is**
   A. Septic.
   B. Anaphylactic.
   C. Neurogenic.
   D. Cardiogenic.

5. **Spinal shock is defined as**
   A. Areflexia at or below the spinal cord injury.
   B. Hyperreflexia and spasticity after spinal cord injury.
   C. Areflexia that rises above the site of injury.
   D. Spasticity below the site of injury.

6. **What is myasthenia gravis?**
   A. A neuromuscular disorder in which myelin is destroyed at varying rates
   B. A neuromuscular disorder that affects the neuromuscular junction
   C. A neuromuscular disorder seen after viral infections
   D. A fatal neuromuscular disorder of upper motor neurons and lower motor neurons that causes muscle wasting

7. **What are some common symptoms of myasthenia gravis?**
   A. Ptosis, proximal muscle weakness, spasticity
   B. Dysphonia, sialorrhea, atrophy
   C. Fatigue, proximal muscle weakness, respiratory weakness
   D. Generalized weakness, hyperreflexia, dyspnea

8. **Betty is a 50-year-old lady admitted to the telemetry unit for acute coronary syndrome. She also has myasthenia gravis and is allowed to keep her pyridostigmine at her bedside so she does not miss a dose. Suddenly, her monitor alarms with a severe bradycardia. You suspect an overdose of pyridostigmine. If that is true, Betty's problem is**
   A. Cholinergic crisis.
   B. Acetylcholine crisis.
   C. Myasthenia gravis crisis.
   D. The bradycardia is related to the acute coronary syndrome, not myasthenia gravis.

9. **Fredrick, 18 years old, was injured while skateboarding and had a T8 spinal cord injury one month ago. He had been diagnosed with spinal shock while in the intensive care unit. Fredrick is now in the progressive care unit. As his nurse, you know the symptoms of spinal shock include**
   A. Areflexia, autonomic dysfunction, loss of sensation, and eliminatory dysfunction.
   B. Areflexia, peripheral vasodilatation, decreased SVR, and loss of sensation.
   C. Areflexia, heightened sensation, and cardiovascular shock.
   D. Areflexia, bowel and bladder dysfunction, and bradycardia.

10. **Grace has a C6 spinal cord injury for which she spent 45 days in intensive care due to neurogenic shock. Neurogenic shock differs from spinal shock in which of the following ways?**
    A. It is a less severe form of shock with spinal cord injury that causes a brief decrease in blood pressure.
    B. It is a more severe form of shock that causes cardiovascular collapse in patients with a spinal cord injury above T6.
    C. It is a more severe shock that increases the risk of paralysis and death.
    D. It is a more severe form of shock that occurs within hours after a spinal cord injury and causes increased sympathetic outflow.

11. **Amy, a 36-year-old secretary, is transferred to DOU after recovering from a subarachnoid hemorrhage due to a ruptured anterior communicating artery aneurysm. Cerebral aneurysms are most often found in which of the following anatomical areas?**
    A. Internal carotid arteries
    B. Bifurcations of the anterior–posterior circle of Willis
    C. Temporal artery
    D. Vertebral arteries

12. **The most common first symptom of a rupturing cerebral aneurysm is**
    A. Fever.
    B. Nuchal rigidity.
    C. Nausea and vomiting.
    D. Explosive headache, often described as "the worst headache of my life."

13. **A patient's family member asks you about the arteriovenous malformation (AVM) that caused her brother's stroke. You explain that AVMs are**
    A. Commonly found misshapen blood vessels.
    B. More common in women than in men.
    C. A complex tangle of misshapen blood vessels susceptible to hemorrhage.
    D. Never seen in children.

14. **Nursing management of a patient with a cerebral aneurysm includes**
    A. Ambulation and monitoring of vital and neurologic signs.
    B. Glasgow Coma Scale assessments and monitoring for cerebral vascular spasm.
    C. Maintaining normal intracranial pressure.
    D. Maintaining systolic blood pressure less than 120 mm Hg.

15. **Randall is a 79-year-old patient with a long history of alcohol abuse. He is in hepatic failure due to cirrhosis and is experiencing encephalopathy. The hallmark of encephalopathy of any cause is**
    A. Altered mental state.
    B. Liver failure.
    C. Renal failure.
    D. Infection.

16. **Continuing with the scenario from Question 15, the treatment of Randall's hepatic encephalopathy should include**
    A. Antibiotics.
    B. High-dose steroids.
    C. Treatment of the underlying cause.
    D. Electrolyte replacement.

17. **Diagnostic tests for a patient with encephalopathy could include**
    A. BMP, CRP, and CXR.
    B. Blood tests, CSF evaluation, and EEG.
    C. EEG and Dilantin levels.
    D. Lumbar puncture and renal ultrasound.

18. **Tom, a 25-year-old baseball player, is admitted to the progressive care unit after being struck by a baseball bat during a game. He has blunt force trauma to the left side of his head. Nursing management of this patient includes frequent assessments. Which of the following parameters is the most sensitive indicator of Tom's status?**
    A. Vital signs
    B. Glasgow Coma Scale score
    C. Level of consciousness
    D. Intracranial pressure

19. Frances, a 28-year-old mother of three, has been diagnosed with multiple sclerosis (MS). She was admitted to the telemetry care unit after an acute exacerbation in which she experienced left-side weakness. Multiple sclerosis is which type of disease?
    A. A motor disorder of the spinal cord
    B. A demyelinating disorder of the brain and spinal cord
    C. A motor disorder of the brain and spinal cord
    D. A demyelinating disease of the spinal cord

20. Continuing with the scenario from Question 19, Frances is very depressed. She states, "I don't want to die like my mother did with MS." She is currently experiencing which Kübler-Ross stage of grief?
    A. Denial
    B. Bargaining
    C. Anger
    D. Acceptance

21. Susan was an unrestrained passenger in a motor vehicle accident. She was admitted to the PCCU after a basilar skull fracture. Which of the following signs differentiate a fracture of the middle fossa?
    A. Rhinorrhea
    B. Raccoon's eyes
    C. Battle's sign
    D. Subconjunctival hemorrhage

22. While assessing a patient with a basilar skull fracture, the PCCU nurse notices a stain on the patient's pillow. The stain is a small amount of blood encircled by a pale yellow stain. This stain is called
    A. Halo sign.
    B. Battle's sign.
    C. Grey–Turner's sign.
    D. Ludwig's sign.

23. Your patient suffered a closed head injury. Which of the following parameters would require immediate intervention?
    A. EKG showing borderline sinus tachycardia without ectopy at 100
    B. Oral temperature of 37.2°C
    C. Profound respirations at 26 per minute
    D. Blood pressure 146/86, left arm

24. Normal intracranial pressure is
    A. 0–5 mm Hg.
    B. 4–15 mm Hg.
    C. 16–20 mm Hg.
    D. 20–40 mm Hg.

25. What are the two major types of multiple sclerosis?
    A. Progressive and relapsing–resolving
    B. Relapsing–remitting and static
    C. Progressive and relapsing–relapsing
    D. Relapsing–remitting and progressive

26. **What is the function of the myelin sheath in the central nervous system?**
    A. It protects the dendrites from injury.
    B. It allows for faster transmission of nerve impulses.
    C. Its purpose has not yet been determined.
    D. It creates the gray matter in the brain and spinal cord.

27. **Mary is a "no code" patient in your PCCU. She has suffered an acute hemorrhagic stroke and is not expected to survive long. You know that her intracranial pressure is rising and she is developing Cushing syndrome. Which signs and symptoms would you expect to see?**
    A. Increased systolic blood pressure, widening pulse pressure, bradycardia
    B. Elevated blood pressure, narrow pulse pressure, tachycardia
    C. Bradycardia, low blood pressure, narrow pulse pressure
    D. Tachycardia, increased systolic blood pressure, widening pulse pressure

28. **While you are teaching Frances about her multiple sclerosis (MS), you explain that some common symptoms of an exacerbation of multiple sclerosis can include which of the following symptoms?**
    A. Hyperthesia, fatigue, hyporeflexia
    B. Parasthesias, urinary incontinence, constipation
    C. Diplopia, ataxia, emotional lability
    D. Ataxia, dementia, temporal neuralgia

29. **When should a lumbar puncture be done on a patient with, or suspected of having, increased intracranial pressure?**
    A. Once the patient has undergone a CT or MRI scan
    B. Always, to check intracranial pressure
    C. Done on a case-by-case basis
    D. Never

30. **Which of the following physiological responses decreases intracranial pressure?**
    A. CO_2 retention
    B. PaO_2 less than 50 mm Hg
    C. Increased cerebrospinal fluid absorption
    D. Increased metabolic activity

31. **Mrs. B. has a closed head injury secondary to a fall. As a PCCU nurse, you know which of the following assessments is the most important indicator of neurologic deterioration in this patient?**
    A. Blood pressure
    B. Cranial nerve testing
    C. Level of consciousness
    D. Glasgow Coma Scale score

32. **Mrs. B., a closed head injury patient, has a Foley catheter. In one hour, her urine output increases from 30 mL/h to 1,000 mL of very pale, clear urine. The PCCU nurse knows this change is probably due to**
    A. A volume shift from the third space.
    B. Syndrome of inappropriate antidiuretic hormone.
    C. Diabetes insipidus.
    D. Diuresis from steroids.

33. **As a progressive care nurse, you know the treatment of diabetes insipidus includes the following possible treatment:**
    A. Fluid restriction.
    B. Intravenous replacement to cover the increased urine output.
    C. Diuretics.
    D. Demeclocycline.

34. **What is the "Triple H" therapy for cerebral aneurysm rupture?**
    A. Hypertension, hypervolemia, hemodilution
    B. Hypertension, hypovolemia, hemodilution
    C. Hypovolemia, hypotension, hemoconcentration
    D. Hemoconcentration, hypertension, hypervolemia

35. **Why is it important to stop seizure activity in status epilepticus?**
    A. Oxygen depletion can occur due to an impeded airway.
    B. There is increased risk of cerebrovascular accident.
    C. Continued seizure activity causes lactic acidosis and cerebral edema.
    D. Injury risk increases with continued seizures.

36. **Frank, an 87-year-old retired school teacher, is recovering from cerebral hemorrhage. He has been diagnosed with communicating hydrocephalus. Communicating hydrocephalus is caused by which mechanism?**
    A. Closed head injury
    B. Subarachnoid hemorrhage
    C. Epidural bleed
    D. Cerebrovascular accident

37. **What is the formula for calculating cerebral perfusion pressure (CPP)?**
    A. CPP = SBP − MAP − ICP
    B. CPP = MAP − ICP
    C. CPP = ICP − MAP
    D. CPP = MAP − CVP − ICP

38. **What is the goal for cerebral perfusion pressure (CPP)?**
    A. 50–80 mm Hg
    B. 20–40 mm Hg
    C. 10–20 mm Hg
    D. 70–90 mm Hg

39. **Joy had a small basilar skull fracture after a motor vehicle accident. Which of the cranial nerves (CN) are affected by a basilar skull fracture?**
    A. I, VII, VIII
    B. I, II, III
    C. I, V, VIII
    D. II, III, VIII

40. **What is the cause of multiple sclerosis?**
    A. Heredity
    B. Unknown
    C. Chemical exposure
    D. Heavy metal poisoning

41. **Your previously stable head injured patient has just developed nystagmus. As a nurse, you know nystagmus is**
    A. Eyes deviated to the side of the injury.
    B. A convergent gaze.
    C. Rhythmic tremor or shaking of the eyes.
    D. A divergent gaze.

42. **Your patient who has oat-cell lung cancer has decreased urinary output to less than 10 mL/h. This may be caused by**
    A. Dehydration.
    B. Syndrome of inappropriate antidiuretic hormone.
    C. Diabetes insipidus.
    D. Third spacing.

43. **What are the most common causes of syndrome of inappropriate antidiuretic hormone?**
    A. Bronchogenic (oat-cell) carcinoma, pneumonia, head injury
    B. Pneumonia, COPD, tuberculosis
    C. Brain tumors, pneumonia, polycystic kidney disease
    D. Polycystic kidney disease, cerebrovascular accident, oat-cell carcinoma

44. **Spinal reflexes indicate which of the following physiological states?**
    A. Functional upper motor neurons
    B. Nonfunctional lower motor neurons
    C. Nonfunctional upper motor neurons
    D. Functional lower motor neurons

45. **You are caring for Gene, a new paraplegic in the PCCU. The neurologist wants to test Gene's spinothalamic tract responses. How is the spinothalamic tract tested?**
    A. Deep tendon reflexes
    B. Babinski reflex
    C. Pinprick or monofilament testing
    D. Patellar tendon reflex

46. **Lab studies for multiple sclerosis identification include**
    A. Cerebral spinal fluid evaluation, sedimentation rate, and fluorescent treponomal antibody absorption.
    B. Cerebral spinal fluid evaluation, syphilis, and drug screen.
    C. Cerebral spinal fluid evaluation, CBC, and HIV.
    D. Cerebral spinal fluid evaluation, lipids, and sedimentation rate.

47. **Jerri is a quadriplegic with a C6 spinal injury. She is admitted to the step-down unit for a possible myocardial infarction. While there, Jerri develops severe hypertension and headache. The hospitalist diagnoses autonomic hyperreflexia. What is one cause of autonomic hyperreflexia?**
   A. Diarrhea
   B. Suctioning
   C. Constipation
   D. Warm breeze

48. **What is autonomic hyperreflexia?**
   A. A malfunction of the autonomic nervous system seen with head injury
   B. A malfunction of the autonomic nervous system seen with spinal cord injury
   C. A malfunction of the autonomic nervous system seen with pituitary tumor removal
   D. A malfunction of the autonomic nervous system seen with epidural bleeds

49. **The nurse should anticipate which of the following treatments for syndrome of inappropriate antidiuretic hormone (SIADH)?**
   A. Fluid replacement, potassium chloride, Declomycin
   B. Fluid restriction, diuretics, sodium replacement, Declomycin
   C. Declomycin, vasopressin, diuretics
   D. Fluid restriction, potassium chloride, diuretics

50. **Part of the criteria for brain death is an absent doll's eyes reflex. Which of the following responses is seen as a normal response to the doll's eyes maneuver?**
   A. Disconjugate gaze with head turn
   B. Conjugate gaze in the opposite direction as the head is turned
   C. Conjugate gaze in the same direction as the head is turned
   D. Nystagmus with head turning

51. **What does the Glasgow Coma Scale measure?**
   A. Verbal response, orientation, activity
   B. Eye opening, motor response, verbal response
   C. Eye opening, orientation, motor response
   D. Verbal response, orientation, eye opening

52. **Sonia is comatose after cardiopulmonary resuscitation. Which Glasgow Coma Scale score indicates coma?**
   A. 8–10
   B. 6–7
   C. 5–6
   D. 4–5

53. **Susan P., an 18-year-old college student, was injured in a motor vehicle accident. This morning she began decerebrate posturing. As the PCCU nurse, you will anticipate which symptoms?**
   A. One arm flexed, one arm flaccid, legs flaccid
   B. Both arms fully extended and internally rotated, legs flaccid
   C. Both arms fully extended and internally rotated, legs fully extended with toes pointed
   D. Flaccid arms and legs extended

54. Felix has been transferred from the ICU to PCCU after a gunshot wound to his T11–T12 spine. Upon assessment, you find motor paralysis on the same side as the gunshot wound but loss of pain and temperature sensation on the opposite side. This is called
    A. Grey–Turner syndrome.
    B. Cushing syndrome.
    C. Syndrome X.
    D. Brown–Sequard syndrome.

55. Your telemetry patient suddenly develops right pupil dilation. What does this change indicate?
    A. Basilar skull fracture
    B. Uncal herniation
    C. Brain stem herniation
    D. Cerebrovascular accident

56. What is the most common bacteria causing meningococcal meningitis?
    A. *Streptococcus pneumoniae*
    B. *Neisseria meningitidis*
    C. *Staphylcoccus aureus*
    D. *Haemophilus influenzae*

57. What is the hallmark symptom of meningococcal meningitis?
    A. Headache
    B. Petechiae
    C. Malaise
    D. Vomiting

58. Ted was ill 4 days ago with a slight cold. Now he is experiencing ascending weakness in both legs. This symptom is suggestive of which of the following illnesses?
    A. Guillain-Barré syndrome
    B. Chronic fatigue syndrome
    C. Tetanus
    D. *Clostridium botulinum* infection

59. A positive Babinski or plantar reflex indicates a problem in which area?
    A. A reflex elicited with a reflex hammer to the Achilles tendon
    B. Normal neurologic functioning
    C. Upper motor neuron lesion of the pyramidal tract
    D. Lower motor neuron lesion of the pyramidal tract

60. What is the proper technique for eliciting a Babinski response?
    A. Stroke the sole of the foot from side to side
    B. Stroke the sole of the foot along the lateral sole from the heel up toward toes and across the ball of the foot
    C. Strike the heel and the ball of the foot
    D. Strike the Achilles tendon with a reflex hammer

61. Cerebrospinal fluid is formed in which location in the brain?
    A. Lateral ventricles
    B. Choroid plexus
    C. Subarachnoid space
    D. Arachnoid villi

62. What volume of cerebrospinal fluid is produced each day?
    A. 1,000–1,200 mL
    B. 600–700 mL
    C. 400–800 mL
    D. 800–900 mL

63. Henry is a 23-year-old with Guillain-Barré syndrome. When teaching this patient about his condition, you explain the differences between the various types of Guillain-Barré syndrome. Which of the following are the four types of Guillain-Barré syndrome?
    A. Ascending, progressive, relapsing–remitting, pure motor
    B. Ascending, descending, Miller–Fischer variant, pure motor
    C. Ascending, descending, relapsing, pure sensory
    D. Ascending, relapsing–remitting, pure motor, pure sensory

64. Amelia has had progressive symptoms of weakness, diplopia, and difficulty swallowing. Her neurologist suspects myasthenia gravis. Which one of the following tests is indicative of a myasthenia gravis diagnosis?
    A. Weber test
    B. Rinne test
    C. Tensilon test
    D. Clonus test

65. George B. is a 55-year-old high school teacher with meningitis. Today he is having a lumbar puncture. As his PCCU nurse, you know the cerebrospinal fluid (CSF) should be
    A. Hazy, with a glucose level of 85.
    B. Clear, with RBCs present.
    C. Clear and colorless, with less than 45 mg/dL of protein.
    D. Clear and colorless, with a white blood cell count more than 150 cells/mm^2.

66. While performing a neurologic examination, the six cardinal eye directions (cranial nerves) to assess for eye movement are
    A. CN II, III, and IV.
    B. CN III, IV, and VI.
    C. CN II, V, and VII.
    D. CN V, VI, and VII.

67. Your patient was an unrestrained driver in a motor vehicle crash where he struck and fractured the windshield. He has a left frontal lobe injury. Which symptoms would you expect with this patient?

A. Hearing and balance impairment
B. Sensory and memory problems
C. Personality changes, poor short-term memory
D. Loss of motor function, hearing problems

68. **Gwen, an 84-year-old female, has had a RIND. What does the acronym RIND stand for?**
    A. Recurrent ischemic neurologic default
    B. Reversible intracerebral neurologic deficit
    C. Recurrent intracerebral neurologic default
    D. Reversible ischemic neurologic deficit

69. **What differentiates a transient ischemic attack (TIA) from a reversible ischemic neurologic deficit (RIND)?**
    A. A TIA lasts less than 24 hours, a RIND lasts more than 24 hours.
    B. A TIA lasts less than 6 hours, a RIND lasts more than 48 hours.
    C. A TIA lasts more than 24 hours, a RIND lasts less than 24 hours.
    D. A TIA lasts less than 24 hours, a RIND lasts less than 6 hours.

70. **Your patient has had a major left-side stroke. What is the most common cause of stroke in the United States?**
    A. Uncontrolled diabetes mellitus
    B. Cocaine abuse
    C. Uncontrolled hypertension
    D. Tobacco addiction

71. **You are educating your patient and their family about stroke. Part of your talk involves modifiable risk factors for stroke. Which of the following are modifiable risk factors for stroke?**
    A. Alcohol use, obesity, family history
    B. Alcohol use, smoking, obesity
    C. Alcohol use, family history, smoking
    D. Alcohol use, family history, hypertension

72. **What are the two major types of stroke?**
    A. Ischemic and lacunar
    B. Ischemic and hemorrhagic
    C. Hemorrhagic and transient ischemic attack
    D. Hemorrhagic and reversible ischemic neurologic deficit

73. **Javier has newly diagnosed diabetes mellitus with an HgbA$_{1c}$ level of 10.3. You are explaining the long-term effects of uncontrolled diabetes, including the increased risk of stroke. Why does diabetes mellitus increase the risk of stroke?**
    A. Increased risk of hypertension
    B. Decreased neuroreceptor response in cerebral circulation
    C. Accelerated atherosclerosis of the large arteries
    D. Increased risk of clot formation

74. **Your patient with uncontrolled hypertension is most likely to have which type of stroke?**
    A. Ischemic
    B. Lacunar
    C. Transient ischemic attack
    D. Reversible neurologic deficit

75. **Which cerebral or cerebellar hemisphere is likely to be affected by stroke?**
    A. Right cerebellar hemisphere
    B. Right cerebral hemisphere
    C. Left cerebral hemisphere
    D. Left cerebellar hemisphere

76. **You are caring for a 72-year-old man with a left-sided cerebrovascular accident. Which symptoms do you expect to see?**
    A. Hearing deficits, left vision problems, left facial droop
    B. Speech deficits, loss of right visual field, right facial droop
    C. Loss of right visual field, receptive aphasia, left facial droop
    D. Speech deficits, left visual field loss, left facial droop

77. **Your priority in caring for a patient with a cerebrovascular accident is**
    A. Preventing decubitus ulcers.
    B. Preventing aspiration of food or fluid.
    C. Preventing contractures.
    D. Preventing depression.

78. **Jeremy has had a stroke and is now unable to communicate. Which area in the cerebrum controls verbal expression?**
    A. Wernicke's area
    B. Broca's area
    C. Limbic area
    D. Pontine area

79. **Fred F., an 80-year-old African-American man, has experienced a left temporal cerebrovascular accident due to uncontrolled hypertension. As the PCCU nurse, you know that Fred is likely to have which of the following deficits?**
    A. Motor deficits
    B. Expressive aphasia
    C. Receptive aphasia
    D. Balance deficits

80. **What is the homunculus?**
    A. A strip of the frontal lobe that affects motor skills
    B. A strip of the parietal lobe that affects sensory reception
    C. A strip in the cerebellum that affects balance and fine motor coordination
    D. A strip of cerebral cortex that involves the sensory and motor functioning

81. **Georgia, a 35-year-old woman, has Guillain-Barré syndrome. What is the most important measurement or test for this patient?**
    A. Blood pressure
    B. Negative inspiratory force (NIF)
    C. Pain level
    D. Cerebrospinal fluid study results

82. **Which results would you expect in the evaluation of the cerebrospinal fluid in a patient with Guillain-Barré syndrome?**
    A. Increased white blood cells
    B. Increased protein levels
    C. Increased glucose levels
    D. Anaerobic bacteria

83. **Which of the following nursing diagnoses would be the most appropriate for a patient with Guillain-Barré syndrome?**
    A. Impaired motor weakness, impaired respiratory function, acute pain
    B. Impaired respiratory function, impaired nutrition, acute pain
    C. Impaired motor weakness, impaired bowel function, acute pain
    D. Impaired respiratory function, impaired bowel function, acute pain

84. **Your patient with Guillain-Barré syndrome is experiencing a great deal of pain. Why is this occurring?**
    A. Parasympathetic function
    B. Sympathetic inactivity
    C. Autonomic dysfunction
    D. Sympathetic function

85. **Nursing management of a patient with Guillain-Barré syndrome includes which of the following measures?**
    A. Monitoring lab results and neurologic signs
    B. Monitoring respiratory status and neurologic signs
    C. Monitoring respiratory status and lab results
    D. Monitoring lab results and urinary output

86. **A nursing diagnosis for a patient with Guillain-Barré syndrome includes**
    A. Impaired nutrition.
    B. Risk for impaired respiratory function.
    C. Impaired fluid balance.
    D. Impaired body image.

87. **What is the vector for West Nile virus?**
    A. Fleas
    B. Field mice
    C. Birds
    D. Cockroaches

88. **What differentiates West Nile virus from other forms of vector-borne encephalitis?**
    A. Extreme fatigue and a diffuse papular rash
    B. Lymphadenopathy and extreme fatigue
    C. Erythematous rash and lymphadenopathy
    D. Bull's-eye rash and lymphadenopathy

89. **Jenny B. has had a transsphenoidal resection of a pituitary tumor. Her postoperative care should include**
    A. Monitoring vital signs, I&O, and neurologic signs.
    B. Monitoring neurologic signs, urinary output, and moustache dressing changes.
    C. Monitoring I&O, moustache dressing changes, and daily weights.
    D. Changing nasal packing daily, neurologic signs, and daily weights.

90. **Mark H. has three large aneurysms in his Circle of Willis. Which methods are used to treat aneurysms?**
    A. Clipping the aneurysms and endovascular coiling
    B. Clipping of the aneurysms and tPA administration
    C. Medical management of blood pressure and Amicar infusion
    D. Amicar infusion and tPA administration

91. **Death from status epilepticus is usually caused by which mechanism?**
    A. Airway blockage that leads to severe cerebral hypoxia
    B. Creation of a hypermetabolic state within the brain
    C. Falls from seizure, causing head trauma
    D. Aspiration pneumonia

92. **Nancy is a patient with new-onset grand mal seizures. While at the bedside you witness a seizure. What should you do first?**
    A. Hold the patient down to prevent injury
    B. Roll Nancy to her right side and protect her airway
    C. Insert an oral airway and call for help
    D. Hit the Code Blue button

93. **Jerry had a grand mal seizure lasting 70 seconds. As soon as the seizure passed, he was fully awake and asked for food. The PCCU nurse should**
    A. Tell the patient she knows he faked the seizure.
    B. Feed the patient.
    C. Notify the attending physician and anticipate a psychological evaluation.
    D. Give Dilantin 1 gram slowly.

94. **John Doe is admitted to the PCCU for seizure activity. The nurse should anticipate which of the following laboratory tests?**
    A. CBC, lipid panel, toxicology screen
    B. CBC, toxicology screen, LFTs
    C. CBC, CMP, lipid panel
    D. CBC, CMP, sedimentation rate, CRP, RPR, toxicology screen

95. **Continuing with the scenario from Question 94, which diagnoses should be considered for causing John Doe's seizures?**
    A. Alcohol abuse and hypertension
    B. Panic attack and psychological illness
    C. Panic attacks and transient ischemic attack
    D. Cardiac arrhythmias and hypertension

96. **The brain utilizes what percentage of the total resting cardiac output to maintain levels of glucose?**
    A. 30%
    B. 15–20%
    C. 40–50%
    D. 5–10%

97. **Which of the following potential causes of stroke is not a trait identified in Virchow's triad?**
    A. Hypocoagulopathy
    B. Hypercholesterolemia
    C. Flow disturbances
    D. Blood vessel wall abnormalities

98. **Stroke risk is increased if the patient has all of the following except**
    A. Sickle cell disease.
    B. Thrombocytosis.
    C. Polycythemia.
    D. Hypothermia.

99. **The type of imaging that utilizes radionucleotides, sugar, and a computer to help identify small blood vessels is**
    A. Computerized tomography (CT) scan.
    B. Digital subtraction angiography.
    C. Magnetic resonance imaging (MRI).
    D. Positron emission tomography (PET) scan.

100. **A nursing action prior to the patient undergoing an MRI is to ascertain if the patient has any _____ that would prevent the test from occurring.**
    A. autograft heart valves
    B. metal dental fillings
    C. unremoved bullets
    D. burn grafts

101. **A patient with a right brain injury may exhibit**
    A. Aphasia and partial paralysis of the face.
    B. Difficulty judging distance.
    C. Cautious behavior.
    D. Loss of pain sensation on the right side.

102. The most common type of stroke is the _____ stroke.
    A. lacunar
    B. subarachnoid
    C. hemorrhagic
    D. thrombotic

103. The most common lacunar syndrome is
    A. Sensory area blockage.
    B. Thalamic infarct.
    C. Pure motor stroke with hemiparesis.
    D. Dysarthria.

104. On the Hunt–Hess Grading System, a patient with some stupor and moderate hemiparesis is classified as
    A. Grade 2.
    B. Grade 3.
    C. Grade 4.
    D. Grade 5.

105. Using the NIH Scale, which score would you give to a patient with a severe total sensory loss?
    A. 0
    B. 1
    C. 2
    D. 3

You have completed the PCCN Neurology Questions section.

ANSWERS

1. **Correct Answer: A**
   There are many responses to sympathetic stimuli as the body prepares for "flight, fright, or fight." Also included are dilated pupils for increased visual acuity, increased heart rate, increased myocardial contractility, increased blood pressure, increased respiratory rate, decreased gastric motility, decreased gastric secretion, decreased urine output, decreased insulin production, and decreased renal blood flow.

2. **Correct Answer: D**
   Glaucoma is characterized by complications of increased intraocular pressure (IOP) and resulting damage to the ocular nerve. Coughing increases intracranial pressures and, therefore, intraocular pressures, resulting in further damage to the optic nerve. Nursing staff should take precautions to avoid any increase in intracranial or intraocular pressures.

3. **Correct Answer: C**
   Meniere's disease is a disease of the inner ear characterized by vertigo, tinnitus, sweating, nausea, and sensorineural hearing loss. Symptoms may incapacitate the person, because vertigo with nausea and vomiting may occur suddenly. Although symptoms usually begin between ages 30 and 60, some cases have been diagnosed as early as the late teens to early twenties.

4. **Correct Answer: C**
   Neurogenic shock is a distributive shock (or maldistribution of blood flow shock) characterized by massive vasodilation with blood pooling in the vessels without compensation. Spinal cord injury at the fifth thoracic (T5) vertebra or above, from spinal anesthesia or severe pain, may result in neurogenic shock. Treatment is based on the cause of the neurogenic shock, and includes spinal stabilization, fluid resuscitation, and vasoactive drug therapy to maintain blood pressure.

5. **Correct Answer: A**
   Spinal shock occurs hours to weeks after an injury to the spinal cord. The patient develops flaccidity, loss of sensation, and loss of bowel and bladder function. Answer B occurs after spinal shock resolves.

6. **Correct Answer: B**
   Myasthenia gravis is a pure motor disorder that occurs when an autoimmune response at the neuromuscular junction destroys acetylcholine receptors on the muscle membrane. Answer A is multiple sclerosis, answer C is Guillain-Barré syndrome, and answer D is amyotrophic lateral sclerosis (ALS).

7. **Correct Answer: C**
   Most myasthenia gravis symptoms are the result of the weakness caused by the lack of acetylcholine receptors at the neuromuscular junction. These symptoms include ptosis, diplopia, facial weakness, dysphagia, dysarthria, dysphagia, neck weakness, proximal limb weakness, respiratory weakness, and generalized weakness.

8. **Correct Answer: A**

Cholinergic crisis is a life-threatening problem with any overdose, accidental or otherwise. It causes bradycardia, severe weakness, cardiac arrest, and occasionally respiratory arrest.

9. **Correct Answer: A**

Spinal shock occurs hours to weeks after a spinal cord injury causing autonomic loss. The severity of the spinal cord injury cannot be fully assessed until the shock has resolved. The level of function for a patient with a spinal cord injury to T8 would include no abdominal reflexes and spastic paraplegia of the lower limbs, but the patient could be functionally independent.

10. **Correct Answer: B**

Neurogenic shock is a much more severe form of shock that may occur with spinal cord injuries at or above T6. The autonomic dysfunction causes increased vagal tone, which results in severe bradycardia, decreased cardiac output and peripheral dilatation.

11. **Correct Answer: B**

Approximately 85% of cerebral aneurysms are located at the anterior bifurcations of the circle of Willis and 15% at the posterior bifurcations.

12. **Correct Answer: D**

Explosive headache is the most common symptom of a rupturing cerebral aneurysm. "This is the worst headache of my life" is frequently the last thing patients say before losing consciousness.

13. **Correct Answer: C**

AVMs, in addition to being a complex tangle of misshapen blood vessels, lack the normal blood flow. In an AVM, arterial flow to venous flow occurs without going through a capillary bed. This high-pressure flow makes the AVM more likely to bleed. While AVMs are not common, they occur slightly more often in men. AVMs are the most common cause of stroke in children younger than 12 years of age.

14. **Correct Answer: B**

Glasgow Coma Scale assessment is imperative in monitoring for vascular spasm, a potentially life-threatening problem for a patient with a cerebral aneurysm. Vascular spasms occur secondary to meningeal irritation caused by the presence of blood in the subarachnoid space. The earliest sign of vasospasm is a change in the level of consciousness in the patient.

15. **Correct Answer: A**

"Encephalopathy" is an umbrella term for a collection of symptoms of other illnesses, which can include liver or renal failure, infection, brain tumors, increasing hydrocephalus, and environmental hazard exposure.

16. **Correct Answer: C**

Because it has so many potential causes, encephalopathy must be treated based on its cause. Examples of treatments include antibiotics, hemodialysis, and electrolyte replacement. Managing this patient's ammonia levels by the use of lactulose is another form of treatment.

17. **Correct Answer: B**
    Blood tests can include CMP, CBC, sedimentation rate, and tests for a specific illness or toxin. A lumbar puncture may also be performed to rule out neurologic infection. Other tests include electroencephalogram and imaging studies of specific structures (e.g., hepatic or renal imaging).

18. **Correct Answer: C**
    Level of consciousness is the most sensitive indicator of neurologic status in a patient. Brain tissues are extremely sensitive to even minute changes in oxygen and glucose levels. When cerebral edema occurs, as in a closed head injury, these levels very quickly affect the patient's level of consciousness.

19. **Correct Answer: B**
    Multiple sclerosis is a demyelinating disorder of the white matter of the brain and spinal cord. It can be intermittent, progressive or relapsing. MS follows either an acute or a progressive course. It is the major cause of disability in young adults age 16–40. It affects more females than males.

20. **Correct Answer: C**
    Frances is angry at her diagnosis and afraid she will suffer the same fate as her mother. The five stages of grief identified by Kübler-Ross in 1969 are denial, anger, bargaining, depression, and acceptance. The patient can move through these stages in any order and can revisit a stage at any time. The nurse should try to encourage the patient to express her feelings. The physician should also be notified, and the patient should receive counseling. Antidepressants may be considered.

21. **Correct Answer: C**
    Battle's sign is seen as ecchymosis over the mastoid bone 12–24 hours after the injury. Rhinorrhea, Raccoon eyes, and subconjunctival hemorrhage are all signs of an anterior fossa fracture.

22. **Correct Answer: A**
    The halo sign is indicative of a basilar skull fracture. It can be a dangerous sign for the patient, as meningitis can easily develop if bacteria enter the brain from the oropharynx.

23. **Correct Answer: B**
    Changes in intracranial pressure can be ominous and any change in the respiratory rate or pattern requires immediate assessment and intervention.

24. **Correct Answer: B**
    Normal intracranial pressure is 4–15 mm Hg.

25. **Correct Answer: D**
    Relapsing–remitting and progressive are the most common forms of multiple sclerosis. The frequency of relapsing–remitting episodes is related to stress and illness. Progressive disease may follow a continuous but slow route, or it may advance quickly to the patient's death. Relapsing–remitting disease may worsen to progressive MS.

26. **Correct Answer: B**
    The myelin sheath is produced by the oligodendrocytes in the brain and by the Schwann cells in the peripheral nervous system. Myelin is responsible for the rapidity

of nerve impulses from neuron to neuron and from the brain to the spinal cord. Impulses can travel as fast as 25,000 miles per second along an axon coated with myelin. This is why diseases such as multiple sclerosis affect mobility due to the destruction of myelin.

27. **Correct Answer: A**
Cushing syndrome is also known as the "triad of symptoms." These are late indicators of a serious deterioration of neurologic status. This patient is at very high risk for herniation and imminent death.

28. **Correct Answer: C**
Multiple sclerosis produces a wide variety of symptoms depending on the white matter that is affected by the exacerbation. These symptoms include both motor and sensory problems. Symptoms may include ataxia, Babinski reflex, vision disturbances, clumsiness, emotional lability, fatigue, parasthesias, paralysis, hyperactive deep tendon reflexes, loss of proprioception, loss of vibratory sense, impotence in men, and urinary problems in women.

29. **Correct Answer: D**
Lumbar punctures in a patient with increased intracranial pressure can lead to herniation of the tentorium or brain stem and death.

30. **Correct Answer: C**
Cerebrospinal fluid, when absorbed at an increased rate, decreases intracranial pressure. The other answers contribute to increased intracranial pressure.

31. **Correct Answer: C**
Changes in level of consciousness are seen before other symptoms develop because the cerebral cortex is extremely sensitive to oxygen pressure changes. Signs can be subtle at first, such as mild confusion.

32. **Correct Answer: C**
Diabetes insipidus (DI) is a serious decrease in antidiuretic hormone (ADH). The most common causes of neurogenic DI are closed head injury and posterior pituitary tumor removal. ADH is produced by the posterior pituitary gland. Closed head injury and cerebral edema lead to pressure on the pituitary gland, thereby decreasing ADH production. Other common causes of DI are lung cancer (small- or oat-cell carcinoma), leukemia, and lymphoma.

33. **Correct Answer: B**
Intravenous replacement with D_5W ½NS and 20 mEq potassium is titrated to replace hourly urine output. Other therapies include DDAVP (desmopressin) nasal spray or a pitressin infusion. Strict I&O, daily weights, monitoring electrolytes, serum and urine osmolalities, are also done.

34. **Correct Answer: A**
Triple H therapy reduces the chance of vasospasm of the affected arteries by maintaining full vessels. Cerebral vasospasm after an aneurysm bleed greatly increases the patient's mortality risk. These patients should be transferred to the intensive care unit as soon as possible.

35. **Correct Answer: C**

   Continued seizures deplete glucose and oxygen in the brain. The hypoxia causes cerebral edema, and increased lactic acidosis can lead to damage of the neurons.

36. **Correct Answer: B**

   Communicating hydrocephalus is caused when the blood cells from a subarachnoid hemorrhage block the arachnoid villi from reabsorbing the cerebrospinal fluid. This condition may be transient. If the condition is permanent, a ventriculo-peritoneal (VP) shunt will be placed.

37. **Correct Answer: B**

   Cerebral perfusion pressure (CPP) is a calculated measurement of the pressure gradient that allows blood to flow to the brain. The CPP may also be calculated using the central venous pressure (CVP) instead of the ICP because it is a measure of vascular resistance. The formula is CPP = MAP − ICP.

38. **Correct Answer: A**

   The goal is a CPP of 50–80 mm Hg.

39. **Correct Answer: A**

   Cranial nerve (CN) I is the frequently affected cranial nerve in a basilar skull fracture and leads to a loss of sense of smell. CN VII and CN VIII are less likely to be affected unless the patient suffers a severe head injury. CN VII (facial nerve) injury causes ipsilateral (same-side) paralysis. CN VIII (acoustic nerve) injury can interrupt balance and hearing.

40. **Correct Answer: B**

   Although the exact cause of multiple sclerosis is unknown, it is thought to be an autoimmune disorder triggered by environmental exposure or viral illness. Disease clusters in Northern European families have been identified, and there is a higher incidence in people who work with manganese.

41. **Correct Answer: C**

   Nystagmus indicates pressure or damage to cranial nerve VIII (acoustic) in the vestibular portion. Shaking is usually stronger on one side and may occur in any of the cardinal eye directions.

42. **Correct Answer: B**

   Syndrome of inappropriate antidiuretic hormone (SIADH) is caused by interrupted feedback of the osmotic stimuli and continuous antidiuretic hormone secretion. It causes fluid intoxication and electrolyte imbalance. Oat-cell carcinoma is a common cause due to its high rate of metastasis to the brain.

43. **Correct Answer: A**

   Syndrome of inappropriate antidiuretic hormone (SIADH) has many causes. The most common include bronchogenic (oat-cell) cancer, pneumonia, and head injury. Less common causes include stroke, tuberculosis, Guillain-Barré syndrome, meningitis, encephalitis, multiple sclerosis, subarachnoid hemorrhage, pancreatic cancer, and lymphoma.

44. **Correct Answer: D**

   The knee jerk, also known as the patellar reflex, is an example of a functional lower motor neuron. This reflex is also known as a deep tendon reflex. The nerve impulse makes an arc from the tendon to the sensory portion of the spinal cord to the motor root and back to the patella, causing extension of the lower leg.

45. **Correct Answer: C**
The spinothalamic tract carries impulses from the spine to the thalamus; thus it is a sensory motor tract. The lateral spinothalamic senses pain and temperature, whereas the anterior tract senses light touch and pressure. The spinal tracts can be identified by their names. For example, in the name "spinothalamic tract," "spino" means the tract starts in the spinal cord and "thalamic" means it terminates in the thalamus. By comparison, a cerebrospinal tract goes from the cerebral cortex to the spinal cord.

46. **Correct Answer: A**
Cerebral spinal fluid evaluation includes negative syphilis (RPR), abnormal colloid gold curve, increased IgG, myelin debris, and slightly increased protein. Other tests include FTA-ABS, sedimentation rate, HTLV-1 serology, and a check for vasculitic disorders. Neurologic testing includes evoked responses that are highly predictive for MS. MRI scans shows plaques as white spots in the brain.

47. **Correct Answer: C**
Autonomic hyperreflexia (also known as autonomic dysreflexia) is caused by numerous stimuli, such as bowel or bladder dysfunction, cool breezes, a clogged urinary catheter, and constipation.

48. **Correct Answer: B**
Autonomic hyperreflexia is a potentially life-threatening response to a minor stimuli seen after spinal cord injury at T6 or higher. It occurs after the initial spinal shock has resolved. Symptoms can include severe hypertension, dysrhythmias, severe headache, and photophobia.

49. **Correct Answer: B**
SIADH causes hemodilution therefore the treatment centers on normalizing serum and urine osmolality.

50. **Correct Answer: B**
The normal doll's eyes (oculocephalic) reflex results when the eyes appear to move to the opposite direction from the head turn. For example, if the head is turned quickly to the patient's left, the eyes normally appear to move to the far right side. If this reflex is absent, the eyes appear fixed and do not move. This is a poor neurologic sign. It represents pontine and midbrain damage. The doll's eyes reflex may be utilized in determining brain death.

51. **Correct Answer: B**
The Glasgow Coma Scale measures eye opening, motor response and verbal response. It rates each element on a total scale that ranges from 3 to 15, where 15 is a fully responsive patient. A score of 6–7 is comatose level. The longer that the patient remains in the lower score ranges, the worse the projected outcome.

52. **Correct Answer: B**
A score of 6–7 is comatose level on the Glasgow Coma Scale. A score of 15 is a patient who is fully awake. A score of 3 means there is no eye, motor, or verbal response from the patient.

53. **Correct Answer: C**
Decerebrate posturing demonstrates pressure on the midbrain and pons. It is a very poor neurologic sign, especially if it continues for more than 4 hours.

54. **Correct Answer: D**
Brown–Sequard syndrome causes ipsilateral (same-side) motor paralysis and contralateral (opposite-side) loss of pain and temperature sensation. This syndrome occurs because of the way the pyramidal tracts cross in the spinal column.

55. **Correct Answer: B**
Ipsilateral (same-side) pupil dilation is the symptom seen with uncal herniation across the tentorium. The tentorium is a fold of dura mater that supports the temporal and occipital lobes. This herniation puts pressure directly on CN III, causing pupil dilation.

56. **Correct Answer: B**
Neisseria meningitides is the causative agent for meningococcal meningitis. *Streptococcus pneumoniae* causes pneumococcal meningitis. *Haemophilus influenzae* causes *Haemophilus* meningitis. *Staphylococcus aureus* is not likely to cause meningitis but can cause infection in the brain if the patient has an open head injury.

57. **Correct Answer: B**
Petechiae are the hallmark symptom of meningococcal meningitis. The other symptoms can be seen with any form of meningitis.

58. **Correct Answer: A**
Guillain-Barré syndrome is a demyelinating autoimmune process that affects the spinal and cranial nerves. It is seen after viral infections. The most common form is the ascending variety, which demonstrates bilateral ascending weakness.

59. **Correct Answer: C**
A positive Babinski or plantar reflex is a sign of an upper motor neuron lesion. It can be seen with spinal cord compression, head injury and stroke. It is a pathologic sign.

60. **Correct Answer: B**
The proper technique follows the lateral sole of the foot from the heel up to and across the ball of the foot. It should be done in one motion with a relatively sharp instrument such as the end of a reflex hammer.

61. **Correct Answer: B**
Cerebrospinal fluid is formed by the choroid plexus of the third ventricle. The arachnoid villi, projections from the subarachnoid space, reabsorb the cerebrospinal fluid.

62. **Correct Answer: C**
The choroid plexus in the third ventricle produces 400–800 mL of cerebrospinal fluid (CSF) each day. There is approximately 125–150 mL of CSF circulating in the ventricular system and spinal column at one time.

63. **Correct Answer: B**
Ascending, descending, Miller–Fischer variant, and pure motor are the four types of Guillain-Barré syndrome. Ascending Guillain-Barré syndrome is the classic form of weakness and numbness that starts in the legs and moves up the trunk to involve the

cranial nerves in some patients; the weakness is symmetrical. Descending Guillain-Barré syndrome affects the cranial nerves first, and then the weakness progresses caudally; respiratory failure is a major problem for these patients. Miller–Fischer variant is a very rare form of Guillain-Barré syndrome that is characterized by a triad of symptoms that include ophthalmoplegia, areflexia, and pronounced ataxia. The pure motor form of Guillain-Barré syndrome is identical to the ascending form, but there is limited sensory involvement and, therefore, no pain.

64. **Correct Answer: C**
The Tensilon test is often used to test for myasthenia gravis because of the ease of administration. This medication, which is given as 10 mg intravenously, has a quick onset and short half-life. If there is improvement in a weak muscle, it is considered a positive Tensilon test. The Weber and Rinne tests are for hearing. Clonus is a reflex used to test spasticity.

65. **Correct Answer: C**
The cerebrospinal fluid should be clear and colorless, with a protein count of 16–45 mg/dL. The WBCs should be 0–5 cells/mm^2, and the glucose level is approximately 80% of the serum glucose.

66. **Correct Answer: B**
The six cardinal eye movements test CN II (oculomotor), CN IV (trochlear), and CN VI (abducens). CN III is assessed by having the patient follow the examiner's finger or a light up and out, up and in, down and out, and inward toward the nose. CN IV is assessed by having the patient follow the examiner's finger down and in toward the tip of the nose. CN VI is assessed by following the examiner's finger out toward the ear.

67. **Correct Answer: C**
The frontal lobe is responsible for personality, memory, motor function, Broca's area functions, and critical thinking skills.

68. **Correct Answer: D**
RIND stands for "reversible ischemic neurologic deficit." It is similar to a TIA but RIND symptoms last more than 24 hours; the patient then recovers completely.

69. **Correct Answer: A**
TIAs typically last a very short time, sometimes less than one hour, but no longer than 24 hours; they do not produce any permanent neurologic deficits. With a RIND, the symptoms last more than 24 hours but the patient still has a complete recovery. Both are possible precursors of a major stroke within a year.

70. **Correct Answer: C**
Uncontrolled hypertension is the most common cause of stroke in the United States. More than 360,000 strokes per year are attributed to hypertension. Stroke is the first symptom of hypertension for many patients. Diabetes mellitus can lead to cardiovascular disease and hypertension, but it is a less common cause of stroke than hypertension alone.

71. **Correct Answer: B**
Alcohol use, smoking, and obesity are all modifiable risk factors in preventing stroke.

72. **Correct Answer: B**
Hemorrhagic strokes are usually caused by hypertension and may include aneurysm rupture. Ischemic strokes are usually caused by an occlusion of an atherosclerotic cerebral artery secondary to an embolus or occlusion.

73. **Correct Answer: C**
Diabetes mellitus causes accelerated atherosclerosis in the large arteries of the cerebral circulation, thereby narrowing the lumen. This makes the diabetic patient much more likely to have a vascular event such as a stroke or myocardial infarction.

74. **Correct Answer: B**
A lacunar infarction is caused by thrombosis of the small arteries that penetrate the cerebrum. It leads to facial, arm, and leg deficits.

75. **Correct Answer: C**
The dominant side of the brain is the most likely site for a cerebrovascular accident. Because more than 90% of the population is right-side dominant, the left hemisphere is more likely to suffer a stroke.

76. **Correct Answer: B**
A left-sided cerebrovascular accident causes right-side deficits because of crossing of the cerebrospinal tracts in the brain and spinal cord.

77. **Correct Answer: B**
Prevention of aspiration should be the nurse's priority. The other answers are also a part of caring for a patient with a cerebrovascular accident, but the ABCs (airway, breathing, circulation) are always the first priority.

78. **Correct Answer: B**
Broca's area, found at the lower edge of the frontal lobe, is responsible for verbal expression. A deficit in this area is called expressive aphasia. The patient can comprehend what is said but lacks the ability to form the words due to loss of motor skills.

79. **Correct Answer: C**
This patient has had a stroke affecting Wernicke's area in the temporal lobe, which governs verbal reception. Damage to this area causes an inability to interpret speech and can also affect comprehension of written words.

80. **Correct Answer: D**
The homunculus is the outer strip of the cerebral cortex that governs the motor functioning of the frontal lobe and the sensory functioning of the parietal lobe. It demonstrates how much of the cortex controls each body part. For example, in the parietal lobe, very large sections of the cortex are devoted to the face, hands, and feet due to the complexity of the sensations necessary for protection. In the frontal lobe, larger portions of the motor cortex are devoted to the face, hands, and tongue.

81. **Correct Answer: B**
The negative inspiratory force measures the ability of the patient to take a deep breath to a pressure of minus 28 mm Hg. Once the effort is less than 28 mm Hg, the patient should be evaluated for intubation to prevent respiratory arrest.

82. **Correct Answer: B**
Protein in the CSF is always increased with Guillain-Barré syndrome due to the destruction of the myelin sheath. Because Guillain-Barré syndrome is an autoimmune disorder, WBCs, abnormal glucose levels, and bacteria would not be present in the CSF.

83. **Correct Answer: A**
Patients with Guillain-Barré syndrome experience motor weakness, impaired respiratory function, and acute pain—these are the most important nursing diagnoses. The pain is due to accentuated sympathetic response secondary to loss of parasympathetic counterbalance.

84. **Correct Answer: C**
Autonomic dysfunction in Guillain-Barré syndrome is caused by lack of balance in the autonomic nervous system. The sympathetic nervous system is unopposed, causing heightened sensitivity and over-response to even minor stimuli.

85. **Correct Answer: B**
Respiratory status and neurologic signs are the most important nursing management issues, especially in the early onset of the demyelinating process.

86. **Correct Answer: B**
Risk for impaired respiratory function is the most important nursing diagnosis. Other nursing diagnoses include acute pain, risk for impaired verbal communication, and potential for neuromuscular weakness related to demyelination.

87. **Correct Answer: C**
Crows are a well-known vector for the mosquitoes that spread West Nile virus. Fleas are the vector for bubonic plague, and field mice vector the Hantavirus.

88. **Correct Answer: C**
Erythematous rash and lymphadenopathy are indicative of infection with West Nile virus. Other common signs of any type of vector-borne viral encephalitis include flu-like symptoms such as fever, chills, malaise, headache, nausea, and vomiting.

89. **Correct Answer: B**
Monitoring neurologic signs, urinary output and moustache dressing changes are the most important postoperative care for the patient with a transsphenoidal resection of a pituitary tumor. Daily weights are important, as is monitoring of vital signs. Patients who undergo this surgery are at increased risk for diabetes insipidus due to a lack of ADH.

90. **Correct Answer: A**
Clipping of the aneurysm and endovascular coiling are the two most common methods of managing aneurysms. Tissue plasminogen activator (tPA) is a thrombolytic and would not be given to this patient. Controlling the blood pressure involves maintaining a good cerebral perfusion pressure to reduce the risk of vasospasm. Amicar inhibits plasminogen activator, allowing fibrin production.

91. **Correct Answer: B**
Status epilepticus decreases oxygen and glucose levels in the brain, leading to the release of glutamate. The increased production of glutamate causes an influx of calcium into the neurons, destabilizing them electronically, which leads to cell injury and death.

92. **Correct Answer: B**
    The best action is to turn the patient to her right side and protect her airway. Because the seizure has already started, it would be impossible to safely insert an oral airway. Never try to restrain a patient who is having a seizure. Hitting the Code Blue button is certainly an option but it doesn't help the patient immediately. Precipitating events, aura, onset, duration, nursing actions, and postictal state should be included in the nursing notes.

93. **Correct Answer: C**
    This patient should be given a psychological evaluation. If he had a genuine grand mal seizure, the postictal state would be expected to last several hours and the patient would not be able to request food.

94. **Correct Answer: D**
    CBC, CMP, sedimentation rate, CRP, RPR, and toxicology screen are the tests that need to be performed to establish the cause of John Doe's seizures. Seizures can be caused by illness, infection, overdose on drugs or alcohol, tertiary syphilis, dehydration, electrolyte imbalance, and cardiac arrhythmia.

95. **Correct Answer: C**
    Panic attacks, transient ischemic attacks, cardiac arrhythmias, and syncope are some causes of seizures.

96. **Correct Answer: B**
    The brain is the most metabolically active tissue in the body. It may utilize 15–20% of the total resting cardiac output to maintain glucose and oxygen levels necessary for metabolism. An ischemic event stops or slows blood flow and can be caused by embolism, low perfusion secondary to other states, or thrombosis. At a blood flow rate of less than 18 mL per 100 mg/min, irreversible damage occurs. This process is called the ischemic cascade.

97. **Correct Answer: B**
    Virchow's triad was identified almost two centuries ago. Blood vessel wall abnormalities, flow disturbances and coagulation disturbances were all found to be potential causes of stroke.

98. **Correct Answer: D**
    Sickle cell disease, thrombocytosis, and polycythemia all increase the risk of stroke because of how they alter blood flow, change blood viscosity, or affect coagulation. Hypothermia is sometimes used as a treatment for stroke to decrease the metabolic demands of the brain.

99. **Correct Answer: D**
    A positron emission tomography (PET) scan measures brain cell metabolism. In this test, a radionucleotide is combined with sugar. Tumors will utilize sugar faster than normal or healthy tissue does, so the computer can identify higher concentrations of nucleotides attached to the sugar in tumor tissue as compared to abnormal tissue. PET scans can determine if brain tissue is functioning even if blood flow to that area appears to be diminished.

100. **Correct Answer: C**
Any metal within the patient will be attracted to the MRI magnet, causing internal damage as the metal moves within the tissues. Metal heart valves, bullets, shrapnel, pacemakers, surgical clips, ear implants, metal rods and clips, metal plates, and BB shot all pose a risk with this type of imaging. Metal dental fillings are not prone to magnetic pull and are not a contraindication to MRI.

101. **Correct Answer: B**
Right-sided brain injuries exhibit left-sided paralysis. In addition to difficulty judging distance, the right brain stroke victim may have an altered sense of touch, pain, and temperature of the left side; partial or complete left-sided paralysis of the face, arm, and leg; and may act impulsively and without concern for safety.

102. **Correct Answer: D**
Thrombotic and embolic strokes are the two types of ischemic strokes that account for approximately 80% of all strokes. Patients usually have a significant history of hypertension, hyperlipidemia, and/or smoking. Thrombotic strokes account for approximately 52% of all ischemic strokes. They occur when blood clots block blood flow to the brain. Atherosclerosis increases the risk of clot formation around the plaque within the vessel, and carotid and vertebral arteries are at greatest risk. Most thrombotic strokes occur at night or early morning and are typically preceded by transient ischemic attacks (TIAs).

103. **Correct Answer: C**
Pure motor stroke with hemiparesis accounts for 33–50% of lacunar syndromes. Hemiparesis or hemiplegia typically affects the face, arms, and legs equally. Transient sensory symptoms may be evident, as well as dysarthria and dysphagia.

104. **Correct Answer: C**
Grade 4 indicates that the patient is stuporous, with moderate to severe hemiparesis and possibly early decerebrate rigidity. Grade 2 patients have severe headaches associated with nuchal rigidity and possible cranial nerve deficit. Grade 3 patients exhibit drowsy or confused mentation and may have a mild focal neurologic deficit. At Grade 5, the patient is typically comatose with decerebrate rigidity or flaccidity.

105. **Correct Answer: C**
NIHSS grades the patient on multiple factors: level of consciousness, ability to answer level of consciousness questions, ability to follow commands, visual gaze, visual field, facial palsy, motor function of the arms and legs, limb ataxia, sensory response, language, dysarthria, and extinction and inattention. Function in each section is assigned a score of 0, 1, or 2 points. The higher the score (in each category and total score), the more impaired the patient's function. A patient with total sensory loss would be scored at 2 points as the patient is totally unaware of being touched in the face, arms, or legs. Any sensation scores a 1 if the sensation is abnormal. Zero points are assigned if sensory function is normal and intact.

BIBLIOGRAPHY

Ahrens, T. (2006). *Critical care nursing certification.* Columbus, OH: McGraw-Hill.

Akopian, G., Gaspard, D. J., & Alexander, M. (2007). Outcomes of blunt head trauma without intracranial pressure monitoring. *American Surgeon, 73*(5), 447–450.

Alspach, J. G. (2006). *American Association of Critical-Care Nurses: Core curriculum for critical care nursing* (6th ed.). Philadelphia: Saunders.

American Association of Critical-Care Nurses. (2006). *Core curriculum for critical care nursing* (6th ed.). Philadelphia: Saunders.

American Association of Critical-Care Nurses. (2007). *AACN certification and core review for high acuity and critical care* (6th ed.). Philadelphia: Saunders.

American Heart Association. (2007). *Guidelines 2005 for cardiopulmonary resuscitation and emergency cardiovascular care.* Retrieved July 24, 2008, from http://circ.ahajournals.org/content/vol112/24_suppl

Bader, M. K., & Littlejohns, L. R. (2004). *AANN core curriculum for neuroscience nursing* (4th ed.). St. Louis: Saunders.

Ball, C., & Westhorpe, R. N. (2006). Muscle relaxants: Reversal agents. *Anaesthesia and Intensive Care, 34*(4), 415.

Barker, E. (Ed.). (2002). *Neuroscience nursing: A spectrum of care* (2nd ed.). St Louis: Mosby.

Bickley, L. S., & Szilagyi, P. G. (2003). *Bates' guide to physical examination and history taking* (8th ed.). Philadelphia: Lippincott, Williams & Wilkins.

Brain Injury Association of America. (2006). *Facts about traumatic brain injury.* Retrieved January 15, 2008, from http://www.biausa.org/aboutbi.htm

Braunwald, E., Fauci, A. S., Kasper, D. L., Hauser, S. L., Longo, D. L., & Jameson, J. L. (Eds.). (2001). *Harrison's principles of internal medicine* (15th ed.). New York: McGraw-Hill.

Britton, E., Harris, N., & Turton, A. (2008). An exploratory randomized controlled trial of assisted practice for improving sit-to-stand in stroke patients in the hospital setting. *Clinical Rehabilitation, 22*(5), 458–468.

Burns, S. M. (Ed.). (2007). *American Association of Critical-Care Nurses (AACN): AACN protocols for practice: Healing environments* (2nd ed.). Sudbury, MA: Jones and Bartlett.

Centers for Disease Control and Prevention. (2008). *Spinal cord injuries: Acute injury care.* Retrieved March 23, 2008, from http://www.cdc.gov/ncipc/dir/AcuteInjuryCare.htm

Chen, H., Richard, M., Sandler, D. P., Umbach, D. M., & Kamel, F. (2007). Head injury and amyotrophic lateral sclerosis. *American Journal of Epidemiology, 166*(7), 810–816.

Chernecky, C. C., & Berger, B. J. (2001). *Laboratory tests and diagnostic procedures* (3rd ed.). Philadelphia: Saunders.

Chieregato, A., Tanfani, A., Compagnone, C., Turrini, C., Sarpieri, F., Ravaldini, M., et al. (2007). Global cerebral blood flow and CPP after severe head injury: A xenon-CT study. *Intensive Care Medicine, 33*(5), 856–862.

Cho, S. J., Minn, Y. K., & Kwon, K. H. (2007). Stroke after burn. *Cerebrovascular Diseases, 24*(2–3), 261–263.

Copstead, L., & Banasik, J. L. (2000). *Pathophysiology: Biological and behavioral perspectives* (2nd ed.). Philadelphia: Saunders/Elsevier.

Crawford-Faucher, A. (2008). When is CT indicated after minor head injury? *American Family Physician, 77*(2), 228, 231.

Curley, M. A. Q. (1998). Patient–nurse synergy: Optimizing patients' outcomes. *American Journal of Critical Care, 7,* 64–72.

Delye, H., Verschueren, P., Depreitere, B., Verpoest, I., Berckmans, D., Vander Sloten, J., et al. (2007). Biomechanics of frontal skull fracture. *Journal of Neurotrauma, 24*(10), 1576–1586.

Dossey, B. M., Keegan, L., & Guzzetta, C. (2003). *Holistic nursing: A handbook for practice* (3rd ed.). Sudbury, MA: Jones and Bartlett.

Edwards, D. F. (1999). The Synergy Model: Linking patient needs to nurse competencies. *Critical Care Nurse, 19*(1), 88–98.

Eide, P. K., Bentsen, G., Stanisic, M., & Stubhaug, A. (2007). Association between intracranial pulse pressure levels and brain energy metabolism in a patient with an aneurysmal subarachnoid haemorrhage. *Acta Anaesthesiologica Scandinavica, 51*(9), 1273–1276.

Emergency Nurses Association & Newberry, L. (2003). *Sheehy's emergency nursing: Principles and practice* (5th ed.). St. Louis, MO: Mosby/Elsevier.

Flachenecker, P. (2007). Autonomic dysfunction in Guillain-Barré syndrome and multiple sclerosis. *Journal of Neurology, 254*(suppl), II96–II101.

Frank, J. (2008). Managing hypertension using combination therapy. *American Family Physician, 77*(9), 1279–1281, 1284–1286.

Gilman, S., & Newman, S. W. (2003). *Manter and Gatz's essentials of clinical neuroanatomy and neurophysiology* (10th ed.). Philadelphia: F. A. Davis.

Greim, B., Engel, C., Apel, A., & Zettl, U. K. (2007). Fatigue in neuroimmunological diseases. *Journal of Neurology, 254*(suppl), II102–II106.

Hardin, S. R., & Kaplow, R. (Eds.). (2004). *Synergy for clinical excellence: The AACN Synergy Model for Patient Care.* Sudbury, MA: Jones and Bartlett.

Hickey, J. V. (2002). *The clinical practice of neurological and neurosurgical nursing* (5th ed.). Philadelphia: Lippincott, Williams & Wilkins.

Hitzeman, N., & Applebaum, S. (2008). Oral anticoagulants vs. antiplatelet therapy. *American Family Physician, 77*(9), 1250–1252.

Hoge, C. H., McGurk, D., Thomas, J. L., Cox, A. L., Engel, C. C., & Castro, C. A. (2008). Mild traumatic brain injury in U.S. soldiers returning from Iraq. *New England Journal of Medicine, 358*(5), 453–463.

Hughes, R. A. C., Swan, A. V., Raphaël, J. C., Annane, D., van Koningsveld, R., & van Doorn, P. A. (2007). Immunotherapy for Guillain-Barré syndrome: A systematic review. *Brain, 130*(9), 2245–2257.

Information from your family doctor: Hypertension: What you should know. (2008). *American Family Physician, 77*(9), 1289.

Iseki, K., Mezaki, T., Kawamoto, Y., Tomimoto, H., Fukuyama, H., & Shibasaki, H. (2007). Concurrence of non-myasthenic symptoms with myasthenia gravis. *Neurological Sciences, 28*(2), 114–115.

Juurlink, D. N., Stukel, T. A., Kwong, J., Kopp, A., McGeer, A., Upshur, R. E., et al. (2006). Guillain-Barré syndrome after influenza vaccination in adults. *Archives of Internal Medicine, 166*(20), 2217–2221.

Kelsberg, G., Rubenstein, C., & St. Anna, L. (2008). Differential diagnosis of tremor. *American Family Physician, 77*(9), 1305–1306.

Keris, V., Lavendelis, E., & Macane, I. (2007). Association between implementation of clinical practice guidelines and outcome for traumatic brain injury. *World Journal of Surgery, 31*(6), 1352–1355.

Kilpatrick, A. M., LaDeau, S. L., & Marra, P. P. (2007). Ecology of West Nile virus transmission and its impact on birds in the Western hemisphere. *Auk, 124*(4), 1121–1136.

Labuz-Roszak, B., & Pierzchala, K. (2007). Difficulties in the diagnosis of autonomic dysfunction in multiple sclerosis. *Clinical Autonomic Research, 17*(6), 375–377.

Lipson, J. G., Dibble, S. L., & Minarik, P. A. (Eds.). (1996). *Culture and nursing care: A pocket guide.* San Francisco, CA: UCSF Nursing Press.

Logullo, F., Manicone, M., Di Bella, P., & Provinciali, L. (2006). Asymmetric Guillain-Barré syndrome. *Neurological Sciences, 27*(5), 355–359.

McCance, K. L., & Huether, S. E. (2002). *Pathophysiology: The biologic basis for disease in adults and children* (4th ed.). St. Louis, MO: Mosby.

McQuillan, K. A., Von Rueden, K. T., Hartsock, R. L., Flynn, M. B., & Whalen, E. (Eds.). (2002). *Trauma nursing: From resuscitation through rehabilitation* (3rd ed.). Philadelphia: Saunders/ Elsevier.

Medina, J., & Puntillo, K. (2006). *AACN protocols for practice: Palliative care and end-of-life issues in critical care.* Sudbury, MA: Jones and Bartlett.

Pagana, K. D., & Pagana, J. (2005). *Mosby's manual of diagnostic and laboratory tests* (3rd ed.). St. Louis, MO: Mosby/Elsevier.

Papadakis, M., Fee, P., Wilhelm, T., Davenport, A., & Connolly, J. (2007). Facial weakness in a haemodialysis patient. *Lancet, 369*(9562), 714.

Parker, T. M., Osternig, L. R., van Donkelaar, P., & Chou, L. S. (2007). Recovery of cognitive and dynamic motor function following concussion. *British Journal of Sports Medicine, 41*(12), 868.

Pascual, J. L., Maloney-Wilensky, E., Reilly, P. M., Sicoutris, C., Keutmann, M. K., Stein, S. C., et al. (2008, March). Resuscitation of hypotensive head-injured patients: Is hypertonic saline the answer? *American Surgeon, 74*(3), 253–259.

Ruff Dirksen, S., Mantik Lewis, S., & McLean Heitkemper, M. (2004). *Clinical companion to medical surgical nursing* (3rd ed.). St. Louis, MO: Mosby.

Ruts, L., van Koningsveld, R., Jacobs, B. C., & van Doorn, P. A. (2007). Determination of pain and response to methylprednisolone in Guillain-Barré syndrome. *Journal of Neurology, 254*(10), 1318–1323.

Sammarco, C. L. (2007). A case study: Identifying alcohol abuse in multiple sclerosis. *Journal of Neuroscience Nursing, 39*(6), 373–376.

Sejvar, J. J. (2007). The long-term outcomes of human West Nile virus infection. *Clinical Infectious Diseases, 44*(12), 1617.

Seneviratne, J., Mandrekar, J., Wijdicks, E. F. M., & Rabinstein, A. A. (2008). Noninvasive ventilation in myasthenic crisis. *Archives of Neurology, 65*(1), 54.

Siedel, H. M., Ball, J. W., Dains, J. E., & Benedict, G. W. (2003). *Mosby's physical examination handbook* (3rd ed.). St. Louis, MO: Mosby.

Siegel, A., & Siegel, H. (2002). *Neuroscience: Pretest self-assessment and review* (5th ed.). New York: McGraw-Hill.

Skidmore-Roth, L. (2004). *Mosby's 2004 nursing drug reference.* St. Louis, MO: Mosby/Elsevier.

Smeltzer, S., & Bare, B. G. (2003). *Brunner and Suddarth's textbook of medical–surgical nursing* (10th ed.). Philadelphia: Lippincott, Williams & Wilkins.

Sole, M. L., Hartshorn, J., & Lamborne, M. L. (2001). *Introduction to critical care nursing* (3rd ed.). Philadelphia: Saunders/Elsevier.

Stewart-Amidei, C., & Kunkel, J. A. (2001). *AANN's neuroscience nursing: Human responses to neurologic dysfunction* (2nd ed.). Philadelphia: Saunders.

Stocchetti, N., Colombo, A., Ortolano, F., Videtta, W., Marchesi, R., Longhi, L., et al. (2007). Time course of intracranial hypertension after traumatic brain injury. *Journal of Neurotrauma, 24*(8), 1339–1346.

Swinton, F., & Schuster-Bruce, M. (2007). Epidural haematomas. *Anaesthesia, 62*(12), 1299.

Takahashi, M., Tsunemi, T., Miyayosi, T., & Mizusawa, H. (2007). Reversible central neurogenic hyperventilation in an awake patient with multiple sclerosis. *Journal of Neurology, 254*(12), 1763–1764.

Tiemstra, J. D., & Khatkhate, N. (2007). Bell's palsy: Diagnosis and management. *American Family Physician, 76*(7), 997–1002.

Urden, L. D., Stacy, K. M., & Lough, M. E. (2007). *Thelan's critical care nursing: Diagnosis and management* (5th ed.). St. Louis, MO: Mosby.

van de Beek, D., Kremers, W., Daly, R. C., Edwards, B. S., Clavell, A. L., McGregor, C. G. A., et al. (2008). Effect of neurologic complications on outcome after heart transplant. *Archives of Neurology, 65*(2), 226.

Venes, D. (2001). *Taber's cyclopedic medical dictionary* (19th ed.). Philadelphia: F.A. Davis.

Wiegand, D. J. L., & Carlson, K. K. (Eds.). (2005). *AACN procedure manual for critical care* (5th ed.). Philadelphia: Elsevier.

Woods, S., Sivarajan Froelicher, E. S., & Motzer, S. U. (2000). *Cardiac nursing* (4th ed.). Philadelphia: Lippincott, Williams & Wilkins.

World Health Organization. (2006). Meningococcal vaccine and Guillain-Barré syndrome. *WHO Drug Information, 20*(4), 247–248.

Zhao, X., Rizzo, A., Malek, B., Fakhry, S., & Watson, J. (2008). Basilar skull fracture: A risk factor for transverse/sigmoid venous sinus obstruction. *Journal of Neurotrauma, 25*(2), 104–111.

Gastrointestinal

QUESTIONS

1. **A regular diet would be inappropriate for a stroke patient with which of the following cranial nerve(s) directly involved?**
   A. Cranial nerve I
   B. Cranial nerves II and III
   C. Cranial nerves V and VII
   D. Cranial nerve VIII

2. **Assessment of the abdomen should occur in which order?**
   A. Inspection, palpation, auscultation, percussion
   B. Auscultation, inspection, palpation, percussion
   C. Percussion, inspection, palpation, auscultation
   D. Inspection, auscultation, percussion, palpation

3. **Your patient has been diagnosed with chronic liver disease. In addition to a venous hum or murmur, you may note this finding during abdominal auscultation:**
   A. An aortic bruit
   B. A hepatic bruit
   C. An iliac artery bruit
   D. A renal artery bruit

4. **Your patient is suspected to have a biliary obstruction. Which of the following diagnostic procedures would confirm this diagnosis?**
   A. Flexible sigmoidoscopy
   B. Colonoscopy
   C. Angiography
   D. Endoscopic retrograde cholangiopancreatography (ERCP)

5. **Melena stools may indicate bleeding from which area?**
   A. Mouth
   B. Upper gastrointestinal
   C. Descending colon
   D. It is not from bleeding, but from iron ingestion.

6. **Normal portal pressures are**
   A. 5–10 mm Hg.
   B. 10–20 mm Hg.
   C. 5 mm Hg below the inferior vena cava pressure.
   D. 10 mm Hg above the inferior vena cava pressure.

7. Your patient has acute esophageal and gastric varices. Which esophagogastric tamponade tube is the best choice for differentiating bleeding from the esophagus and bleeding from the stomach?
   A. A Minnesota tube
   B. A Sengstaken–Blakemore tube
   C. A Linton–Nachlas tube
   D. A standard nasogastric tube

8. Your patient has a history of transsphenoidal hypohysectomy. Which of the following procedures is absolutely contraindicated?
   A. Nasal placement with gastric tube
   B. Oral placement with gastric tube
   C. Oral intubation with endotracheal tube
   D. Tracheal intubation

9. You have just assisted with the insertion of an esophageal and gastric balloon. Tamponade therapy duration should be carefully documented because
   A. Prolonged inflation may lead to necrosis or ulceration.
   B. Comfort increases 24 hours after placement.
   C. Hgb and Hct should drop after placement.
   D. Enteral feeding may be given via the tube after 36 hours.

10. Your patient with a Minnesota tube has a sudden drop in oral secretions and esophageal balloon pressures. You should
    A. Provide oral care and check the patient again in 2 hours.
    B. Document pressures and check the patient again in 2 hours.
    C. Check for bleeding and notify the physician.
    D. Attempt to reinflate the balloon to 70 mm Hg.

11. Your 18-year-old patient overdosed on Valium and Paxil. Gastric lavage is ordered. This is best accomplished if
    A. Done within 60 minutes of ingestion.
    B. 0.45% normal saline is used.
    C. Lavage is not recommended for this type of overdose.
    D. The ingestion is liquefied first.

12. The wife of your 60-year-old patient with newly diagnosed acute hepatitis A asks if her husband is getting better. The AST, ALT, alkaline phosphate, and GGT levels are returning to normal after being severely high. The PT, INR, and bilirubin levels are still rising. You tell her:
    A. "Of course. The important labs are improving."
    B. "I can't talk to you. You don't have power of attorney."
    C. "No, but you have to wait for the doctor."
    D. "Although some of the labs are stabilizing, the increasing PT, INR, and bilirubin levels indicate that your husband is still very ill."

13. **What is the most common postoperative complication following an appendectomy?**
    A. Wound infection
    B. Pancreatic abscess
    C. Fecal fistula
    D. Impacted bowel

14. **The daughters of your patient with severe biliary obstruction notice that their father has multiple scratches and excoriations over his skin. They are concerned that their father is being abused. You explain:**
    A. "Do not panic, we are not abusing him."
    B. "I understand you are concerned. Because of the high bilirubin levels, he scratches unconsciously."
    C. "He must have gotten out of the restraints."
    D. "He did it to himself as a result of PCCU psychosis."

15. **The most common cause of death related to acute hepatic failure is**
    A. Brain stem herniation.
    B. Anemia.
    C. Pulmonary embolism.
    D. Pulmonary edema.

16. **The family of your 41-year-old patient with chronic liver failure would like to know what they can do to make him more comfortable. You tell them that they can**
    A. Provide deep tissue massage every 2 hours.
    B. Apply a moisturizing lotion when visiting.
    C. Assist with rapid range-of-motion exercises every 4 hours.
    D. Limit visitation to once a day.

17. **Hepatic encephalopathy has _____ grades based on _____ clinical findings.**
    A. 3; 4
    B. 4; 4
    C. 4; 5
    D. 5; 5

18. **James is a 45-year-old crane operator who was admitted tonight to your unit with jaundice and profound ascites. He has a significant history for alcohol abuse. James is diagnosed with hepatorenal syndrome. Hepatorenal syndrome is a complication of hepatic failure due to**
    A. Increased circulating plasma.
    B. Vasodilatation.
    C. Increased renal circulation.
    D. Release of mediators.

19. Your 19-year-old patient was involved in a motor vehicle accident with blunt abdominal trauma related to the seat belt placement. He begins complaining of severe abdominal pain around the epigastric area that is knife-like and twisting. You also note a low-grade fever with diaphoresis, abdominal distention, decreased bowel tones, and rebound tenderness. You suspect
    A. Pancreatitis.
    B. Acute liver failure.
    C. Gastrointestinal bleeding.
    D. Abdominal bruising.

20. A patient with acute pancreatitis had labs drawn this morning. A result you would expect to see would be
    A. Elevated serum amylase.
    B. Decreased serum lipase.
    C. Elevated albumin.
    D. Decreased trypsin level.

21. Cullen's sign is
    A. A marbled appearance to the abdomen.
    B. Bruising of the scrotum or labia.
    C. Bluish discoloration of the flanks.
    D. Bluish discoloration of the periumbilical area.

22. Mrs. Jackson has been in the step-down unit for 2 weeks and has developed a stress ulcer. Family members ask why she has developed the ulcer. You acknowledge their concern and explain
    A. There is a decrease in blood flow to the stomach lining.
    B. There is an increase in mucus production.
    C. Ulcers are caused by fungal infections.
    D. Mrs. Jackson had the ulcer before she came into the hospital.

23. Mr. Gonzalez, a non-alcohol-abusing patient, was diagnosed with portal hypertension with direct variceal bleeding. His wedge hepatic venous pressure is less than his portal pressure due to portal vein thrombosis. This result may be caused by
    A. Chronic active hepatitis.
    B. Umbilical vein catheterization as a neonate.
    C. Metastatic carcinoma.
    D. Congestive heart failure.

24. Mr. Jones, who is 86 years old, is a frequent patient to your unit for alcohol-induced coma. Just prior to transfer to his board and care, he begins projectile vomiting bright blood. You would first
    A. Position the patient flat.
    B. Obtain and insert a Linton–Nachlas tube.
    C. Place the patient NPO and verify IV access.
    D. Start dopamine at 5 mcg/kg/min.

25. Mr. Davis is a 33-year-old businessman who is in town for an important conference. He was brought to the hospital after collapsing following complaints to hotel staff of continuous right upper quadrant pain, nausea, vomiting, and fever. He is complaining to you about his work schedule and not being able to take off work. He asks you which course of treatment will result in less hospital time. You tell him:
    A. "I understand your concern; I will ask the physician to speak to you about treatment options."
    B. "Delaying surgery may increase mortality."
    C. "Fifty percent of delayed surgery patients may require emergency surgery."
    D. "Laparoscopic surgery requires even less hospital time and has a decreased risk of bile duct injury."

26. Aaron, an 18-year-old student, was admitted with acute appendicitis four days ago. Antibiotics and morphine have since controlled his symptoms. As you are preparing to transfer him to home, Aaron asks if the pain will ever come back. You tell him:
    A. "No, you should not ever have this problem again."
    B. "Yes, but not for several years."
    C. "Yes, but the pain will not be as severe."
    D. "Possibly—about 33% of patients are readmitted and require surgery within 1 year."

27. Grant, a 21-year-old student, had an appendectomy in another state while on spring break one week ago. He is admitted to the DOU with fever, nausea and vomiting, and abdominal pain with a red, swollen surgical incision. You anticipate
    A. Immediate surgery with IV antibiotics.
    B. Hydration and antibiotics.
    C. Bedside excision of abscess.
    D. Bedside wound debridement.

28. Janice, a 41-year-old homemaker, just had surgery for peritonitis related to diverticulitis. During drug reconciliation, which of the following medications should Janice continue?
    A. Advil for headaches
    B. Prednisone for bronchitis
    C. Morphine for surgical pain
    D. Verapamil for atrial fibrillation

29. Jillian, a 5-foot, 8-inch tall, 20-year-old student, weighs 80 pounds. She was found unconscious by her roommate in the bathroom. She was admitted for severe dehydration and starvation. Which of the following lab results would you anticipate?
    A. Decreased serum lactate
    B. Normal urinary nitrogen excretion
    C. Decreased serum catecholamines, glucagon, and cortisol
    D. Conservation of body fluids with third spacing

30. Sara, an 18-year-old model, is a recovering anorexic. You are preparing to transfer her to her home when you note that she has not touched her lunch. You should tell her:

    A. "It's okay. I know that hospital food is not gourmet, but the dinners are more appetizing."
    B. "If you don't eat, we will have to put a feeding tube in you."
    C. "You need to eat to regain strength and prevent complications. We will work with you to find foods that you like."
    D. "Food is not your enemy. Eating this is not going to make you fat."

31. Wade, a 39-year-old alcoholic diagnosed with chronic pancreatitis, develops respiratory distress with dyspnea and pulmonary edema. These symptoms are probably due to

    A. Pulmonary capillary endothelial damage related to phospholipase A.
    B. Bronchospasm related to stress.
    C. Aspiration.
    D. Atelectasis.

32. Bill, a 58-year-old construction worker with cirrhosis, was admitted yesterday after a weekend party involving alcohol, drugs, and smoking. His A.M. lab results were as follows:

    ALT 250 U/L
    AST 150 U/L
    Bilirubin 10 mg/dL
    PT 23 sec
    PLT $76 \times 10^3/mm^3$
    Hgb 8.2 g/dL
    Hct 32%

    These results would indicate a high risk for

    A. Peptic ulcer disease.
    B. Variceal bleeding.
    C. Gastritis.
    D. Boerhaave's syndrome.

33. Nicolae, a 62-year-old Russian immigrant, is admitted to the DOU with vague epigastric discomfort, vomiting times one week, inability to eat more than a few bites of solid foods, weight loss, weakness, and postprandial fullness. Labs showed a Hgb of 10.8 g/dL and a positive stool guiac. Based on these findings, you would expect to see which of the following results after the upper gastrointestinal studies?

    A. "Unitis plastia" (leather bottle stomach)
    B. Localized ulcer
    C. Esophageal varices
    D. Pyloric stenosis

34. Gordon, a 74-year-old retired teacher, is being admitted for dehydration and malnutrition after collapsing in his apartment. His daughter reports that he has been eating very bland, soft foods for three weeks due to reflux and difficulty swallowing. You suspect

A. Partial tongue paralysis.

B. Gastric cancer.

C. Tracheal neoplasm.

D. Esophageal neoplasm.

35. **Joan's grandmother was diagnosed with colorectal cancer. Joan asks you how the location of the cancer is determined. You tell her:**

    A. "All locations present in the same way."

    B. "Only with an MRI test will we know for certain."

    C. "We will know only based on her lab results."

    D. "The symptoms present differently. A lower gastrointestinal series allows direct internal visualization of the location."

36. **Mort is visiting his mother, who just had colorectal cancer surgery. There is a familial history of polyposis and inflammatory bowel disease. Mort is worried about his risk of developing cancer. Which of the following statements is true regarding colorectal cancers?**

    A. Adenocarcinomas are the least common cancer.

    B. Right colon lesions are rare.

    C. Left colon tumors spread, ulcerate, and erode blood vessels.

    D. Rectal tumors are associated with localized metastasis.

37. **Which form of hepatitis is a DNA virus?**

    A. Hepatitis A

    B. Hepatitis B

    C. Hepatitis C

    D. Hepatitis D

38. **Which form of hepatitis is often misdiagnosed as gastroenteritis?**

    A. Hepatitis A

    B. Hepatitis B

    C. Hepatitis C

    D. Hepatitis E

39. **Peaches, a 22-year-old tattoo artist, complains of flu-like symptoms after a needle stick at work. She has increasing lethargy and decreased appetite with weight loss of 10 pounds. Generally a cheerful and active person, she reports overwhelming malaise with a sense of foreboding. Nursing interventions for Peaches would include**

    A. Weight-bearing physical therapy every 6 hours.

    B. Extended teaching sessions regarding her disease process.

    C. Orders for a low-fat, high-carbohydrate diet.

    D. Allowing visitors 24-hour visitation to cheer Peaches.

40. **Which of the following statements is true about hepatitis D?**

    A. Hepatitis D is detectable only when the patient has concurrent HBV infection.

    B. IgM rises late in hepatitis D infection.

    C. IgG rises slowly and limited to only the acute phase of hepatitis D infection.

    D. Hepatitis D is an RNA virus that is able to self-replicate when present in conjunction with HBV.

41. Georgina, a 24-year-old exchange student from Hungary, is brought in by her roommate after 7 weeks of flu-like symptoms, increasing bruising, headaches, pounding pulses, and fever. Which diagnosis and cause are mostly likely?
    A. DIC related to bacterial infection
    B. Acute liver failure related to unintentional overdose of acetaminophen
    C. Vitamin K deficiency related to poor nutritional intake
    D. Anemia related to Gaucher's disease

42. Which of the following lab tests would support a diagnosis of acute liver failure?
    A. Decreased creatinine and BUN
    B. Increased serum glucose
    C. Negative hepatitis serology
    D. Factors V and VII levels less than or equal to 20% of normal levels

43. Which of the following patients with acute liver failure has the best prognosis if liver transplantation does not occur?
    A. A 51-year-old healthcare worker with hepatitis C
    B. A 32-year-old hippie with *Galerina autumnalis* poisoning
    C. A 79-year-old patient who took an accidental overdose of acetaminophen
    D. A 21-year-old bone marrow transplant recipient with graft-versus-host disease

44. Ascites is a common finding with patients with chronic liver failure. Which of the following statements about ascites is true?
    A. Ascites is a result of an increase in albumin.
    B. Ascites is the result of decreased hydrostatic pressure and increased oncotic pressures in the portal system.
    C. Ascites occurs secondary to aldosteronism.
    D. An increased ventilation/perfusion (V/Q) ratio exists in ascites.

45. Calvin's wife is concerned that her husband with cirrhosis is not urinating. You tell her that this is a common complication of the disease process because there is
    A. An increase in the glomerular filtration ratio.
    B. An increase in renal blood flow.
    C. A decrease in sodium reabsorption, which means the patient's kidneys have shut down.
    D. An increase in renin and aldosterone levels, which causes poor urine output.

46. You are admitting an emergency room patient in the telemetry unit post head injury. As you perform your assessment, you note a stoma to the right iliac fossa in the lower abdomen. There are soft, scattered bowel tones. Output is loose, brownish tinged, without form. You would document your findings as a(n)
    A. Sigmoid colostomy.
    B. Ileostomy.
    C. Loop colostomy.
    D. Ascending colostomy.

47. **Mrs. Chan, a 42-year-old female with severe Crohn's disease and perforation, returns from surgery with an ileostomy. Mrs. Chan is at greatest risk for which of the following complications?**
    A. Prolapsed stoma due to vigorous exercise once discharged
    B. Hypernatremia
    C. Hemorrhage
    D. Dehydration

48. **Mr. H. had abdominal surgery for perforation yesterday. Today's abdominal X-rays show a "double-bubble" appearance. The patient is complaining of nausea with bile-stained emesis, abdominal distention, pain, and fever. The appropriate nursing intervention would be to**
    A. Contact the surgeon and prepare for immediate surgery.
    B. Administer morphine and Tylenol, and then call the physician if there is no improvement.
    C. Position the patient flat and give him Tylenol.
    D. Do nothing; this is normal. The physician should be notified only if the abdomen becomes discolored.

49. **Which of the following methods for measuring intra-abdominal pressures is most commonly used in the progressive care setting?**
    A. Intraperitoneal measuring with a peritoneal dialysis catheter
    B. Measurement of the bladder pressures via indwelling urinary catheter
    C. Intragastric measurement with a nasogastric tube
    D. Rectal measurement with a rectal tube

50. **Mr. K. was diagnosed with pancreatic cancer two weeks ago. A Whipple procedure is recommended. Which of the following health issues may worsen after this procedure is performed?**
    A. Diabetes
    B. Crohn's disease
    C. Hyperbilirubinemia
    D. Obesity

51. **During a Whipple procedure, which of the following organs is removed?**
    A. Gallbladder
    B. Esophagus
    C. Ascending colon
    D. Jejunum

52. **Mrs. P. underwent the Whipple procedure 10 days ago for pancreatic cancer. She was started on clear liquids and then advanced to a soft diet. Two hours after lunch, you enter her room to find her sweating profusely, shaking, and confused. You note tachypnea and tachycardia when assessing her vital signs. You suspect she is experiencing**
    A. An anxiety or panic attack.
    B. Gastroesophageal reflux disease (GERD).
    C. Dumping syndrome.
    D. Hypoglycemia.

53. Lea is experiencing dumping syndrome post gastric bypass surgery after eating any meal. Which of the following medications should Lea stop immediately?
    A. Nitroglycerin
    B. Insulin
    C. Pepcid
    D. Reglan

54. Your patient returned from abdominal surgery two hours ago. Now, you note decreased urine output, increased CVP, increased blood pressure, and restlessness. In addition, the pulse oximeter continuously alarms for low O_2 levels despite your repositioning of the device. Based on these findings, you would expect which intra-abdominal pressure value?
    A. 5 mm Hg
    B. 15 mm Hg
    C. 25 mm Hg
    D. 50 mm Hg

55. Hilda, a 24-year-old mother of six children, is 7 months pregnant when she is admitted to your unit for severe HELLP syndrome. She is also at risk for which of the following conditions?
    A. Intra-abdominal hypertension (IAH) and abdominal compartment syndrome (ACS)
    B. Decreased intracranial pressure (ICP)
    C. Hypocarbia
    D. Increased platelets

56. You just completed intra-abdominal pressure measurements via the bladder measurement method. When documenting the procedure in your notes, you should
    A. Write only "per policy and procedure"; no other documentation is required.
    B. Note the number of stopcocks used in the setup.
    C. Include the patient's position during the procedure.
    D. Indicate when the bladder clamp was released.

57. You are preparing Bill for a paracentesis. Which of the following actions is the first step in assisting with this procedure?
    A. Have the patient void or insert a Foley catheter
    B. Exam the abdomen for dullness
    C. Order an upright X-ray of the abdomen
    D. Position the patient with the affected side up

58. Which of the following lab results would be a contraindication for peritoneal lavage?
    A. RBC 5.2 million/mm^3
    B. PT 12.5 sec and PTT 75 sec
    C. PLT 79,000 mm^3/mL
    D. Hgb 14.7 g/dL and Hct 46%

59. Which of the following types of bowel obstructions leads to infarction or strangulation?

A. Acute

B. Subacute

C. Chronic

D. Intermittent

60. Joab, a 40-year-old Orthodox Jew, presents with an unintentional weight loss of 20 pounds, fatigue, anorexia, and chronic, watery diarrhea with bloody mucus. He is tachycardic, tachypneic, and hyperthermic, with an Hgb of 7 g/dL and Hct of 21%. You suspect

A. Colonic diverticulitis.

B. Ulcerative colitis.

C. Pancreatitis.

D. Cholecystitis.

61. Sam, a 60-year-old computer programmer, was hospitalized for a myocardial infarction with an emergency cardiopulmonary artery bypass graft surgery two days ago. He has been having recurrent uncontrolled atrial fibrillation intermittently for the last 10 hours. This evening he complains of abdominal pain with distention, intolerance for his soft diet, and nausea, vomiting, and fever. The physician orders a plain film of the abdomen. Which of the following results would you expect to see?

A. Air in the biliary tree with signs of small bowel obstruction and calculus in the pelvis

B. Dilated small bowel loops and air–fluid levels

C. Dilation of the entire bowel including the stomach, "thumbprinting," and pneumatosis intestinalis

D. Air under the diaphragm on the right upper chest or over the right lobe of the liver

62. Janet is being treated in the step-down unit for burns sustained to 15% of her body after being trapped in her house during a fire. She is at high risk for developing which of the following conditions?

A. Peptic ulcer

B. Pancreatitis

C. Cholecystitis

D. SRES

63. When checking nasogastric tube placement on your burn patient, you note frank blood returning from the tube. Which of the following therapies would be most effective in managing gastric bleeding in this patient?

A. Vasopressin infusion

B. Endoscopic thermal therapy

C. Endoscopic injection therapy

D. Variceal ligation

64. The physician orders gastric lavage to aid in controlling gastric bleeding in your burn patient. The best fluid choice for gastric lavage is

A. Hot tap water.

B. Iced 3% saline.

C. Iced sterile water.

D. Room-temperature normal saline.

65. During gastric lavage for gastric bleeding from stress-related erosion syndrome (SRES), your patient becomes tachycardic and complains of sudden abdominal pain and abdominal rigidity. You should
    A. Continue with the lavage; these symptoms are normal.
    B. Slow the infusion and change the fluid.
    C. Stop the infusion and rewarm the fluid.
    D. Stop the infusion and contact the physician.

66. Fernando has recurrent gallstones and has been treated medically at home for the last six months. He was brought into the ICU for severe dehydration, vomiting, and fever. On admission, your assessment reveals abdominal distention, guarding, tympany, absent bowel tones, and jaundice. He exhibits Grey–Turner's sign and Cullen's sign. His blood pressure is 75/50, heart rate is 140, and respiratory rate is 40 and shallow. You suspect
    A. Cholecystitis.
    B. Pancreatitis.
    C. Cirrhosis.
    D. Gastritis.

67. Your patient with severe acute pancreatitis now has a blood pressure of 70/40, with a heart rate of 146 and a respiratory rate of 42. You suspect hypovolemic shock. His hypovolemic shock is probably caused by
    A. Blood loss with a ruptured gallbladder.
    B. Third spacing related to capillary leaking.
    C. Insufficient volume intake related to vomiting.
    D. Excessive fluid loss due to diarrhea.

68. Your patient was diagnosed with Barrett's esophagus. Which of the following conditions is your patient at greatest risk for?
    A. Esophageal varices
    B. Gastritis
    C. Esophageal cancer
    D. GERD

69. Luis has been medically treated for GERD for the past three years. He has been admitted to your unit for aspiration pneumonia due to increasing difficulty swallowing and vomiting. He admits to noncompliance with his GERD medication regimen and was diagnosed with Barrett's esophagus six months ago. During his stay in the ICU, Luis is diagnosed with esophageal cancer. Which surgical procedure would Luis likely have to remove his cancer?
    A. Whipple
    B. Modified Whipple
    C. Esophagectomy
    D. Esophagastrectomy

70. Patients considering gastric bypass for weight management control should begin bariatric education
    A. Prior to the decision being made.
    B. When the decision to have surgery is made.
    C. Just prior to surgery.
    D. After surgery.

71. **Which of the following assessments is the most important when caring for a patient considering bariatric surgery?**
    A. Nutritional assessment
    B. Activity or muscular/skeletal assessment
    C. Psychological evaluation
    D. Physiological assessment

72. **You are preparing a patient for gastric bypass surgery when she states, "After surgery I will be able to eat whatever I want and never be fat again." Your response to her should be**
    A. "That's right, you are so lucky."
    B. "You may not be able to eat high-carbohydrate foods, but you won't ever be fat again."
    C. "You will need to modify your diet to avoid high-carbohydrate and sugary foods. You will still need to increase your activity level and control portions to avoid future weight gain."
    D. "You will need to eat fewer, larger meals of whatever you want."

73. **Which of the following bariatric surgical methods does not result in the suturing or removal of gastrointestinal tissue or organs?**
    A. Vertical banding
    B. Gastric banding
    C. Biliopancreatic diversion
    D. Roux-en-Y proximal gastric bypass

74. **Which of the following complications of gastric banding is the most common?**
    A. Stoma obstruction
    B. GERD
    C. Band slippage
    D. Stomach erosion

75. **Your patient underwent the Roux-en-Y gastric bypass procedure three 3 days ago. Which nutritional complication is your patient at greatest risk of developing?**
    A. Hypercalcemia
    B. Vitamin C deficiency
    C. Vitamin B_{12} deficiency
    D. Hyperalbuminism

76. **Which bariatric surgery method allows for a larger, usable stomach pouch?**
    A. Vertical banding
    B. Gastric banding
    C. Biliopancreatic diversion
    D. Roux-en-Y proximal gastric bypass

77. **Anastomotic leaks are common with bariatric surgeries. Symptoms can be subtle and may include hyperthermia, tachycardia, tachypnea, abdominal pain, and anxiety. If undiagnosed, all of the following complications may result except**
    A. Hyperoxia.
    B. Sepsis.
    C. MODS.
    D. Death.

78. Management of pain may be challenging in the bariatric patient. Management with opioids via a patient-controlled analgesic (PCA) pump is necessary to do all of the following except
    A. Prevent pulmonary emboli.
    B. Provide for early mobility.
    C. Prevent atelectasis.
    D. Early transition to oral pain medications.

79. The transjugular intrahepatic portosystemic shunt (TIPS) is used in which of the following types of patients?
    A. Patients with portal hypertension once bleeding has stopped
    B. Patients with a portal pressure gradient of < 10 mm Hg
    C. Transplant patients
    D. Patients with HITS

80. Sandostatin is ordered for your patient with portal hypertension. Which of the following nursing actions is most important to perform when first starting this drug?
    A. Carefully monitor input and output
    B. Check nerve stimulation
    C. Check blood glucose
    D. Check blood pressure every 5 minutes

81. Sarah is admitted to the intensive care unit for abdominal pain. She recently had knee surgery for which she received Tylenol #3 for pain control. She has no bowel sounds, her abdomen is firmly distended, and she is diffusely tender across the abdomen. What is probably wrong with Sarah?
    A. Appendicitis from the pain medications
    B. Pancreatitis from lack of exercise
    C. Gastroenteritis after eating undercooked chicken
    D. Paralytic ileus from the codeine

82. Cimetidine is not compatible with
    A. D_5LR.
    B. Propofol.
    C. Mannitol.
    D. Amphotericin B.

83. Bile is used to _____ triglycerides within the small intestines.
    A. digest
    B. emulsify
    C. transport
    D. compound

This concludes the Gastrointestinal Questions section.

ANSWERS

1. **Correct Answer: C**
    Cranial nerves V and VII control the trigeminal and facial nerves, which are needed for skeletal control during chewing. Cranial nerve I controls the olfactory nerve. Cranial nerves II and III control optic and oculomotor movements. Cranial nerve VIII corresponds with the vestibulocochlear nerve for auditory control.

2. **Correct Answer: D**
    Inspection determines landmarks and appearance, auscultation establishes location and quality of bowel tones, percussion notes whether tones are different for various internal organs, and palpation establishes wall tone, tenderness, and size of organs. Performing percussion and palpation prior to inspection or auscultation could affect the assessment findings. Although you may think this is too basic a concept to test, these simple things are often overlooked by test takers and may cause you to miss a question on the PCCN exam.

3. **Correct Answer: B**
    Hepatic bruits are heard over the liver. They may also indicate primary liver cancer, alcoholic hepatitis, or vascular liver metastases. An aortic bruit over the epigastric area indicates a partial aortic occlusion. Iliac artery bruits are heard over the left and/or right inguinal areas. Renal artery bruits indicate renal artery stenosis.

4. **Correct Answer: D**
    Endoscopic retrograde cholangiopancreatography (ERCP) visualizes the biliary and/or pancreatic ducts by flexible endoscope. Flexible sigmoidoscopy visualizes the rectum, sigmoid colon, and descending colon through the use of a 65-cm flexible scope. Colonoscopy views the colon from the rectum to the ileocecal valve. Angiography involves selective catheterization of the arterial system and venous portal system for blood flow analysis.

5. **Correct Answer: B**
    Melena is black, tarry stool containing 100 to 200 mL of blood from the upper gastrointestinal area or ascending colon. Oral bleeding may result in hematemesis. Descending colon bleeding may lead to bright red stools. Iron, bismuth, and other foods may cause tarry-looking stools that could be mistaken for melena, but an occult blood test of the stool will rule out this possibility.

6. **Correct Answer: A**
    Normal portal pressures are in the range of 5 to 10 mm Hg (7 to 14 cm H_2O). A higher value would indicate portal hypertension. Portal pressures should be 4 to 5 mm Hg higher than the inferior vena cava pressures. An even higher pressure would indicate severe portal hypertension.

7. **Correct Answer: A**
    The Minnesota tube has separate suction and balloons that can function independently. The Sengstaken–Blakemore tube has three lumens with only one suction port. The Linton–Nachlas tube is used for gastric varices only. The standard nasogastric tube has no balloon function to tamponade bleeding.

8. **Correct Answer: A**

   Transsphenoidal hypohysectomy allows for easier access into the cranial vault. Oral gastric tube placement is safe. Oral intubation carries no risk of an increase in complications. Tracheal intubations carry no increased risk of complications related to this history.

9. **Correct Answer: A**

   Maximum therapy time is 24 to 36 hours for esophageal balloons and 48 to 72 hours for gastric balloons. A longer time can lead to increased risk for necrosis, ulceration, erosion of skin around the nares, airway obstruction, and aspiration of gastric or oropharyngeal contents. Patient comfort decreases over time, and the risk of erosion to mucosal lining increases. Hgb and Hct levels should increase or stabilize with cessation of bleeding and blood replacement. The gastrointestinal lining may be inflamed related to blood in the system, and feedings should be held until bleeding is stopped.

10. **Correct Answer: C**

    A sudden drop in the balloon pressure and the patient's ability to swallow may indicate balloon or esophageal rupture, as evidenced by bleeding, and should be reported to the physician immediately. The patient should not be able to swallow when the balloon is inflated properly. An inflation pressure of 70 mm Hg is too high.

11. **Correct Answer: A**

    Unless taken enterically or in sustained-release form, materials are best lavaged within 60 minutes of ingestion and normal saline or tap water should be used. Lavage is contraindicated only if the overdose was from corrosive or hydrocarbon materials. Liquid ingestion would have a faster absorption rate than pill ingestion, so a liquid overdose would require faster treatment.

12. **Correct Answer: D**

    The lab changes indicate near-complete hepatocellular necrosis and indicates a still critical condition without diagnosing a condition. Answer A ignores the serious indicators of impending complete hepatocellular necrosis and gives rise to false hope. As for answer B, his wife has a right to the information as the patient's next of kin. Answer C does answer the question, but fails to provide appropriate information.

13. **Correct Answer: A**

    Wound infection is the postoperative complication most frequently seen following appendectomy. A fecal fistula can occur, but is quite rare.

14. **Correct Answer: B**

    This answer acknowledges the daughters' concerns and provides education. Elevated bilirubin levels deposited in the skin result in unconscious scratching and excoriations. In the presence of increased PT, PTT, and INR levels, hematomas may also form. Answer A provides no explanation for the scratches and decreases communication with the family. Restraints are inappropriate for this patient. ICU/PCCU psychosis can lead to abnormal behavior, but is not the reason for this patient's behavior.

15. **Correct Answer: A**

    Brain stem herniation is the most common cause of death related to increased coagulation times, intracranial hemorrhaging, and hypoxia leading to cerebral edema. Anemia is a complication of prolonged bleeding times, but is not the primary cause of death. Pulmonary impairment is the result of hemorrhaging, not embolism or edema.

16. **Correct Answer: B**
Skin becomes very dry as a result of chronic liver failure, and gentle application of a moisturizer may relieve the patient's discomfort. Deep tissue massage is contraindicated due to the decreased platelet count and increased bruising. Development of orthostatic hypertension prohibits any rapid movement on the patient's part due to dizziness and the increased risk of falls. Both the patient and family members are at risk for depression; visits may decrease this risk and will provide staff with opportunities to assess for and intervene if signs of depression are observed.

17. **Correct Answer: C**
Four grades of hepatic encephalopathy are distinguished based on five clinical findings: level of consciousness, orientation, intellectual function, behavior, mood. and neuromuscular function.

18. **Correct Answer: D**
The release of mediators results in vasoconstriction, which in turn diverts blood flow to the kidneys. The circulating plasma volume decreases as the patient develops ascites. Vasoconstriction, not vasodilatation, occurs in end-stage liver failure. Renal circulation decreases as a result of both the plasma shifting and vasoconstriction.

19. **Correct Answer: A**
Acute pancreatitis may occur as a result of seat belt trauma to the pancreatic duct or abdominal ischemia. Acute liver failure is characterized by flu-like symptoms, jaundice, confusion, and an enlarged liver. Gastrointestinal bleeding is associated with a history of ulcers and/or esophageal varices with hemodynamic changes, narrowing pulse pressures, hematemesis, and hyperactive bowel tones. Abdominal trauma does not produce knife-like and twisting pain, and tenderness and a marbled appearance would be noted if abdominal trauma is present.

20. **Correct Answer: A**
You would see an elevated serum amylase. Serum lipase would be elevated, not decreased. Albumin levels would drop, not increase. Trypsin levels would also increase, not decrease, with the buildup of pancreatic enzymes.

21. **Correct Answer: D**
Cullen's sign refers to the bluish discoloration of the periumbilical area seen in conjunction with pancreatitis and abdominal trauma. A marbled appearance is common with abdominal trauma. Coopernail's sign is bruising of the scrotum or labia. Turner's sign is bruising of the flanks.

22. **Correct Answer: A**
Severe illnesses result in blood shunting to protect cardiac, respiratory, and neurological functions. Any mucosal ischemia may lead to a loss of protective functions within the gastrointestinal system. Mucus acts to protect function within the gastrointestinal system, so a decrease in its production would be harmful. Fungal infections are rare within the gastrointestinal system; instead, bacteria are more commonly the causes of gastric ulcers. Although it is possible to have ulcers on admission to a step-down unit, the diagnosis in this case is a new onset.

23. **Correct Answer: B**

   Prehepatic (pre-sinusoidal) factors lead to hepatic venous pressures less than portal pressures. Umbilical vein catheterizations as a neonate (within the first month of life) due to neonatal illness or prematurity may cause damage to the vessel. Chronic active hepatitis is an intrahepatic (sinusoidal) factor. Wedge hepatic venous pressures are increased or equal to portal pressures. Metastatic carcinoma and cardiac diseases such as CHF can cause portal hypertension and may indirectly cause variceal bleeding.

24. **Correct Answer: C**

   This patient has likely ruptured small varices. Priorities are to maintain the patient's airway, stop bleeding, and verify venous access for blood replacement, fluid management, and homeostasis. Placing the patient NPO and obtaining IV access is the first correct answer listed. You would want to position the patient upright (not flat) to prevent aspiration. You would anticipate the placement of a Minnesota tube, not a Linton–Nachlas tube. Administration of dopamine at 5 mcg/kg/min would better support renal function, not blood pressure, as is needed in this patient.

25. **Correct Answer: A**

   Early surgery (within 7 days of signs and symptoms of onset) usually leads to a shorter hospital stay. It is more appropriate for the nurse to refer treatment options to the physician. A delay in surgery may lead to increased severity of symptoms, although it is not associated with any change in mortality or complications. Only 25% of delayed surgeries may become urgent. Laparoscopic surgeries are associated with shorter hospital stays as compared to open surgeries, but they carry an increased risk of bile duct injuries and 25% of these surgeries may require open surgical interventions related to complications. However, the nurse should not mention the risk of bile duct injury in this case because the patient has yet to be diagnosed.

26. **Correct Answer: D**

   This question requires honest communication with the patient regarding possible reoccurrence of symptoms. Approximately 33% of patients with appendicitis who are treated with antibiotics and pain management are readmitted and require appendectomies within one year. These remaining answers are stated as absolutes and are inappropriate responses for a practitioner. Because his appendix was not removed, this patient may have a reoccurrence of symptoms at a later date. There is no way to predict if and when an appendix may become infected or diseased. There is also no way to predict the severity of pain with appendicitis, as pain is perceived differently by each patient.

27. **Correct Answer: A**

   This patient is exhibiting signs and symptoms of an abscess post surgical intervention for appendicitis. This complication occurs in 5–33% of patients. Surgical debridement of the incision and IV antibiotics are appropriate immediate treatments to prevent sepsis. Hydration and antibiotics alone will not treat the abscess. Bedside excision of the abscess alone may reduce the amount of infected fluid and tissue at the site, but it will not prevent further infection. Bedside wound debridement places the patient at a high risk of further contamination of the site. In approximately 2% of cases, the abscess may be intra-abdominal and may require surgical intervention under anesthesia as well as continued antibiotic treatment.

28. **Correct Answer: D**

    This patient may safely continue Verapamil for atrial fibrillation. Calcium-channel blockers have been found to provide some protection against complications of diverticulae. By contrast, nonsteroidal anti-inflammatory drugs (NSAIDs), corticosteroids, and opiate analgesics have been noted to increase the risk of perforation of diverticulae.

29. **Correct Answer: D**

    Prolonged starvation and protein loss result in fluid shifting and third spacing. Muscle wasting results in an increase in serum lactate levels, not a decrease. Initially, urinary nitrogen excretion increases, but it is eventually followed by a decrease. Serum catecholamine, glucagons, and cortisol levels increase as the body releases elements in an attempt to maintain the amount of energy and glucose available.

30. **Correct Answer: C**

    The goal when working with bulimic and anorexic patients is to support positive nutritional changes while acknowledging and supporting the psychological changes in body and food perception. By acknowledging the difficulties the patient has with food perception and being willing to provide support and counseling with a nutritionist, dietician, and psychologist the patient will find foods that are both appealing and provide needed nutrition. The remaining answers are abrasive or do not address the patient's physiological or psychological struggle with eating.

31. **Correct Answer: A**

    Chronic pancreatitis results in the release of digestive enzymes into the body. Phospholipase A_2 breaks down the cellular structure of the capillary beds, resulting in tissue injury throughout the body. In the lungs, capillary damage is manifested as pulmonary edema and dyspnea leading to respiratory distress. Although stress may lead to bronchospasm in patients with existing respiratory diseases such as asthma, the information given in the question does not provide any evidence of that finding. Aspiration and atelectasis are common complications in patients who require progressive care, but do not explain both symptoms as related to the ongoing disease process.

32. **Correct Answer: B**

    Fifty percent of all deaths of patients with cirrhosis are caused by variceal bleeding. These lab tests are used to differentiate causes of bleeding. The patient's history and lab values lean toward a diagnosis of varices. Although Hgb and Hct levels would be decreased in peptic ulcer disease and gastritis, the other lab changes would not be occurring with those conditions. Boerhaave's syndrome is a full-thickness rupture or perforation of the esophageal wall due to prolonged and frequent vomiting related to eating disorders.

33. **Correct Answer: A**

    This patient is exhibiting both subjective and objective signs and symptoms of stomach cancer. There is a higher incidence of stomach cancer in males 50 to 70 years of age from cultures farthest from the equator. With this diagnosis, an upper gastrointestinal series would show a "leather bottle" stomach. The patient's symptoms do not support a diagnosis of an ulcer. Radiological studies would show ulceration or free air with perforation. Radiological studies for varices would not show any distinct changes. Pyloric stenosis is typically seen in infants and would be manifested as a distended abdomen with nonbilious, projectile vomiting.

34. **Correct Answer: D**

This patient is exhibiting classic signs and symptoms of a developing esophageal neoplasm. Complications that coincide with this disease process are related to changes in nutritional intake. Narrowing of the esophageal lumen results in increasing difficulties and pain when swallowing, which leads to the patient consuming an increasingly softer diet until the patient can swallow only liquids. A diagnosis of partial tongue paralysis would be supported if the patient also had difficulty speaking, but that is not a symptom given here. Gastric cancer is characterized by indigestion and fullness, not difficulty swallowing. Tracheal neoplasm would be associated with more respiratory distress.

35. **Correct Answer: D**

Colorectal neoplasms present differently depending on their location. A lower gastrointestinal series, such as a sigmoidoscopy, allows for direct visualization of the cancer if it is within the lumen. Biopsy provides the definitive diagnosis.

36. **Correct Answer: C**

Left (descending) colon lesions spread, ulcerate, and will erode blood vessels within the colon. Obstruction is a very common complication with this type of lesion. Adenocarcinomas are the most common types of neoplasms. Right (ascending) colon lesions are typically polypoid lesions and are associated with a familial history of polyps. Rectal lesions may spread to the vagina or prostate, but are known for systemic metastasis.

37. **Correct Answer: B**

Hepatitis B is the only DNA virus listed. The other forms of hepatitis are RNA viruses.

38. **Correct Answer: A**

Hepatitis A is often misdiagnosed initially as gastroenteritis because its symptoms are usually self-limiting. Fecal–oral transmission may also be mistaken for food poisoning.

39. **Correct Answer: D**

This patient's history and symptoms are consistent with new-onset hepatitis C. Hepatitis C results in a hypermetabolic state. Nursing interventions should focus on minimizing symptoms and reducing stress on the body. A low-fat, high-carbohydrate diet supports an increase in caloric demand and prevents weight loss. The greater the liver compromise related to infection, the lower the fat and protein intake, as the liver may not be able to assist with effective digestion. This patient should remain on strict bed rest to allow for energy conservation in the acute phase. Light ambulation is permitted as long as the patient is not fatigued with the activity. Although teaching is vital for this patient, extended teaching sessions may tax the patient's ability to concentrate. Teaching should be available in multiple forms that can be utilized at the patient's leisure. Family may be supportive, but planned rest periods should be maintained and supported as patient tolerance allows.

40. **Correct Answer: A**

The hepatitis D virus (HDV) can replicate only when hepatitis B virus (HBV) is present. When HDV is present, either as a co-infection or a super-infection, liver disease and progression are more rapid and severe. The IgM level rises early in infection and may remain chronically high. The IgG level rises slowly during the course of the infection, but the increase will continue for life.

41. **Correct Answer: B**

Acute liver failure related to acetaminophen overdose would be consistent with this patient's presentation. Individuals without full command of the English language are at risk for overdose when self-medicating if the medication label is not read and understood correctly. The patient's symptoms are inconsistent with the presentation of DIC and vitamin K deficiency. Gaucher's disease is a genetic enzyme deficiency disease that is typically diagnosed in childhood; its symptoms are progressive, occurring as glucocerebroside is collected in the spleen and liver. In Gaucher's disease, the patient would present with skeletal weakness, neurological complications, swollen lymph nodes, and pain not related to just the last 7 weeks.

42. **Correct Answer: D**

As the liver becomes compromised, symptoms reflect the inefficiency of the liver functions, with clotting Factors V and VII levels less than or equal to 20% of normal levels. In acute liver failure, creatinine and BUN values will be increased, while serum glucose levels will be decreased. Any patient with new-onset, acute hepatic failure should be tested for all forms of hepatitis. Hepatitis is one of the leading causes of acute liver failure and may be first diagnosed when liver failure presents.

43. **Correct Answer: C**

The patient with acetaminophen overdose has the best prognosis even in the absence of a liver transplant. The patients with viral hepatitis, *Galerina autumnalis* (poisonous mushroom) ingestion, and bone marrow transplant all have very poor prognoses if liver transplants do not become available. Management goals include stabilizing hemodynamics, preventing infection, maintaining stable glucose levels, protecting the airway, and supporting adequate tissue perfusion.

44. **Correct Answer: C**

Aldosteronism initiates sodium retention, thereby increasing portal hypertension. Low albumin levels accompanied by increased hydrostatic pressure and decreased oncotic pressures result in ascites. As a result of fluid shifting, the ventilation/perfusion (V/Q) ratio would decrease.

45. **Correct Answer: D**

Due to the cirrhosis, renal function may be impaired, resulting in poor urine output. Common complications that lead to poor urine output are an increased secretion of renin and aldosterone, leading to sodium retention. Both the glomerular filtration rate and renal blood flow decrease when cirrhosis is present.

46. **Correct Answer: B**

An ileostomy is located at the right ileac fossa just prior to the colon. The majority of water absorption occurs in the colon, so stool from the small intestines is loose and unformed. Sigmoid colostomy stools more closely resemble normal stools because most of the water has been absorbed at this point. Loop, transverse, and ascending colostomies are all characterized by loose stools.

47. **Correct Answer: D**

Dehydration is a severe complication with ileostomy because water reabsorption is accomplished by the colon. This patient may have had a large portion or all of the large intestine removed related to the Crohn's disease process. Oral fluids should be encouraged and IV support maintained to prevent hypovolemic shock. Postoperative teaching should include signs and symptoms of shock and preventive home management. Although a stoma prolapse may occur after discharge home, the stoma can be reopened without major complications. Hyponatremia, not hypernatremia, is a serious complication, as sodium uptake also occurs in the colon. Hemorrhage is not a concern unless the stoma is scratched or damaged during care. Light pressure should be applied until the bleeding stops, but it is not a life-threatening complication.

48. **Correct Answer: A**
The patient is exhibiting signs and symptoms of malrotation and duodenal obstruction related to a volvulus. The nurse should contact the physician immediately and prepare for surgery before necrosis of the bowel occurs. Tylenol and morphine will mask these serious symptoms. Pain is related to the ischemia experienced by the intestines when the malrotation cuts off the blood supply. Fever may indicate perforation or necrosis of the intestines impacted by the volvulus. The patient will need to sit upright to prevent aspiration post vomiting. These symptoms are not normal, and discoloration of the abdomen indicates greater ischemia and a higher risk of perforation.

49. **Correct Answer: B**
The method most commonly used to measure intra-abdominal pressure is via the bladder. A specialized catheter with transducer allows for direct measurement of pressures with equipment that is usually found in the critical care unit.

50. **Correct Answer: A**
If a patient has been diagnosed with diabetes or has uncontrolled blood glucose levels, then removal of the pancreatic head may result in diabetes or worsening symptoms. It is imperative that the patient's blood glucose levels be monitored closely. Even with removal of only part of the pancreas, the pancreas may not produce and release insulin at previous levels; as a consequence, insulin injections may be required. The Whipple procedure removes part of the bile duct, which may improve bilirubin levels. With removal of part of the stomach and pancreas, patients are at risk of long-term malnutrition and weight loss.

51. **Correct Answer: A**
The Whipple procedure removes the tip or head of the pancreas, the gallbladder, the duodenum, and part of the bile duct. Occasionally, part of the stomach may also be removed. The extent of the cancerous pancreatic tumor will dictate the extent of removal.

52. **Correct Answer: C**
Mrs. P.'s symptoms are consistent with late dumping syndrome, related to the partial gastrectomy during the Whipple procedure. With late dumping syndrome, symptoms occur 1 to 3 hours after meals. Additional symptoms include weakness, fatigue, dizziness, anxiety, palpitations, and fainting. Patients may also exhibit early signs of dumping syndrome approximately 15 to 30 minutes after a meal: nausea, vomiting, cramps or abdominal pain, diarrhea, bloating, tachycardia, dysrhythmias, and dizziness. Although anxiety may be exhibited with dumping syndrome, an alteration in mental status when combined with the patient's food consumption and history support a dumping syndrome diagnosis. Hypoglycemia is a greater risk for patients who have undergone a simple gastrectomy or bypass. GERD presents with heartburn and epigastric pain.

53. **Correct Answer: D**
Reglan increases gastric emptying by increasing peristalsis, thereby exacerbating the effects of dumping syndrome. Reglan may be used post gastrectomy when gastroparesis is present. Once peristalsis has resumed, this medication should be stopped.

54. **Correct Answer: C**
Intra-abdominal pressures of 5 to 15 mm Hg indicate a low to moderate pressure problem. When respiratory function is impaired, values may range as high as 25 mm Hg. You would expect to see increased respiratory distress and compromise. Severe compromise is seen with intra-abdominal pressures exceeding 40 mm Hg. Thoracic pressures increase as intra-abdominal pressures increase, inhibiting lung expansion and diaphragm movement and resulting in hypoventilation and hypoxia.

This question is intended more to convey information than to test your knowledge. Some progressive care units have the capability of measuring intra-abdominal pressures, but most do not. We wanted you to know which values are normal and what might affect these values, just in case a future exam contains a similar question.

55. **Correct Answer: A**
Because of the patient's pregnancy and resulting HELLP syndrome, she is at increased risk for fluid buildup in the abdominal cavity and for tissue edema. Signs and symptoms of IAH and ACS include increased ICP, hypercarbia, decreased platelet values, decreased cardiac output, poor or absent urinary output, and abdominal wall rigidity.

We deliberately made this mother quite young to serve as a distracter of sorts. You probably found yourself thinking, "How can this mother be so young and already have all these kids and be pregnant again?" That line of thought keeps you from focusing on the point of the question, which is HELLP syndrome.

56. **Correct Answer: C**
Documentation for IAP should include vital signs prior to the procedure, patient position and abdominal values, vital signs during and after the procedure, changes in patient assessment, amount of fluid into the bladder, output amount subtracted from input, any outcomes, interventions, reportable conditions, and any education provided. (This is another FYI question.)

57. **Correct Answer: A**
The correct order for these interventions when assisting with a paracentesis is (1) have the patient void or insert a Foley catheter, (2) order an upright X-ray of the abdomen, (3) position the patient with the affected side up, and (4) examine the abdomen for dullness.

58. **Correct Answer: C**
A patient with a platelet count of 79,000 mm^3/mL is thrombocytopenic and at risk for coagulation complications. Heparin is normally added to the solution to prevent clotting and can lead to further complications of bleeding. The other lab values are within normal ranges for either males or females.

59. **Correct Answer: A**
Acute bowel obstruction is the only type of obstruction that leads to infarction or strangulation. Obstruction occurs rapidly and may inhibit blood flow to a portion of the bowel. The other types of obstructions permit limited or intermittent blood flow that sustains but compromises tissue function.

60. **Correct Answer: B**

    Based on his presenting symptoms and ethnicity, Joab has ulcerative colitis. He may also have leukocytosis and cachexia. Colonic diverticulitis presents with left upper quadrant pain, hyperthermia, vomiting, chills, diarrhea, and tenderness over the descending colon. Pancreatitis presents with left upper quadrant pain that radiates to the back or chest, hyperthermia, rigidity, rebound abdominal tenderness, nausea and vomiting, jaundice, Cullen's sign, Grey–Turner's sign, abdominal distention, and diminished bowel sounds. Cholecystitis presents with right upper quadrant or epigastric pain, pain that lasts as long as 6 hours after a fatty meal, vomiting, and increased white blood cell counts.

61. **Correct Answer: B**

    This patient is exhibiting signs of early ischemic bowel. At this time, there will be some dilation of the bowel, with loops forming behind the ischemic bowel because the ischemic bowel is not performing peristaltic actions. Late signs, if the condition is not diagnosed and treated early, include dilation of the entire bowel including the stomach. "Thumbprinting" occurs when edema of the bowel wall shows the convex indentations of the lumen. In pneumatosis intestinalis, the bowel wall demonstrates a mottled gas pattern. Air in the biliary tree is indicative of a gallbladder emergency, and air under the diaphragm is a sign of pneumoperitoneum.

62. **Correct Answer: D**

    Stress-related erosive syndrome (SRES) was once cited as an explanation for gastric complications related to critical care illnesses. The stress response within the patient may lead to rapid erosion of the mucosal lining and result in ulcerations. Patients suffering from severe physiological illnesses are at high risk of SRES and, if SRES is left untreated, of gastric bleeding.

63. **Correct Answer: A**

    This patient is likely having gastric bleeding related to stress-related erosion syndrome (SRES). Due to the generalized bleeding associated with this condition, endoscopic therapies are not as effective in treating SRES as arginine vasopressin infusion into the gastric artery to cause splanchnic vasoconstriction. There is no indication that this patient has varices that would require ligation.

64. **Correct Answer: D**

    In the past, iced solutions were used in controlling gastric bleeding, but more recent research has shown that the iced solutions may cause additional bleeding by irritating both the healthy and compromised mucosal lining. The temperature may also result in core hypothermia and a shift in the oxyhemoglobin dissociation curve, resulting in a decrease in oxygen delivery to the tissues. Administration of a 3% saline solution would cause a fluid shift. Use of tap water should be avoided because it may increase the risk of systemic infection if the water is contaminated.

65. **Correct Answer: D**

    The patient is exhibiting signs and symptoms of gastric perforation, which is a surgical emergency. The lavage should be stopped, fluid aspirated, and the physician notified immediately. Additional actions should include placing at least two large-bore IVs, preparing to administer IV fluid replacement if hypovolemic shock occurs, and preparing the patient for immediate surgery.

66. **Correct Answer: B**

Although his initial symptoms and history may indicate cholecystitis, this patient's symptoms are the classic presentation of pancreatitis. Abdominal rigidity, Grey–Turner's sign, and Cullen's sign are late indicators of pancreatitis. This patient is also presenting with severe hypovolemic shock. Immediate fluid resuscitation should be initiated to support cardiovascular function.

67. **Correct Answer: B**

Patients with pancreatitis undergo massive fluid shifting as part of the body's inflammatory response to pancreatic self-digestion. The release of mediators during the inflammatory response leads to vasodilation and increased capillary permeability. Fluid may shift into the bowel, mucosal lining, and within the lungs, leading to acute lung injury (AJI). The drop in blood pressure may lead to acute kidney injury (AKI) and renal failure. Immediate fluid replacement with crystalloids and colloids is required to maintain intravascular volume. A history of poor volume intake certainly worsens the hypovolemia, but it is not the primary and most severe cause of the hypovolemic shock.

68. **Correct Answer: C**

Barrett's esophagus is a result of mucosal changes in the esophagus that occur after repeated and prolonged exposure to the gastric secretions seen in untreated gastro-esophageal reflux disease (GERD). Because of cellular changes in the esophageal lining, the patient is at increased risk for esophageal cancer.

69. **Correct Answer: C**

An esophagectomy involves removal of the damaged esophagus to the proximal portion of the stomach. The stomach is then resectioned to form a new esophagus. If the stomach is also cancerous, it is removed and the small bowel is resectioned to create a new esophagus.

70. **Correct Answer: A**

Gastric bypass surgery can lead to permanent gastric changes and places the obese patient at risk for both surgical and anesthesia-related complications. For many bariatric patients, the initial gastric bypass surgery is not the only surgery required. Often cosmetic surgery to remove loose skin around the stomach, back, thighs, arms, and chest is required to improve self-image. Each surgery carries additional risk.

Given these risks, complete bariatric education should be provided to any patient who is considering bariatric surgery. Education should include preoperative changes in diet, nutritional consultation, psychological evaluation, and full medical evaluation including lab work and cardiovascular testing. Education and support for the bariatric surgery patient should continue throughout the surgical process, with ongoing education, nutritional support, and physiological support continuing for years after surgery.

71. **Correct Answer: C**

Although each of these assessments is vital prior to bariatric surgery, psychological evaluation assesses the patient's psychological health regarding weight management, food, diet, nutrition, activity, exercise, health, surgery, coping mechanisms, self-image, and self-esteem, and it may estimate the long-term success of surgery. Obesity has many different causes, and assessing the patient's psychological health may reveal dangerous beliefs and behaviors related to food and nutrition that need to be addressed prior to surgery.

72. **Correct Answer: C**

   Regardless of which type of bariatric surgery is performed, the stomach size is always altered or restricted. Some forms of bypass also alter the normal pathway of food through digestion or malabsorption. Either method results in a poor tolerance for large volumes of food and fluids, requiring patients to eat more frequent, smaller meals. Foods that are high in carbohydrates and sugar are also more difficult to digest when malabsorptive surgical methods are used. The resulting "dumping syndrome" can be extremely physically painful. This effect provides a level of behavior modification meant to deter patients from consuming carbohydrates or sugary foods.

   Patients must understand the mandatory changes in diet that come with bariatric surgery. The leading cause of failure with restrictive surgical techniques is that patients consume foods in ever-increasing amounts that lead to stomach stretching of the pouch. Over time, the stomach can be restretched to almost its original size.

73. **Correct Answer: B**

   In gastric banding, an adjustable band is placed around the upper portion of the stomach, creating a 1- to 2-ounce area to act as the stomach. Because the size is restricted without suturing of the stomach or removal of any tissue, the procedure may be reversed for medical reasons such as pregnancy. Vertical banding, biliopancreatic diversion, and Roux-en-Y proximal gastric bypass all make some permanent change to the normal gastric pathway.

74. **Correct Answer: B**

   Gastroesophageal reflux disease (GERD) is a common complication of gastric banding. Due to the smaller gastric size and the close proximity of the band to the sphincter, the patient may experience reflux, nausea, and vomiting after eating. Deflation of the band with slower reinflation adjustments made every two weeks will ease symptoms. Stoma obstruction may occur if the patient fails to chew food properly and thoroughly. Band slippage may lead to erosion and perforation of the stomach or a folding of the larger portion of the stomach over the smaller portion.

75. **Correct Answer: C**

   Because the gastric size is greatly reduced, less intrinsic factor is available to assist in vitamin B_{12} absorption, which is necessary to prevent pernicious anemia. Oral supplements are not recommended, as they may not be absorbed quickly enough. Instead, sublingual or injected vitamin B_{12} may be required. Iron, thiamin, and calcium are all absorbed in the duodenum. In gastric bypass, the duodenum is also bypassed greatly limiting the absorption of these vitamins and minerals. Careful supplementation is mandatory to prevent malnutrition. Protein deficiencies are also common, and protein supplementation is necessary, especially in the early postoperative recovery period to prevent muscle wasting during the rapid weight loss period.

76. **Correct Answer: C**

   Biliopancreatic diversion uses a 5-ounce stomach pouch and wide anastomosis. The biliary branch or limb connects a portion of the small bowel to the biliary tract, allowing for normal biliary excretion. To prevent further preoperative or postoperative complications associated with cholecystitis, the gallbladder may be removed during the procedure.

77. **Correct Answer: A**
    Hyperoxia is not a complication of bariatric surgery and anastomosis leakage. Symptoms may present as an acute abdomen. If the symptoms are subtle, sepsis may set in, leading to multiple-organ dysfunction or failure, and ultimately death.

78. **Correct Answer: D**
    Pain management via a PCA pump should allow for a transition to oral pain medications only after anastamoses have healed. Effective pain management allows for early ambulation, which improves lung expansion and blood circulation. The pain management will help prevent atelectasis, pneumonia, and pulmonary embolism. Because of bariatric patients' high fat ratio, pain medications may need to be adjusted for greatest effectiveness.

79. **Correct Answer: C**
    TIPS is used in transplant procedures to bridge between the two livers in a hemodynamically unstable patient and increase the patient's stability. TIPS can be used during active bleeding via varices. Patients must have a directly measured portal pressure gradient of >10 mm Hg. This procedure should be postponed if the patient's bleeding is caused by heparin-induced thrombocytopenia (HITS), but may be performed when the patient is stabilized.

80. **Correct Answer: C**
    Glycemic emergencies may occur with Sandostatin, especially in patients with diabetes. It is important to monitor these patients' blood glucose to prevent hyperglycemia and/or hypoglycemia. Blood pressure and urinary function may also be affected, but do not reach life-threatening status as quickly as glucose levels.

81. **Correct Answer: D**
    Codeine slows gastric motility throughout the GI tract. This patient needs a nasogastric tube and motility medications such as metoclopramide.

82. **Correct Answer: D**
    Cimetidine is compatible with most drugs, but is *not* compatible with amphotericin B. Dilution is not required, although the drug can be diluted with 0.9% normal saline. Whenever the chance for drug interactions is unknown, seek expert opinion from pharmacy staff or check the manufacturer's insert.

83. **Correct Answer: B**
    Bile does not contain any digestive enzymes. Instead, bile salts emulsify (beat) triglycerides or fats into their smallest forms, so that digestive enzymes can function. Once digested or broken into fatty acids and monoglycerides, the digestive enzymes bind again with bile salts for transport into epithelial cells.

BIBLIOGRAPHY

Ahmed, I., & Beckingham, I. J. (2007). Liver trauma. *Trauma, 9*(3), 171–180.

Ahrens, T. (2006). *Critical care nursing certification.* Columbus, OH: McGraw-Hill.

American Association of Critical-Care Nurses. (2006). *Core curriculum for critical care nursing* (6th ed.). Philadelphia: Saunders.

American Association of Critical-Care Nurses. (2007). *AACN certification and core review for high acuity and critical care* (6th ed.). Philadelphia: Saunders.

American Heart Association. (2007). *Guidelines 2005 for cardiopulmonary resuscitation and emergency cardiovascular care.* Retrieved July 24, 2008 from http://circ.ahajournals.org/content/vol112/24_suppl

Barry, M., Cahill, R. A., & O'Connor, J. (2006). Duodenal hematoma secondary to blunt abdominal trauma. *European Journal of Trauma, 32*(6), 576–577.

Betz, T. G., Lee, P., & Victor, J. C. (2008). Hepatitis A vaccine versus immune globulin for post-exposure prophylaxis. *New England Journal of Medicine, 358*(5), 531–532.

Britt, R. C., Gannon, T., Collins, J. N., Cole, F, J., Weireter, L. J., & Britt, L. D. (2005). Secondary abdominal compartment syndrome: Risk factors and outcomes. *American Surgeon, 71*(11), 982–985.

Brolin, R. E., & Cody, R. P. (2007). Adding malabsorption for weight loss failure after gastric bypass. *Surgical Endoscopy, 21*(11), 1924–1926.

Burns, S. M. (Ed.). (2007). *American Association of Critical-Care Nurses (AACN): AACN protocols for practice: Healing environments* (2nd ed.). Sudbury, MA: Jones and Bartlett.

Cho, Y. P., Kwon, Y. M., Kwon, T. W., & Kim, G. E. (2003). Mesenteric Buerger's disease. *Annals of Vascular Surgery, 17*(2), 221–223.

Conover, M. B. (2003). *Understanding electrocardiography* (8th ed.). St. Louis, MO: Mosby/Elsevier.

Copstead, L., & Banasik, J. L. (2000). *Pathophysiology: Biological and behavioral perspectives* (2nd ed.). Philadelphia: Saunders/Elsevier.

Curley, M. A. Q. (1998). Patient–nurse synergy: Optimizing patients' outcomes. *American Journal of Critical Care, 7,* 64–72.

De laet, I., Hoste, E., Verholen, E.. & De Waele, J. J. (2007). The effect of neuromuscular blockers in patients with intra-abdominal hypertension. *Intensive Care Medicine, 33*(10), 1811–1814.

Dossey, B. M., Keegan, L., & Guzzetta, C. (2003). *Holistic nursing: A handbook for practice* (3rd ed.). Sudbury, MA: Jones and Bartlett.

Edwards, D. F. (1999). The Synergy Model: Linking patient needs to nurse competencies. *Critical Care Nurse, 19*(1), 88–98.

Emergency Nurses Association & Newberry, L. (2003). *Sheehy's emergency nursing: Principles and practice* (5th ed.). St. Louis, MO: Mosby/Elsevier.

Finkelmeier, B. A. (2000). *Cardiothoracic surgical nursing* (2nd ed.). Philadelphia: Lippincott, Williams & Wilkins.

Hamza, S. M., & Kaufman, S. (2007). Effect of mesenteric vascular congestion on reflex control of renal blood flow. *American Journal of Physiology: Regulatory, Integrative and Comparative Physiology, 293*(5), R1917.

Hanchanale, V. S., Rao, A. R., & Gilbert, J. M. (2007). What caused this massive GI hemorrhage? *Contemporary Surgery, 63*(11), 566–568.

Hardin, S. R., & Kaplow, R. (Eds.). (2004). *Synergy for clinical excellence: The AACN Synergy Model for Patient Care.* Sudbury, MA: Jones and Bartlett.

Hickey, J. V. (2002). *The clinical practice of neurological and neurosurgical nursing* (5th ed.). Philadelphia: Lippincott, Williams & Wilkins.

Hiraga, N., Aikata, H., Takaki, S., Kodama, H., Shirakawa, H., Imamura, M., et al. (2007). The long-term outcome of patients with bleeding gastric varices after balloon-occluded retrograde transvenous obliteration. *Journal of Gastroenterology, 42*(8), 663–672.

Horng, M. S. (2006). Beta blockers failed in primary prevention of gastroesophageal varices. *Journal of Clinical Outcomes Management, 13*(1), 15–16.

Jain, P., & Nijhawan, S. (2007). Acute viral hepatitis with pancreatitis: Is it due to the viruses or sludge? *Pancreatology, 7*(5–6), 544–545.

Khan, F., & Morad, N. (2006). Cytomegalovirus enteritis in a mechanically ventilated patient with chronic obstructive pulmonary disease. *Indian Journal of Critical Care Medicine, 10*(1), 40–43.

Knaapen, H. K. A., & Barrera, P. (2007). Therapy for Whipple's disease. *Journal of Antimicrobial Chemotherapy, 60*(3), 457–458.

Köklü, S., Çoban, S., Yüksel, O., & Arhan, M. (2007). Left-sided portal hypertension. *Digestive Diseases and Sciences, 52*(5), 1141–1149.

Lipson, J. G., Dibble, S. L., & Minarik, P. A. (Eds.). (1996). *Culture and nursing care: A pocket guide.* San Francisco, CA: UCSF Nursing Press.

Lisman, T., & Leebeek, F. W. G. (2007). Hemostatic alterations in liver disease: A review on pathophysiology, clinical consequences, and treatment. *Digestive Surgery, 24*(4), 250–258.

Maharaj, D., Perry, A., Ramdass, M., & Naraynsingh, V. (2003). Late small bowel obstruction after blunt abdominal trauma. *Postgraduate Medical Journal, 79*(927), 57–58.

Mayo Clinic Staff. (2007). Dumping syndrome. *Mayo Foundation for Medical Education and Research.* Retrieved August 26, 2008, from http://www.mayoclinic.com/health/dumping-syndrome/DS00715/

McNally, P. (2001). *GI/liver secrets* (2nd ed.). Philadelphia: Hanley & Belfus/Elsevier.

McQuillan, K. A., Von Rueden, K. T., Hartsock, R. L., Flynn, M. B., & Whalen, E. (Eds.). (2002). *Trauma nursing: From resuscitation through rehabilitation* (3rd ed.). Philadelphia: Saunders/Elsevier.

Medina, J., & Puntillo, K. (2006). *AACN protocols for practice: Palliative care and end-of-life issues in critical care.* Sudbury, MA: Jones and Bartlett.

Morales, C. H., Villegas, M. I., Villavicencio, R., et al. (2004). Intra-abdominal infection in patients with abdominal trauma. *Archives of Surgery, 139*(12), 1278–1285, discussion 1285.

Morgan, M. Y. (2007). The treatment of hepatic encephalopathy. *Metabolic Brain Disease, 22*(3–4), 389–405.

Okuse, C., Yotsuyanagi, H., & Koike, K. (2007). Hepatitis C as a systemic disease: Virus and host immunologic responses underlie hepatic and extrahepatic manifestations. *Journal of Gastroenterology, 42*(11), 857–865.

Olson, M. M., Ilada, P. B., & Apelgren, K. N. (2003). Portal vein thrombosis. *Surgical Endoscopy, 17*(8), 1322.

Oncel, D., Malinoski, D., Brown, C., Demetriades, D., & Salim, A. (2007). Blunt gastric injuries. *American Surgeon, 73*(9), 880–883.

Pagana, K. D., & Pagana, J. (2005). *Mosby's manual of diagnostic and laboratory tests* (3rd ed.). St. Louis, MO: Mosby/Elsevier.

Reesink, H. W., Engelfriet, C. P., Henn, G., Mayr, W. R., Delage, G., Bernier, F., et al. (2008). Occult hepatitis B infection in blood donors. *Vox Sanguinis, 94*(2), 153–166.

Rogula, T., Yenumula, P. R., & Schauer, P. R. (2007). A complication of Roux-en-Y gastric bypass: Intestinal obstruction. *Surgical Endoscopy, 21*(11), 1914–1918.

Schaefer, P. J., Schaefer, F. K. W., Mueller-Huelsbeck, S., & Jahnke, T. (2007). Chronic mesenteric ischemia: Stenting of mesenteric arteries. *Abdominal Imaging, 32*(3), 304–309.

Shah, V. H., & Kamath, P. (2006). Management of portal hypertension. *Postgraduate Medicine, 119*(3), 14–18.

Shawcross, D., & Jalan, R. (2005). Dispelling myths in the treatment of hepatic encephalopathy. *Lancet, 365*(9457), 431–433.

Shawcross, D. L., Wright, G., Olde Damink, S. W. M., & Jalan, R. (2007). Role of ammonia and inflammation in minimal hepatic encephalopathy. *Metabolic Brain Disease, 22*(1), 125–138.

Shebrain, S., Zelada, J., Lipsky, A. M., & Putnam, B. (2006). Mesenteric injuries after blunt abdominal trauma: Delay in diagnosis and increased morbidity. *American Surgeon, 72*(10), 955–961.

Skidmore-Roth, L. (2004). *Mosby's 2004 nursing drug reference*. St. Louis, MO: Mosby/Elsevier.

Smeltzer, S., & Bare, B. G. (2003). *Brunner and Suddarth's textbook of medical–surgical nursing* (10th ed.). Philadelphia: Lippincott, Williams & Wilkins.

Sole, M. L., Hartshorn, J.. & Lamborne, M. L. (2001). *Introduction to critical care nursing* (3rd ed.). Philadelphia: Saunders/Elsevier.

Sonfield, J., Robison, J., & Leon, S. M. (2007). Occult aortic injury after penetrating abdominal trauma. *American Surgeon, 73*(3), 239–242.

Stewart, C. A., & Cerhan, J. (2005). Hepatic encephalopathy: A dynamic or static condition. *Metabolic Brain Disease, 20*(3), 193–204.

Sun, D., & Fang, J. (2007). Two common reasons of malabsorption syndromes: Celiac disease and Whipple's disease. *Digestion, 74*(3–4), 174–183.

Tseng, Y., Wu, M., Lin, M., & Lai, W. (2004). Massive upper gastrointestinal bleeding after acid-corrosive injury. *World Journal of Surgery, 28*(1), 50–54.

University of Southern California, Department of Surgery. (2005). Whipple operation. *USC Center for Pancreatic and Biliary Disease*. Retrieved February 20, 2005, from http://www.surgery.usc.edu/divisions/tumor/PancreasDiseases

Urden, L. D., Stacy, K. M., & Lough, M. E. (2007). *Thelan's critical care nursing: Diagnosis and management* (5th ed.). St. Louis, MO: Mosby.

Warwick, M., Goonewardene, K., Burton, P. R., Usatoff, V., & Evans, P. M. (2007). HP38P management of traumative pancreatic injury. *ANZ Journal of Surgery, 77*(s1), A48.

Wiegand, D. J. L., & Carlson, K. K. (Eds.). (2005). *AACN procedure manual for critical care* (5th ed.). Philadelphia: Elsevier.

Williams, O. M., Nightingale, A. K., Hartley, J., Bramkamp, M., Ruggieri, F., Schneemann, M., et al. (2007). Whipple's disease. *New England Journal of Medicine, 356*(14), 1479–1481.

Woods, S., Sivarajan Froelicher, E. S., & Motzer, S. U. (2000). *Cardiac nursing* (4th ed.). Philadelphia: Lippincott, Williams & Wilkins.

Wright, B. E., Reinke, T., & Aye, R. A. (2005). Chronic traumatic diaphragmatic hernia with pericardial rupture and associated gastroesophageal reflux. *Hernia, 9*(4), 392–396.

Zeller, J. L. (2007). Risk of gastric cancer after Roux-en-Y gastric bypass. *Journal of the American Medical Association, 298*(22), 2600.

Zeller, J. L. (2007). Spectrum and risk factors of complications after gastric bypass. *Journal of the American Medical Association, 298*(21), 2461.

Renal

QUESTIONS

1. After being resuscitated following a cardiac arrest, Myra spent a week recovering in the MICU. This morning she was admitted to your progressive care unit. Because the resuscitation was prolonged, Myra developed acute renal failure. The definition of acute renal failure is
   A. Trauma to one or both kidneys.
   B. Decrease in renal perfusion from shock or anaphylaxis.
   C. A sudden or rapid decline in renal filtration function.
   D. An obstruction to passage of urine.

2. Myra was diagnosed with intrinsic AKI as a result of resuscitation. Intrinsic AKI is most commonly caused by
   A. Arteriolar vasoconstriction.
   B. Acute ischemic or cytotoxic injury.
   C. Amphotericin.
   D. Hypercalcemia.

3. Phillip was admitted to your progressive care unit after two days of unsuccessful attempts to pass a kidney stone. The urologist removed the stone, but Phillip is now anuric. Sudden anuria may be due to
   A. An embolic event.
   B. Congestive heart failure.
   C. Prostate enlargement.
   D. Azotemia.

4. Postrenal AKI may be caused by
   A. Malignant hypertension.
   B. Transplant rejection.
   C. A neurogenic bladder.
   D. DIC, preeclampsia.

5. Susan has been attempting to lose weight utilizing a variety of diets and exercise. Her physician recommended a series of tests because Susan kept complaining of abdominal pain. Susan collapsed while running and was admitted to your care. She has an elevated BUN. As a progressive care nurse, you know that a BUN may be elevated in patients taking:
   A. Steroid treatments.
   B. Streptomycin.
   C. Chloramphenicol.
   D. Low protein supplements .

6. Kyle is a 22-year-old student who underwent a renal transplant one year ago. The physician suspects that the organ is being rejected. You know that a renal transplant that results from humoral rejection or acute cellular rejection may be definitively diagnosed only via
   A. Ultrasound.
   B. Nuclear scan.
   C. Doppler scan.
   D. Renal biopsy.

7. In the polyuric phase of AKI, it is important for the nurse to carefully monitor
   A. Nitrogen balance.
   B. Potassium and phosphorus levels.
   C. Dopamine and mannitol levels.
   D. Desmopressin levels.

8. Anuria is defined as a urine output of
   A. < 30 mL/d.
   B. 200 mL/d.
   C. 300 mL/d.
   D. < 100 mL/d.

9. Oliguria is a urine output of 100–400 mL/d and is usually the result of
   A. Pyelonephritis.
   B. Rhabdomyolitis.
   C. Prerenal syndrome.
   D. Acute glomerular nephritis.

10. Mrs. W. was admitted directly from her physician's office. She had been complaining of fatigue and generalized pain. Her lab results indicated a rapidly rising BUN, and she was admitted for further tests. While assessing Mrs. W., you note that she has severe acne around the face and neck. You suspect that the rise in BUN may be due to
    A. Tetracycline.
    B. HCTZ.
    C. Bumetanide.
    D. Mannitol.

11. Mannitol and loop diuretics may be used in the treatment of AKI. Mannitol is nontoxic but must be used with caution because
    A. Mannitol may damage the eighth cranial nerve.
    B. Mannitol may cause vestibular impairment.
    C. Mannitol may produce a hyperosmolar state.
    D. Mannitol may bind with proteins in the renal tubule.

12. Nephrotoxicity may be caused by administration of
    A. Furosemide.
    B. Aspirin.
    C. Thioguanine.
    D. Acyclovir.

13. **NSAIDs may cause**
    A. Prerenal AKI.
    B. Intrinsic AKI.
    C. Postrenal AKI.
    D. Increased urine osmolality.

14. **Medications that can decrease BUN levels include**
    A. Neomycin, rifampin.
    B. Chloral hydrate, furosemide.
    C. Bacitracin, gentamycin.
    D. Chloramphenicol, streptomycin.

15. **Which of the following statements about creatinine is true?**
    A. A normal range for creatinine would be 0.8 to 1.4 mg/dL.
    B. Creatinine levels are higher in females than in males.
    C. Lower than normal levels of creatinine may indicate pyelonephritis.
    D. Low levels of creatinine are a precursor to eclampsia.

16. **Sally, who is 24 years old, was admitted because of increasing malaise and night sweats. She had various blood tests done to try to determine if her systemic lupus erythematosus caused her allergic nephritis. Allergic nephritis may also be caused by**
    A. Inadequate protein consumption.
    B. Weight loss.
    C. Cimetidine.
    D. Water intoxication.

17. **The primary site for urea synthesis is in the**
    A. Kidneys.
    B. Liver.
    C. Lungs.
    D. Pancreas.

18. **Increased production of urea may be due to**
    A. GI bleeding.
    B. A low protein diet.
    C. Congenital kidney disease.
    D. Hypothermia.

19. **Michael was involved in a head-on collision and had to be freed from under the steering column of his car. Michael has been diagnosed with a ruptured bladder. He was admitted to your unit prior to undergoing surgery to repair the bladder and any other potential injuries. It is important for you to assess him for signs of**
    A. Bowel perforation.
    B. A ruptured spleen.
    C. A shearing injury.
    D. Rectal injury.

20. You notice your patient's hand spasming slightly when the automatic blood pressure cuff inflates. When you attempt a manual blood pressure measurement, the same thing happens when you inflate the cuff to just past the systolic pressure. This carpopedal spasm is indicative of
    A. Hypokalemia.
    B. Hyperphosphatemia.
    C. Hypocalcemia.
    D. Hypernatremia.

21. Your patient is becoming confused, is lethargic, and has muscle weakness. A review of her lab reports shows a calcium level of 11.9. A common way to treat this condition would be to use
    A. D_5W and a Kayexalate enema.
    B. Normal saline and a loop diuretic.
    C. Glucose followed by insulin.
    D. Nothing; this is a normal value.

22. While assessing your patient, you notice significant pretibial and pedal edema. When the patient is weighed, you note that the patient has gained 1 kg of weight in 24 hours. This would be equal to at least _____ of excess fluid.
    A. 2,000 mL
    B. 1,000 mL
    C. 2,200 mL
    D. 500 mL

23. Your patient has a calcium level of 7.8. You would expect which of the following potential EKG changes?
    A. Tall, peaked T waves
    B. A prominent U wave
    C. A first-degree AV block
    D. A prolonged QT interval

24. One way to check for low calcium levels is to tap over a branch of the facial nerve. If the patient is hypocalcemic, the upper lip on the same side (ipsilateral) will twitch. This response is known as
    A. Trousseau's sign.
    B. Chvostek's sign.
    C. Grey–Turner's sign.
    D. Homan's sign.

25. What is the primary acid–base disturbance exhibited by patients with AKI?
    A. Metabolic acidosis
    B. Respiratory acidosis
    C. Metabolic alkalosis
    D. Respiratory alkalosis

26. Herman, a 67-year-old postal worker, is admitted to the progressive care unit for cocaine intoxication. He begins to complain of severe epigastric pain. Lab results are as follows: WBC 17.3 with 77% neutrophils, hematocrit 40%, LDH 341, platelets 226, BUN 7, creatinine 1.0. Urine analysis shows trace proteins, few RBCs, positive urine toxicology for cocaine. What might be the cause of Herman's pain?
    A. Peptic ulcer disease
    B. Renal infarction
    C. Gastroenteritis
    D. Infarcted mesenteric artery

27. Aldosterone is secreted when the extracellular sodium level is _____ and/or when extracellular potassium is _____.
    A. low, low
    B. low, high
    C. high, low
    D. high, high

28. Patrick is a 24-year-old with cystic fibrosis. Because of his condition, he is at high risk for which of the following electrolyte imbalances?
    A. Hypernatremia
    B. Hypocalcemia
    C. Hyponatremia
    D. Hypercalcemia

29. Glenn has a J-tube in place while being treated for peritonitis. Which electrolyte deficit is he probably most at risk for?
    A. Sodium
    B. Magnesium
    C. Manganese
    D. Phosphorus

30. Ada is a 60-year-old with diabetes and congestive heart failure. After 4 days of no contact from her mother, her daughter visited her and found Ada in bed, unresponsive. Ada has a red, dry swollen tongue, a temperature of 102°F, and flushed, dry skin. She is tachycardic, hypotensive, and has decreased reflexes. Her urine specific gravity is 1.050. You suspect
    A. Hypernatremia.
    B. Hypocalcemia.
    C. Hypermagnesemia.
    D. Hypokalemia.

31. _____ is the major extracellular cation, and _____ is the major intracellular cation.
    A. Calcium; magnesium
    B. Sodium; calcium
    C. Potassium; sodium
    D. Sodium; potassium

32. **What percentage of the body's potassium may be found in the extracellular fluid?**
    A. 2%
    B. 5%
    C. 10%
    D. 98%

33. **Potassium is reabsorbed in the**
    A. Proximal tubules.
    B. Distal tubules.
    C. Ascending colon.
    D. Descending colon.

34. **Aldosterone secretions _____ potassium excretion.**
    A. decrease
    B. increase
    C. neutralize
    D. do not affect

35. **Your patient is an alcoholic. What effect will this condition have on the patient's potassium stores?**
    A. Potassium moves from the vascular circulation into the interstitium.
    B. Potassium moves out of the cell into the vascular circulation.
    C. Potassium moves out of the cell into the interstitium.
    D. Potassium from the vascular circulation moves into the cell.

36. **Hypokalemia may cause**
    A. Respiratory alkalosis only.
    B. Metabolic alkalosis only.
    C. Both respiratory and metabolic alkalosis.
    D. Metabolic acidosis only.

37. **Hypokalemia as a result of excessive urinary excretion may be caused by all of the following except**
    A. Oliguria.
    B. Renal disease.
    C. Lasix.
    D. Increased adrenal cortical hormones.

38. **Flo is hypokalemic. Which of the following waveforms would you expect to see on her EKG?**
    A. Peaked T waves
    B. U wave
    C. Shortened QT interval
    D. Absent P wave

39. **Hugh suffered a crush injury when a beam dropped on him. You would expect to see which of the following results on his electrolyte panels?**
    A. Hyperphosphatemia
    B. Hypomagnesemia
    C. Hypocalcemia
    D. Hyperkalemia

40. **It is recommended that adults consume _____ of potassium daily.**
    A. 500 mg
    B. 1,000 mg
    C. 2,000 mg
    D. 3,500 mg

41. **All of the following foods are high in potassium except**
    A. Avocado.
    B. Raisins.
    C. Potatoes.
    D. Carrots.

42. **You are discussing cooking methods of vegetables with your patient's wife. Which of the following cooking techniques leaches the most potassium from vegetables?**
    A. Boiling
    B. Baking
    C. Steaming
    D. Microwaving

43. **Your patient is receiving potassium in his IV fluid and the physician has ordered a potassium rider. What is the maximum rate of infusion for potassium solutions?**
    A. 2 mEq/h
    B. 4 mEq/h
    C. 10 mEq/h
    D. 15 mEq/h

44. **Ian was diagnosed with Addison's disease. In Addison's disease, what happens to the potassium level?**
    A. Hyperkalemia related to the decrease in aldosterone secretion
    B. Hyperkalemia related to the increase in aldosterone secretion
    C. Hypokalemia related to the decrease in aldosterone secretion
    D. Hypocalcemia related to the increase in aldosterone secretion

45. **All of the following are treatments for hyperkalemia except**
    A. Glucose and insulin.
    B. Kaon.
    C. Calcium gluconate.
    D. Bicarbonate administration.

46. Belinda has congestive heart failure and was given Lasix for water retention. Her feet and legs continued to swell, so she took extra Lasix this morning. Now Belinda has profound muscle weakness and flat T waves on her EKG. What might you expect her potassium level to be this morning?
    A. 1.8
    B. 3.8
    C. 4.2
    D. 6.1

47. Current ACLS guidelines recommend the use of magnesium for treatment of polymorphic ventricular tachycardia. The normal magnesium level for an adult is in the range of
    A. 0.5–1.5 mg/dL.
    B. 1.5–2 mg/dL.
    C. 2–3 mg/dL.
    D. 4–5 mg/dL.

48. Magnesium is required for all of the following physiological functions except
    A. To always act as an antagonist with calcium.
    B. For enzyme activation.
    C. Synthesis of nucleic acid and proteins.
    D. For activity of the sodium–potassium pump.

49. Magnesium alters intracellular calcium by affecting which hormone?
    A. Parathyroid
    B. Aldosterone
    C. Cortisol
    D. Glycosol

50. Magnesium is most prevalent in which of the following areas of the body?
    A. Extracellular
    B. In the liver
    C. In the bone
    D. In the spleen

51. As part of his discharge teaching, you are helping Joe to determine which foods are rich in magnesium. He asks you what the recommended daily intake for magnesium for adults is. Your answer should be
    A. 50–100 mg per day.
    B. 100–200 mg per day.
    C. 200–350 mg per day.
    D. 350–420 mg per day.

52. Your patient was admitted and treated for torsades de pointes. You are teaching her about adding foods that are rich in magnesium to her diet. Your patient asks about each of the following foods. Which of the following foods is low or a poor source of magnesium?

A. Honey

B. Broccoli

C. Almonds

D. Chocolate

53. **Kim had gastric bypass surgery two days ago. Which of the following electrolytes is she at the highest risk for a potential imbalance?**
   A. Potassium
   B. Magnesium
   C. Calcium
   D. Sodium

54. **Carla eats a diet high in calcium because her family has a history of osteoporosis. She was admitted status post fractured pelvis and pulmonary embolism when she fell down her stairs. Carla has been experiencing increasing weakness and muscle tremors. She has noted an increase in frequency of "skipping" heartbeats, and stated that she was very dizzy and disoriented just before she fell. Based on her symptoms, which of the following labs should you assess immediately?**
   A. Calcium level
   B. Sodium level
   C. Hemoglobin and hematocrit
   D. Magnesium level

55. **Mrs. D. had major abdominal surgery status post motor vehicle accident. She is now exhibiting signs and symptoms of decreased magnesium levels related to excessive urinary loss. How long will this condition last?**
   A. 12 hours
   B. 24 hours
   C. 36 hours
   D. 48 hours

56. **Your patient was admitted for ketoacidosis. Her magnesium level is 0.5 mEq/L. Which symptoms would you expect to see?**
   A. Convulsions
   B. Lethargy
   C. Negative Babinski sign
   D. Decreased reflexes

57. **Ali was diagnosed with breast cancer 8 years ago. The cancer has now metastasized to the bone. Which of the following changes would you expect to see in Ali's electrolytes?**
   A. Decreased magnesium and increased calcium levels
   B. Decreased magnesium and calcium levels
   C. Increased magnesium and calcium levels
   D. Increased magnesium and decreased calcium levels

58. Your patient is status post cardiac arrest. Magnesium replacement is ordered. What is the fastest rate of infusion that would be considered safe?
    A. 15 mg/min
    B. 30 mg/min
    C. 45 mg/min
    D. 60 mg/min

59. Magnesium is ordered for your patient. While it is infusing, you assess the patient and note flaccidity, absent patellar reflexes, shallow respirations, and a flushed face. You should
    A. Give the magnesium, the patient is just sleeping.
    B. Hold the dose for 1 hour.
    C. Give the dose over 3 hours.
    D. Hold the dose, contact the physician, and obtain a magnesium level.

60. The most common cause of hypermagnesemia is
    A. Gastrointestinal bypass.
    B. Gastrointestinal fistula.
    C. Renal failure.
    D. Overdose.

61. The family of your patient with hypermagnesemia asks why his face is flushed. You answer:
    A. "He has a fever."
    B. "His magnesium level is a little high, which causes his face to look flushed."
    C. "He is embarrassed because the hospital gown does not provide enough coverage."
    D. "He just completed his physical therapy."

62. What percentage of calcium is stored in the bone?
    A. 99%
    B. 85%
    C. 80%
    D. 75%

63. Calcium
    A. Is approximately 40% ionized in the serum.
    B. Cannot be correlated with albumin levels.
    C. Is bonded to protein and so cannot pass through capillary wall.
    D. Is not necessary for coagulation.

64. Serum calcium is decreased by all of the following except
    A. Increase in vitamin D.
    B. Renal tubular excretion.
    C. Gastrointestinal excretion.
    D. Bone demineralization.

65. As calcium levels _____, parathyroid secretions _____.

A. increase; decrease

B. increase; increase

C. decrease; decrease

D. decreases; remain consistent

66. **You are testing for hypocalcemia using Trousseau's sign. How would you elicit this sign?**

A. Tap the cheek

B. Lift the left leg up and look for head lifting to the chest

C. Inflate a BP cuff to greater than the systolic pressure for 3 minutes and wait for a carpal spasm

D. Take a sharp object up from the heel to the toes and watch for the toes to spread

67. **Maria is scheduled to undergo continuous renal replacement therapy (CRRT) this week. Which of the following drugs should be stopped 2–3 days prior to therapy?**

A. Beta blockers

B. ACE inhibitors

C. Heparin

D. Calcium-channel blockers

68. **For non-pumped continuous renal replacement therapy (CRRT) to function appropriately, at a minimum the mean arterial blood pressure must be**

A. 40 mm Hg.

B. 50 mm Hg.

C. 60 mm Hg.

D. 80 mm Hg.

69. **Alice has renal failure and is preparing to have continuous renal replacement therapy (CRRT). She asks if she can have visitors during the procedure. You tell her:**

A. "Of course. There are no restrictions."

B. "No. They would be in the way of the equipment."

C. "No. They will increase your risk of infection."

D. "Yes, but if they are sensitive to the sight of blood, they may want to wait until after the procedure."

70. **Which of the following continuous renal replacement therapies (CRRT) require only venous access and pumping function?**

A. CVVHDF, SCUF

B. CVVH, CVVHD

C. CAVH, CAVHD

D. CVVH, CAVH

71. **Trace is a patient in renal failure post multiple cardiac arrests. He has recovered from cardiogenic shock but has continued cardiovascular instability. The best method for removal of Trace's excess fluid is**

A. Hemodialysis.

B. Peritoneal dialysis.

C. Continuous renal replacement therapy (CRRT).

D. Plasmapheresis.

72. Floyd is undergoing hemodialysis for renal failure as a result of uncontrolled Type II diabetes. His wife asks you how you know the hemodialysis is effective. As a nurse, you know the adequacy of dialysis is measured by
    A. Urine creatinine clearance.
    B. Sodium, chloride, and potassium levels.
    C. Blood pressure.
    D. Urea clearance.

73. You are assessing your patient's vascular access prior to hemodialysis. You note that there is no thrill or bruit. Your next nursing action would be to
    A. Call the surgeon to do a new graft.
    B. Use a Doppler to determine graft patency.
    C. Administer a bolus of heparin.
    D. Continue with the hemodialysis, there is nothing wrong.

74. Hemodialysis is used to treat many metabolic abnormalities as well as renal failure. One possible treatment is:
    A. Vitamin C and calcium carbonate for osteoporosis.
    B. Erythropoietin for excessive iron.
    C. Phosphate binders for hyperphosphatemia.
    D. Glucose for hyperglycemia.

75. Communication between all staff is vital. When transferring your patient with a graft, which information is a priority to communicate to all staff that may come in contact with this patient?
    A. Last dialysis date
    B. Location of the graft
    C. Type of dialysis machine used
    D. Total fluid removed with last dialysis

76. The usual amount of dialysate used in peritoneal dialysis is
    A. 0.5–1 L.
    B. 1–2 L.
    C. 2–3 L.
    D. 3–4 L.

77. Which of the following is the correct fluid exchange sequence in peritoneal dialysis?
    A. Dump, dwell, drain
    B. Instillation, dwell, drain
    C. Drain, instillation, dwell
    D. Instillation, drain, dwell

78. Peritoneal dialysis functions by using which two principles?
    A. Diffusion and ultrafiltration
    B. Osmotic pressure and osmosis
    C. Ultrafiltration and oncotic pressure
    D. Diffusion and osmosis

79. **You are preparing Louise for her first peritoneal dialysis session. It is important to tell her which of the following findings is normal?**
   A. During the instillation phase, the insertion site may leak.
   B. During the dwell phase, she may feel abdominal fullness and shortness of breath.
   C. During the dwell phase, subcutaneous fluid may be seen in the groin.
   D. During the drain phase, she may feel dizzy and have palpitations.

80. **During the drain phase of a peritoneal dialysis session, you note only 50% return in the collection bag. What is your first action?**
   A. Position the patient prone
   B. Check for kinks, bends, or cracks in the tubing
   C. Double-check the amount instilled
   D. Assess for subcutaneous fluid

81. **You are providing discharge teaching to the family and patient receiving peritoneal dialysis. As part of the discharge procedure, your patient will receive a home glucometer. The daughter questions this because her mother is not a diabetic. You would tell her:**
   A. "Peritoneal dialysis can cause diabetes."
   B. "She didn't tell you? Your mother was just diagnosed with diabetes."
   C. "The dialysate contains glucose and can lead to hyperglycemia."
   D. "Peritoneal dialysis may lead to pancreatitis."

82. **For which of the following disease processes is immunoadsorption used as a treatment?**
   A. Paraneoplastic neurologic syndromes
   B. Multiple sclerosis
   C. Cutaneous T-cell lymphomas
   D. Heart transplant rejection

83. **Apheresis is best defined as**
   A. The removal of plasma and/or proteins from the blood.
   B. The selective removal of cells, plasma, and other substances from the blood.
   C. The selective removal of cellular components from the blood.
   D. The removal of an antigen in the blood.

84. **The exchange plasma volume used in apheresis is usually at a ratio of**
   A. 1.5:1.
   B. 2:1.
   C. 2.5:1.
   D. 3:1.

85. **Holly, a 24-year-old teacher, is undergoing lymphocytopheresis and plasma exchange for progressive multiple sclerosis with citrate as the anticoagulant. She begins to feel tingling. Which of the following lab results should you check first?**
   A. ABG, ionized calcium, PT/PTT levels
   B. Potassium, magnesium, PT/PTT levels
   C. INR, potassium, sodium, chloride levels
   D. ACT, ionized calcium level and ABG

86. Jeff has been diagnosed with hypertension. He states that to control his blood pressure he "will never eat another thing with salt." You would tell him instead:

    A. "That is not easy. Most fresh vegetables and fruit have tons of sodium."
    B. "Great. Sodium plays only a minor part in water balance and cellular activity, so your body won't know the difference."
    C. "You cannot completely eliminate sodium from your diet. Your body has an intricate system of safety measures to protect the level of sodium in your body."
    D. "Okay. Sodium is controlled by aldosterone, which is released by the pituitary gland."

87. The recommended daily sodium intake for someone limiting sodium in their diet should range between

    A. 100–900 mg.
    B. 1,000–2,000 mg.
    C. 3,000–5,000 mg.
    D. 4,000–6,000 mg.

88. Hannah was put on a limited-sodium diet and has been working with a nutritionist. She was admitted to your unit for chest pain (angina) and pulmonary edema. Hannah reports that she has stopped all additional sodium intake, has been following her diet regimen closely, stopped eating out, is drinking eight to ten 8-ounce glasses of tap water every day, and is voiding well. Her sodium level is 155 mEq/L. What is the likely cause of Hannah's hypernatremia?

    A. Renal failure
    B. Hypotonic fluids
    C. Diabetes mellitus
    D. Water softener system

89. Which of the following fruits has the lowest sodium content per 3.5-ounce serving?

    A. Cantaloupe
    B. Grapes
    C. Peaches
    D. Blackberries

90. Henry is trying to limit his salt intake. Which of the following meat products would you recommend for Henry to eat?

    A. Chicken without the skin
    B. Canned beef hash
    C. Fresh pike
    D. Canned crab

91. Edward loves cheese, but must limit his sodium intake. Which of the following cheeses has the highest sodium content per 3.5-ounce serving?

    A. Swiss cheese
    B. Mozzarella cheese
    C. Cheddar cheese
    D. Parmesan cheese

92. You are receiving report on Dale, who was injured when he suffered a seizure while working on his roof. His sodium level on admission was 120 mEq/L. Which symptoms of hyponatremia would you expect to see?
    A. Twitching
    B. Tachypnea
    C. Lethargy
    D. Flattened T waves

93. A common cause of hyponatremia is
    A. Salt water drowning.
    B. Over-hydration.
    C. Administration of hypertonic solutions.
    D. Hyperoxia.

94. The primary diagnostic studies for bladder cancer include
    A. Open loop resection and MRI.
    B. Intravenous pyelogram (IVP), ultrasound, and CT.
    C. Laser photocoagulation.
    D. CT and cystectomy.

95. A disadvantage of peritoneal dialysis is
    A. Migration of the catheter.
    B. Hypotension during the procedure.
    C. The dietary and fluid restrictions.
    D. Increased cardiovascular stress.

This concludes the Renal Questions section.

ANSWERS

1. **Correct Answer: C**
   Acute renal failure is now known as acute renal injury (AKI) and can be classified as prerenal, intrinsic, or postrenal. Because material covered on the PCCN exam reflects practice up to two years ago, we introduced the new terminology here. Some item writers may use this new terminology on the exam.

2. **Correct Answer: B**
   Other causes of intrinsic AKI include cell detachment, dilatation of the lumen, and injury to the distal nephron. Answers A, C, and D are causes of prerenal AKI.

3. **Correct Answer: A**
   Anuria is usually due to postrenal AKI and involves mechanical obstruction of the urinary collection system. The collection system is comprised of the renal pelvis, the ureters, the bladder, and the urethra. Phillip may have a clot from the procedure required to remove the kidney stone.

4. **Correct Answer: C**
   Other causes of postrenal AKI include tumor, tricyclic antidepressants, fibrosis, BPH, prostate CA, urethral obstruction, stone disease, and ligation during surgery. Answers A, B, and D are causes of intrinsic failure/injury.

5. **Correct Answer: A**
   The BUN may also be elevated in cases of GI or mucosal bleeding or when the patient has excessive protein intake.

6. **Correct Answer: D**
   Ultrasound results may be difficult to obtain or interpret due to ascites, obesity or fluid in the retroperitoneal area. Doppler scans measure blood flow, which is diminished due to prerenal and intrinsic AKI. Nuclear scans are of limited value because the excretion rates may be slowed by disease. Renal biopsy is the gold standard for diagnosing rejection.

7. **Correct Answer: B**
   Potassium and phosphorus levels must be diligently monitored because of the potential for dysrhythmias.

8. **Correct Answer: D**
   Anuria is defined as a urine output of less than 100 mL per day.

9. **Correct Answer: C**
   Answers A, B, and D are causes of non-oliguria (> 400 mL/d of urine output). Hepatorenal syndrome is another cause of oliguria.

10. **Correct Answer: A**
    Tetracycline decreases anabolism, thereby increasing the BUN. It is the only medication listed as an option that would be used for treatment of acne.

11. **Correct Answer: C**
    Answers A, B, and D are characteristics of loop diuretics such as furosemide, bumetadine, and torsemide.

12. **Correct Answer: D**

    Acyclovir can crystallize in the kidney and cause AKI. It is important for the progressive care nurse to carefully monitor the infusion time and the amount of fluid used to dilute intravenous drugs. Other drugs that can crystallize in the kidney include sulfonamides, idinivir, and triamterine.

13. **Correct Answer: A**

    NSAIDs block prostaglandin production and, in turn, alters glomerular arteriolar perfusion.

14. **Correct Answer: D**

    Answers A, B, and C are medications that increase BUN levels.

15. **Correct Answer: A**

    Females have less muscle mass than males, so they have lower levels of creatinine. Abnormally high levels of creatinine may indicate pyelonephritis or eclampsia.

16. **Correct Answer: C**

    Cimetidine interferes with creatinine excretion in the renal tubule. Renal function does not decrease, but the creatinine level does rise. If the patient has diminished renal function, an allergic nephritis may develop.

17. **Correct Answer: B**

    More than 99% of urea synthesis occurs in the liver. Dietary protein is converted into amino acids and peptides. Approximately 90% of these molecules are absorbed and transfer to the liver. Any excess nitrogen is converted into urea.

18. **Correct Answer: A**

    Approximately 500 mL of whole blood equals 100 g of protein. The extra protein must be converted to urea.

19. **Correct Answer: D**

    Individuals who become trapped under the steering column often have rectal injuries, pelvic fractures, and injured iliac vessels.

20. **Correct Answer: C**

    This procedure elicits Trousseau's sign, an indication of hypocalcemia. You can also elicit this response by having the patient hyperventilate. When the patient becomes alkalotic, the serum calcium level decreases and a carpopedal spasm will occur when the blood pressure cuff is inflated.

21. **Correct Answer: B**

    The patient is hypercalcemic. A loop diuretic prevents reabsorption of calcium, and normal saline is used to increase the patient's glomerular filtration rate. Administering a thiazide diuretic would actually decrease calcium excretion. Glucose, insulin and Kayexalate are not indicated because they are treatments for hyperkalemia.

22. **Correct Answer: B**

    1 kilogram = 2.2 pounds = 1,000 milliliters. Although you may think this is too basic a piece of information for a PCCN review, it is the little pieces of information like this that trip up individuals when they are taking the exam.

23. **Correct Answer: D**

This patient is hypocalcemic. Lack of calcium slows cardiac contractility (leading to a prolonged QT interval), and the patient might develop torsades de pointes (polymorphic ventricular tachycardia). Torsades is also caused by hyperkalemia.

24. **Correct Answer: B**

Eliciting Trousseau's sign requires using a BP cuff to elicit a carpopedal spasm indicative of hypocalcemia. Grey–Turner's sign consists of ecchymosis around the umbilicus indicating abdominal issues. Homan's sign may indicate DVT.

25. **Correct Answer: A**

The patient with AKI cannot excrete ammonium or acid ions in quantities necessary to aid in the excretion of hydrogen. The buildup of hydrogen causes the acidosis.

26. **Correct Answer: B**

Renal infarction can occur with cocaine intoxication. Cocaine abuse can lead to any type of infarction, including MI. The proteinuria and RBCs in the urine are indicative of the renal infarction. Always consider the obvious assessment. Patients of all ages are at risk for substance abuse.

27. **Correct Answer: B**

Aldosterone is a hormone secreted by the adrenal glands. Aldosterone will also be secreted if the individual's blood pressure is too low and when a person is under extreme physical stress.

28. **Correct Answer: C**

Because of a defect in chromosome 7, patients with cystic fibrosis lose sodium through their skin and mucous membranes. This results in a thickening of the mucous layers leading to infection and hyponatremia.

29. **Correct Answer: A**

Large amounts of extracellular fluids are in the peritoneal cavity. If sodium is lost here, then it is no longer available to be absorbed into the vasculature.

30. **Correct Answer: A**

Due to her medical condition, Ada was unable to drink leading to dehydration, and subsequent hemoconcentration. Her diabetes may have caused additional renal injury. This injury, coupled with the decreased blood flow through the kidneys from the CHF, meant that her kidneys were unable to filter the excess sodium from Ada's body.

31. **Correct Answer: D**

Sodium is the major extracellular cation, and potassium is the major intracellular cation.

32. **Correct Answer: A**

Approximately 2% of potassium is extracellular while the remaining 98% is intracellular. Intracellular levels of electrolytes cannot be directly measured, but extracellular levels can be measured. Normal values for extracellular electrolytes range from 3.5 to 5.0 mEq/L.

33. **Correct Answer: B**

Regulated excretion of potassium occurs in the distal tubules.

34. **Correct Answer: B**

    As aldosterone is secreted, potassium excretion increases. The opposite is also true: As aldosterone secretion slows, potassium excretion decreases and more potassium is retained.

35. **Correct Answer: D**

    Alcohol intake leads to an alkalotic state. Since potassium has a positive charge, hydrogen (a negatively charged ion) moves opposite of potassium. As potassium moves into the cell, hydrogen moves out to correct the alkalosis.

36. **Correct Answer: C**

    Potassium and hydrogen move in opposite directions. In hypokalemia, hydrogen moves into the extracellular fluid, leading to both respiratory and metabolic alkalosis.

37. **Correct Answer: A**

    Oliguria is result of hyperkalemia. Renal disease, Lasix, and increased adrenal cortical hormones lead to hypokalemia.

38. **Correct Answer: B**

    A U wave is seen in hypokalemia. A peaked T wave, a shortened QT interval, and an absent P wave may be seen in hyperkalemia.

39. **Correct Answer: D**

    The patient will become hyperkalemic as the potassium from the cells is released into the vasculature during the crush injury.

40. **Correct Answer: C**

    Some people may take in 800 to 11,000 mg of potassium per day through their diet.

41. **Correct Answer: D**

    Carrots have the lowest amount of potassium (233 mg per serving) as compared to avocados (1,484 mg), raisins (751 mg), and potatoes (610 mg).

42. **Correct Answer: A**

    Boiling leaches out most of the nutrients into the water. Baking is the best method for allowing the vegetables to retain most of their potassium and other nutrients.

43. **Correct Answer: C**

    Potassium should not be infused at a rate faster than 10 mEq/h to prevent extravasation, pain, or spasms related to rapid electrolyte changes.

44. **Correct Answer: A**

    Addison's disease results in a decrease in aldosterone secretion. This leads to hyperkalemia and hyponatremia, as sodium cannot be retained and potassium cannot be removed.

45. **Correct Answer: B**

    Kaon is another name for potassium gluconate, a common potassium replacement medication. It is an herbal supplement. Glucose and insulin, calcium gluconate, and bicarbonate all bind or push the potassium back into the cell from the intravascular space, which results in decreased extracellular potassium levels.

46. **Correct Answer: A**
    Belinda is exhibiting signs and symptoms of hypokalemia. Hypokalemia is defined as a potassium level less than 3.5 mEq/L. It is important to teach patients who are given new medications how those medications will affect their electrolyte levels.

47. **Correct Answer: C**
    The current recommended serum magnesium level is 2–3 mg/dL, though it may be higher for patients with cardiac disease or women in the third trimester of pregnancy. Magnesium is also used to treat pregnancy-induced hypertension and to control premature contractions.

48. **Correct Answer: A**
    Magnesium usually acts synergistically with calcium to control neuromuscular function within all muscle groups.

49. **Correct Answer: A**
    The parathyroid controls the calcium level within the body. Magnesium has been found to influence the secretion rate of the parathyroid and, therefore, calcium levels.

50. **Correct Answer: C**
    Approximately 50% of the body's magnesium is found within the bone marrow. The measured serum magnesium reflects only approximately 1% of the body's magnesium, and the remaining 49% is found in the intracellular area.

51. **Correct Answer: D**
    The recommended adult intake of magnesium is 350–420 mg per day. For pregnant women, the preferred intake is at the higher end of this range. The recommended intake for children is less and is based on age.

52. **Correct Answer: A**
    Honey has the lowest amount of magnesium. It is better to recommend foods such as leafy vegetables that have a deep, green color; whole grains, nuts, legumes, seafood, cocoa, and chocolate.

53. **Correct Answer: B**
    Because magnesium is absorbed in the small intestines, surgeries such as gastric bypass or procedures that remove or alter the small intestines place patients at risk for hypomagnesemia. Gastric surgeries also affect water reabsorption, the amount of time needed for processing in the intestines, calcium level, and the amount of lactose in the diet.

54. **Correct Answer: D**
    Carla is exhibiting signs and symptoms of hypomagnesemia related to her high calcium intake. Calcium and magnesium are absorbed in the small intestines. Calcium in extremely high doses competes with magnesium absorption. Carla will need nutritional teaching to balance her diet.

55. **Correct Answer: B**
    Abdominal surgery and trauma place increased stress on the body and stimulate increased secretion of aldosterone. This increase in aldosterone secretion leads to increased magnesium excretion that contributes to hypomagnesemia. This condition lasts for approximately 24 hours. There is an additional risk with any abdominal injury or surgery that impairs small bowel absorption of magnesium.

56. **Correct Answer: A**

    Ketoacidosis leads to excessive urinary secretion of magnesium as a result of osmotic diuresis caused by the elevated glucose concentration. In addition, the use of insulin to treat the hyperglycemia forces magnesium into the cells, which further lowers the extracellular concentration of magnesium. As magnesium levels drop, cellular irritability increases and the risk of convulsions increases. You would expect to see greater overall irritability, a positive Babinski sign, and increased reflexes.

57. **Correct Answer: A**

    As cancer spreads through bone, calcium is released into the serum. When the individual is in a hypercalcemic state, magnesium secretion increases, leading to hypomagnesemia.

58. **Correct Answer: B**

    Only if a patient is in cardiopulmonary arrest would you infuse magnesium at a rate of 1–2 g over 5–10 minutes. IV infusions should be administered at a rate no faster than 30 mg/min. Careful monitoring should be implemented, along with venous access and EKG changes. If using stock magnesium or ampules, be aware that multiple concentrations are available. Solutions come in 10%, 20%, and 50%. To prevent medication errors, physician orders should specify the milliliters of a concentration in a specific amount of fluid to be given over a specified time frame. For example, 2 mL of 50% magnesium sulfate (do not use abbreviation $MgSO_4$, it may be confused with MS or morphine) to be diluted in 100 mL of normal saline (or 9% sodium chloride) over 2 hours.

59. **Correct Answer: D**

    The patient is exhibiting signs and symptoms of hypermagnesemia. The dose should be held, the physician contacted, and the patient's magnesium level evaluated.

60. **Correct Answer: C**

    Renal failure is one of the most common causes of hypermagnesemia. The patient is unable to excrete excess magnesium via the urine. Gastrointestinal bypass and fistulas will lead to hypomagnesemia.

61. **Correct Answer: B**

    Magnesium levels greater than 5 mEq/L lead to vasodilation of the facial vessels.

62. **Correct Answer: A**

    Approximately 99% of the body's calcium is stored in the bone.

63. **Correct Answer: C**

    If calcium is bonded with protein, the resulting molecule is too large to pass from the extracellular fluid into intracellular areas due to restrictive capillary permeability. Approximately 50–70% of serum calcium is ionized in the serum. Because of the protein-binding ability of calcium, albumin and calcium levels can be directly correlated. Calcium plays a role in coagulation.

64. **Correct Answer: A**

    Vitamin D increases serum calcium.

65. **Correct Answer: A**

    Parathyroid is the hormone most closely related to serum calcium management. In response to rising calcium levels, the parathyroid gland decreases secretion of this hormone in an effort to decrease or stabilize calcium levels.

66. **Correct Answer: C**

   The technique for eliciting Trousseau's sign is to inflate a blood pressure cuff to greater than the systolic blood pressure for three minutes. A positive sign is elicited when the carpal nerve spasms, causing the hand to curve inward with all fingers touching.

67. **Correct Answer: A**

   Beta blockers may cause an anaphylactic reaction with the membranes or the filter in the CRRT filter. Bradykinins are released as a result, causing systemic anaphylaxis.

68. **Correct Answer: C**

   The patient's blood pressure provides the gradient on which the system functions. If the blood pressure is too low, the system will not filter appropriately. The minimum MAP should be 60 mm Hg.

69. **Correct Answer: D**

   Some individuals do not tolerate the sight of blood. Because CRRT occurs outside the body, blood is in full sight. To improve communication between both patient and visitors, it is best for the patient to let visitors know when procedures are planned so that they may visit at a time when a CRRT procedure is not occurring.

   There are some restrictions to how many people may fit in one room with the equipment, though this number will vary by facility. The more people in a room, the higher the risk that the equipment could be touched and/or disconnected. Visitors should be informed not to touch equipment while in the room.

   Simple hand washing prevents many infections. Other infection control measures should be used on a per patient, per disease process basis.

70. **Correct Answer: B**

   The "C" in the acronyms stands for "continuous." The second two letters refer to the access and return sites. CVV types of dilution require a pump function as the blood must be pumped through the system. CAV types of filtration use arterial pressures to drive the flow and the filtration. H, HD, and HDF refer to the type of filtration: hemofiltration, hemodialysis, and hemodiafiltration, respectively. Slow continuous ultrafiltration (SCUF) is used to remove fluid from the patient and no replacement is given.

71. **Correct Answer: C**

   Continuous renal replacement therapy (CRRT) results in slower volume regulation to avoid rapid shifts in volume. This method results in continuous removal and/or regulation of solutes and volume.

72. **Correct Answer: D**

   Urea clearance in the blood is the best indicator for monitoring the effectiveness of dialysis. Electrolytes may be altered due to fluid shifting and the type of distillate used. Blood pressure may fluctuate with fluid removal, so it is not the best measurement method. Urine creatinine clearance indicates residual renal function.

73. **Correct Answer: B**

   Lack of thrill and/or bruit may indicate that the graft is occluded and dialysis is not possible. It is best to use a Doppler to determine graft patency prior to any calls or administration of any medication. Although you may not hear or feel the thrill and bruit, the graft may still be patent. The surgeon should be notified if the Doppler study is negative. Heparin will not lyse an existing clot.

74. **Correct Answer: C**
Hemodialysis is used to administer phosphate binders for patients with hyperphos-phatemia. In addition, it may be used to provide vitamin D and calcium carbonate therapy for osteoporosis. Erythropoietin is used to treat iron deficiencies (anemia), and glucose is given for hypoglycemia.

75. **Correct Answer: B**
It is imperative that all staff are made aware of the graft site location. This includes lab technicians, nursing assistants, student nurses, medical staff, physical therapists, and respiratory therapists. All personnel should avoid any lab or blood draws, blood pressures, or occlusions in the grafted limb.

76. **Correct Answer: C**
Approximately 2–3 L of dialysate is used in peritoneal dialysis.

77. **Correct Answer: B**
The correct sequence for fluid exchange in peritoneal dialysis is (1) instill the dialysate, (2) allow the fluid to dwell within the abdomen for a predetermined time, and (3) drain the fluid. The number of exchanges is determined by the physician and the desired outcomes.

78. **Correct Answer: D**
Peritoneal dialysis functions by the principles of diffusion and osmosis. Diffusion is the passive movement of solutes across a membrane. Its direction is determined by concentration (solutes move from areas of higher concentration to areas of lower concentration), heat, and pressure. The speed at which diffusion occurs is based on the grade or steepness of the differences in concentrations on each side of the membrane and the characteristics of the molecules (e.g., size, polarity) moving across the membrane.

Osmosis is the passive movement of a solvent (i.e., water) over a permeable membrane. Movement of the solvent is dependent on the permeability of the membrane. The more permeable the membrane, the more passive the movement of solutes and solvents. Permeability may dictate which types of solutes are able to (intentionally or unintentionally) cross the membrane.

79. **Correct Answer: B**
Patients often experience a feeling of abdominal fullness related to the 2–3 L of dialysate that is instilled in the abdomen and allowed to dwell there. Leaking at the insertion site must be reported to the physician, as the patient may develop peritonitis and the patient should be monitored closely. Dialysis cannot continue until the insertion site is repaired.

If fluid is felt or seen in the groin, its presence indicates a hernia. A hernia may lead to strangulation of any bowel that enters the groin during the dwell phase and is trapped there when the dialysate is drained.

If a patient feels dizzy or has palpitations during the drain phase, this reaction indicates a too-rapid fluid shift or triggering of the vagus nerve. The drain time may need to be lengthened.

80. **Correct Answer: B**
Kinking, bends, and cracks in the tubing are the most likely causes of a decreased dialysate return. If eliminating these mechanical problems does not correct fluid flow,

then reposition the patient and assess for any subcutaneous fluid or fluid within the groin. Double-check the amount of fluid instilled and complete an assessment prior to reporting the situation to the physician.

81. **Correct Answer: C**
The dialysate often contains at least some glucose. During diffusion, glucose may cross the membranes and lead to hyperglycemia. It is important for the patient to monitor for this complication at home. Careful education will assist the family in managing any complications and knowing when to notify the physician.

82. **Correct Answer: A**
Each of the answer options is a condition often treated with apheresis. Paraneoplastic neurologic syndromes are often treated with immunoadsorption. Multiple sclerosis is treated with plasma lymphocyte a. Cutaneous T-cell lymphomas are treated using a combination of photopheresis and leukopheresis. Heart transplant rejections are treated with a combination of photopheresis and plasmapheresis.

83. **Correct Answer: B**
Apheresis is a general term used to describe all pheresis techniques. This term encompasses any selective removal of cells, plasma, and substances from blood, which is then followed by the return of the remaining components and volume to the patient. Plasmapheresis is the removal of plasma and/or proteins from the blood or as a plasma exchange. Cytapheresis is the selective removal of cellular components from the blood (e.g., WBCs). Leukapheresis is the removal of WBCs. Erythrocytapheresis is the removal of RBCs. Plateletpheresis is the removal of platelets. Plasma adsorption/perfusion is the filtering and treatment of plasma via adsorptive fiber filters. Immunoadsorption is the removal of an antigen via an antibody filter. Photopheresis is the removal and return of blood after exposure to ultraviolet light to destroy specific cells (used in solid-organ transplant rejection).

84. **Correct Answer: A**
Replacement of plasma volume in plasmapheresis is usually at a 1:1 or 1.5:1 ratio. Replacement fluids may include FFP, thawed plasma, albumin, and electrolytes, with the selection of the fluids based on the patient's condition.

85. **Correct Answer: D**
Citrate binds with calcium in the blood and metabolizes into sodium bicarbonate, thus increasing sodium and phosphate alkaline. Tests such as ACT, ionized calcium levels, and ABG will show the extent of binding. The tingling is caused by the decrease in the amount of calcium in the tissues.

86. **Correct Answer: C**
Sodium cannot be completely eliminated from the diet. A major cation in the extracellular fluid within the body, sodium plays a key part in driving the sodium–potassium pump and stabilizing polarization of cells and water balance. The body attempts to protect sodium levels by titrating aldosterone and antidiuretic hormone (ADH), and by changing filtration within the kidneys.

   Fresh fruits and vegetables contain minimal amounts of salt. Canned vegetables use sodium to preserve the food's flavor and will have the highest sodium levels.

87. **Correct Answer: B**
    The daily recommended sodium intake for someone limiting sodium consumption should be between 1,000 and 2,000 mg per day. This challenges the body to use sodium efficiently without overstressing the body's systems. A low-sodium diet aims for sodium intake of less than 1,000 mg per day.

88. **Correct Answer: D**
    Many water softener systems filter out calcium and magnesium (these minerals make water hard) and replace them with sodium. The longer the filter has been in place, the greater the sodium content of the water. Not all water softeners use sodium, so patients should be instructed to check their systems before assuming this source is the problem. Instead of drinking tap water, Hannah might be told to drink and prepare food using distilled or bottled water. She might also consider replacing her water filter with a reverse-osmosis system.

    Hannah is following her diet as prescribed and does not exhibit any signs of renal failure. Hypertonic fluids would lead to higher sodium levels. Diabetes insipidus would lead to elevated sodium levels due to the lack of ADH.

89. **Correct Answer: D**
    Blackberries contain 1 mg of sodium per 3.5-ounce serving. Peaches have 2 mg per serving, grapes have 3 mg per serving, and cantaloupe has 12 mg per serving.

90. **Correct Answer: C**
    Most fresh fish will be low in sodium. Pike contains only 51 mg sodium per 3.5-ounce serving—much less than chicken (60–80 mg), canned beef hash (540 mg), and canned crab (1,000 mg). Any canned or processed meat will contain some type of preservative. If the product is not labeled as being low in sodium, the patient should check the sugar content—it may be high. For most people, eating fresh or fresh frozen meats, vegetables, and fruits will aid in limiting sodium, fat, and sugar intake.

91. **Correct Answer: D**
    Parmesan cheese contains 1,862 mg of sodium per 3.5-ounce serving, whereas Swiss cheese has 260 mg per serving, cheddar cheese has 620 mg per serving, and mozzarella has 373 mg per serving.

92. **Correct Answer: A**
    With hyponatremia, sodium levels drop below 135 mEq/L. Twitching and seizures are common, as are apnea (not tachypnea), irritability (lethargy is seen with hypernatremia), and generalized muscle weakness (late sign). Flattened T waves are seen with hypokalemia.

93. **Correct Answer: B**
    Overhydration is a common cause of hyponatremia. It is not a real hyponatremia, in that the level is below normal because of dilution and not a disease process or injury. Intake, whether orally or intravenously, has caused an artificial drop in the patient's sodium level. Correction is achieved by restricting fluids or decreasing IV rates. Other causes of hyponatremia include loss of sodium through sweating or vomiting, shock, bleeding, SIADH, renal failure (inability to save sodium), hypoxia, freshwater drowning, and overadministration of hypotonic fluids.

94. **Correct Answer: B**

    Intravenous pyelogram (IVP), ultrasound, and CT are used as primary diagnostic procedures to detect bladder cancer. Confirmation of the diagnosis is then made by cystoscopy and biopsy. Bladder cancer has a higher incidence in men than in women between 60 and 70 years of age. The majority of diagnoses are malignant tumors of the transitional cells of the bladder. Open loop resection, laser photocoagulation, and transurethral resection with fulguration are surgical procedures used to treat and manage bladder cancer.

95. **Correct Answer: A**

    Migration of the catheter during the procedure or between dialysis treatments increases the patient's risk of peritonitis and sepsis. Leakage at the insertion site increases the risk for skin breakdown and localized infections. Careful monitoring and catheter care will prevent these complications associated with peritoneal dialysis.

BIBLIOGRAPHY

Ahrens, T. (2006). *Critical care nursing certification.* Columbus, OH: McGraw-Hill.

American Association of Critical-Care Nurses. (2006). *Core curriculum for critical care nursing* (6th ed.). Philadelphia: Saunders.

American Association of Critical-Care Nurses. (2007). *AACN certification and core review for high acuity and critical care* (6th ed.). Philadelphia: Saunders.

American Heart Association. (2007). *Guidelines 2005 for cardiopulmonary resuscitation and emergency cardiovascular care.* Retrieved July 24, 2008 from http://circ.ahajournals.org/content/vol112/24_suppl

Bossola, M., Giungi, S., Tazza, L., & Luciani, G. (2007). Long-term oral sodium bicarbonate supplementation does not improve serum albumin levels in hemodialysis patients. *Nephron, 106*(1), c51–c56.

Brindley, P. G., Butler, M. S., Cembrowski, G., & Brindley, D. N. (2007). Case report: Falsely elevated point-of-care lactate measurement after ingestion of ethylene glycol. *Canadian Medical Association Journal, 176*(8), 1097–1099.

Burns, S. M. (Ed.). (2007). *American Association of Critical-Care Nurses (AACN): AACN protocols for practice: Healing environments* (2nd ed.). Sudbury, MA: Jones and Bartlett.

Conover, M. B. (2003). *Understanding electrocardiography* (8th ed.). St. Louis, MO: Mosby/Elsevier.

Copstead, L., & Banasik, J. L. (2000). *Pathophysiology: Biological and behavioral perspectives* (2nd ed.). Philadelphia: Saunders/Elsevier.

Curley, M. A. Q. (1998). Patient–nurse synergy: Optimizing patients' outcomes. *American Journal of Critical Care, 7,* 64–72.

Dessap, A. M., Lellouche, N., Audard, V., Roudot-Thoraval, F., Champagne, S., Lim, P., et al. (2008). Effect of renal failure on peak troponin Ic level in patients with acute myocardial infarction. *Cardiology, 109*(4), 217–221.

Dossey, B. M., Keegan, L., & Guzzetta, C. (2003). *Holistic nursing: A handbook for practice* (3rd ed.). Sudbury, MA: Jones and Bartlett.

Eastwood, G., Gardner, A., & O'Connell, B. (2007). Low-flow oxygen therapy: Selecting the right device. *Australian Nursing Journal, 15*(4), 27–30.

Edwards, D. F. (1999). The Synergy Model: Linking patient needs to nurse competencies. *Critical Care Nurse, 19*(1), 88–98.

Emergency Nurses Association & Newberry, L. (2003). *Sheehy's emergency nursing: Principles and practice* (5th ed.). St. Louis, MO: Mosby/Elsevier.

Eslamifar, A., Hamkar, R., Ramezani, A., Ahmadi, F., Gachkar, L., Jalilvand, S., et al. (2007). Hepatitis G virus exposure in dialysis patients. *International Urology and Nephrology, 39*(4), 1257–1263.

Finkelmeier, B. A. (2000). *Cardiothoracic surgical nursing* (2nd ed.). Philadelphia: Lippincott, Williams & Wilkins.

Hardin, S. R., & Kaplow, R. (Eds.). (2004). *Synergy for clinical excellence: The AACN Synergy Model for Patient Care.* Sudbury, MA: Jones and Bartlett.

Herzog, H. A. (2008). Kidney disease in cardiology. *Nephrology, Dialysis, Transplantation, 23*(1), 42–46.

Hickey, J. V. (2002). *The clinical practice of neurological and neurosurgical nursing* (5th ed.). Philadelphia: Lippincott, Williams & Wilkins.

Hodgman, M. J., Horn, J. F., Stork, C. M., Marraffa, J. M., Holland, M. G., Cantor, R., et al. (2007). Profound metabolic acidosis and oxoprolinuria in an adult. *Journal of Medical Toxicology, 3*(3), 119–124.

Kawada, T., Yamazaki, T., Akiyama, T., Li, M., Zheng, C., Shishido, T., et al. (2007). Angiotensin II attenuates myocardial interstitial acetylcholine release in response to vagal stimulation. *American Journal of Physiology: Heart and Circulatory Physiology, 293*(4), H2516.

Komaba, H., Igaki, N., Goto, S., Yokota, K., Takemoto, T., Hirosue, K., et al. (2007). Adiponectin is associated with brain natriuretic peptide and left ventricular hypertrophy in hemodialysis patients with Type 2 diabetes mellitus. *Nephron, 107*(3), c103–c108.

Laine, J., Jalanko, H., Alakulppi, N., & Holmberg, C. (2005). A new tubular disorder with hypokalaemic metabolic alkalosis, severe hypermagnesuric hypomagnesaemia, hypercalciuria and cardiomyopathy. *Nephrology, Dialysis, Transplantation, 20*(6), 1241–1245.

Lankisch, P. G., Weber-Dany, B., Maisonneuve, P., & Lowenfels, A. B. (2008). Frequency and severity of acute pancreatitis in chronic dialysis patients. *Nephrology, Dialysis, Transplantation, 23*(4), 1401–1405.

Lin, S. H., & Halperin, M. L. (2007). Hypokalemia: A practical approach to diagnosis and its genetic basis. *Current Medicinal Chemistry, 14*(14), 1551–1565.

Lipson, J. G., Dibble, S. L., & Minarik, P. A. (Eds.). (1996). *Culture and nursing care: A pocket guide.* San Francisco, CA: UCSF Nursing Press.

Livingston, E. H., & Langert, J. (2006). The impact of age and Medicare status on bariatric surgical outcomes. *Archives of Surgery, 141*(11), 1115–1120, discussion 1121.

Madias, J. E. (2007). Loss of QRS voltage in renal failure. *Journal of Electrocardiology, 40*(5), 400.

McNally, P. (2001). *GI/liver secrets* (2nd ed.). Philadelphia: Hanley & Belfus/Elsevier.

McPhatter, L., & Lockridge, R. S. (2004). Daily dialysis: Nutritional implications and advantages for a state-of-the-art treatment option. *Nephrology Nursing Journal, 31*(2), 223–224.

McQuillan, K. A., Von Rueden, K. T., Hartsock, R. L., Flynn, M. B., & Whalen, E. (Eds.). (2002). *Trauma nursing: From resuscitation through rehabilitation* (3rd ed.). Philadelphia: Saunders/Elsevier.

Medina, J., & Puntillo, K. (2006). *AACN protocols for practice: Palliative care and end-of-life issues in critical care.* Sudbury, MA: Jones and Bartlett.

Mocini, D., Leone, T., Tubaro, M., Santini, M., & Penco, M. (2007). Structure, production and function of erythropoietin: Implications for therapeutical use in cardiovascular disease. *Current Medicinal Chemistry, 14*(21), 2278–2287.

Morgera, S., Haase, M., Ruckert, M., Krieg, H., Kastrup, M., Krausch, D., et al. (2005). Regional citrate anticoagulation in continuous hemodialysis: Acid–base and electrolyte balance at an increased dose of dialysis. *Nephron, 101*(4), c211–c219.

Morris, C. G., & Low, J. (2008). Metabolic acidosis in the critically ill: Part 1. Classification and pathophysiology. *Anaesthesia, 63*(3), 294–301.

Pace, R. C. (2007). Fluid management in patients on hemodialysis. *Nephrology Nursing Journal, 34*(5), 557–559.

Pagana, K. D., & Pagana, J. (2005). *Mosby's manual of diagnostic and laboratory tests* (3rd ed.). St. Louis, MO: Mosby/Elsevier.

Palomar, R., González-Martín, V., Martín, L., Morales, P., de Francisco, A. L. M., & Arias, M. (2007). Is abdominal surgery still a contraindication for peritoneal dialysis? *Nephrology, Dialysis, Transplantation, 22*(8), 2360–2361.

Rosival, V. (2006). Treating metabolic acidosis. *QJM, 99*(12), 881, author reply 881–882.

Sinert, R., Zehtabchi, S., Bloem, S., & Lucchesi, M. (2006). Effect of normal saline infusion on the diagnostic utility of base deficit in identifying major injury in trauma patients. *Academic Emergency Medicine, 13*(12), 1269.

Skidmore-Roth, L. (2004). *Mosby's 2004 nursing drug reference.* St. Louis, MO: Mosby/Elsevier.

Smeltzer, S., & Bare, B. G. (2003). *Brunner and Suddarth's textbook of medical–surgical nursing* (10th ed.). Philadelphia: Lippincott, Williams & Wilkins.

Sole, M. L., Hartshorn, J., & Lamborne, M. L. (2001). *Introduction to critical care nursing* (3rd ed.). Philadelphia: Saunders/Elsevier.

Sood, M. M., & Richardson, R. (2007). Negative anion gap and elevated osmolar gap due to lithium overdose. *Canadian Medical Association Journal, 176*(7), 921–923.

Stookey, J. D., Barclay, D., Arieff, A., & Popkin, B. M. (2007). The altered fluid distribution in obesity may reflect plasma hypertonicity. *European Journal of Clinical Nutrition, 61*(2), 190–199.

Upadya, A., Tilluckdharry, L., Muralidharan, V., Amoateng-Adjepong, Y., & Manthous, C. A. (2005). Fluid balance and weaning outcomes. *Intensive Care Medicine, 31*(12), 1643–1647.

Urden, L. D., Stacy, K. M., & Lough, M. E. (2007). *Thelan's critical care nursing: Diagnosis and management* (5th ed.). St. Louis, MO: Mosby.

Webb, S., & Dobb, G. (2007). ARF, ATN or AKI? It's now acute kidney injury. *Anaesthesia and Intensive Care, 35*(6), 843–844.

Westenbrink, B. D., Visser, F. W., Voors, A. A., Smilde, T. D. J., Lipsic, E., Navis, G., et al. (2007). Anaemia in chronic heart failure is not only related to impaired renal perfusion and blunted erythropoietin production, but to fluid retention as well. *European Heart Journal, 28*(2), 166–171.

Wiegand, D. J. L., & Carlson, K. K. (Eds.). (2005). *AACN procedure manual for critical care* (5th ed.). Philadelphia: Elsevier.

Wiggins, K. J., McDonald, S. P., Brown, F. G., Rosman, J. B., & Johnson, D. W. (2007). High membrane transport status on peritoneal dialysis is not associated with reduced survival following transfer to haemodialysis. *Nephrology, Dialysis, Transplantation, 22*(10), 3005–3012.

Woods, S., Sivarajan Froelicher, E. S., & Motzer, S. U. (2000). *Cardiac Nursing* (4th ed.). Philadelphia: Lippincott, Williams & Wilkins.

QUESTIONS

1. Maria was admitted to the telemetry unit with diffuse abdominal pain and confusion. In the ED, she had generalized seizures and bradycardia. Opioid overdose was suspected, and she was given naloxone with no discernible effect. Maria is now lethargic, but does tell you that she is a "body packer" to help pay for college. Maria becomes hypotensive and bradycardic. Appropriate therapy would include
   A. Bowel irrigations, intubation, mechanical ventilation, and anticonvulsants.
   B. Sodium bicarbonate, activated charcoal, and hemodialysis.
   C. Antiemetics, gastric lavage, and bronchodilators.
   D. Activated charcoal, sodium bicarbonate, and vasopressors.

2. Nancy, age 73, is admitted to your unit with tachycardia (136), RR 34, BP 90/60, T 96.4°F. Her white count is 17,000. Nancy states she was treated for a "kidney infection" two weeks ago. She denies pain at this time. Nancy probably has
   A. MODS.
   B. A kidney stone.
   C. SIRS.
   D. Appendicitis.

3. Cynthia, age 15, was admitted to your unit because of increased respiratory effort and possible pneumonia. The blood culture revealed the presence of *E. coli*. Which of the following antibiotics would have the best effect on the bacteria?
   A. Ganciclovir
   B. Gentamycin
   C. Cytarabine
   D. Cefoxitin

4. Sam is a 19-year-old male admitted to your unit after a burn injury. He was barbequing in the back yard when a sudden flame-up occurred. It caused partial-thickness, first and second degree burns on his chest, right shoulder and caused partial loss of his facial hair. Which finding would be indicative of smoke inhalation in this patient?
   A. PaO_2 81, met Hgb level of 2%
   B. PaO_2 76, pCO_2 26
   C. Increased CO_2
   D. CoHgB of 18%, singed facial hair

5. Continuing with the scenario from Question 4, which treatment would be most appropriate for Sam at this time?
   A. Fluid resuscitation at a rate of 300 cc/h
   B. Monitor pulse oximetry continuously
   C. Intubation and place on FiO_2 100%
   D. Antibiotic therapy

6. Continuing with the scenario from Questions 4 and 5, you have had to intubate Sam and place him on mechanical ventilation. He will be transferred to the MICU within minutes. Sam's urine output drops significantly. This is probably due to
   A. Third spacing.
   B. Sepsis.
   C. Under resuscitation.
   D. MODS.

7. Hypertonic solutions are used frequently to treat burn patients. An advantage of using this type of solution is that it
   A. Minimizes wound edema.
   B. Lessens the chance that sepsis will develop.
   C. Eliminates the need for vitamin replacements.
   D. Has a lower cost.

8. Signs and symptoms of aspirin overdose include
   A. Metabolic acidosis and tachypnea.
   B. Bradycardia and respiratory acidosis.
   C. Bradycardia and metabolic alkalosis.
   D. Tachycardia and metabolic alkalosis.

9. A 36-year-old male was pumping gas when a spark ignited the fumes. He suffered full-thickness burns of the right arm. During your initial assessment, you note that eschar is present and the right radial pulse is not palpable. A Doppler pulse is also not discernible. Which of the following actions would be appropriate at this time?
   A. Move the patient's arm away from his torso and elevate it on a pillow
   B. Escharotomy
   C. Morphine 4 mg IV
   D. Ice packs to reduce swelling

10. During the immediate post-burn period, which of the following fluids would be most beneficial?
    A. Normal saline
    B. 0.45% normal saline
    C. Lactated Ringer's
    D. Albumin

11. The type of burn most likely to cause hemorrhage, thrombus formation, or generalized vascular disruption is a(n)
    A. Chemical burn.
    B. Steam burn.
    C. Direct flame burn.
    D. Electrical burn.

12. Your patient was in full arrest following a root canal. After a successful resuscitation, the patient has developed Ludwig's angina. This type of angina can be defined as

    A. A type of painful bradycardia in which the Q-T interval is lengthened.
    B. An infectious process.
    C. A dysrhythmia with severe pain secondary to inhalation of noxious gases.
    D. Cardiac ischemia post-code syndrome.

13. In sepsis, endotoxins stimulate production of tumor necrosis factor (TNF). The TNF, in turn, stimulates

    A. Neutrophil activation and platelet aggregation.
    B. Parathyroid hormone production.
    C. Increased CO_2 retention.
    D. Increased CPP.

14. Acetaminophen overdose may cause hypoglycemia and should be treated with

    A. Continuous IV of D_5W at 100 cc/h.
    B. Bolus of D_{50}, followed by continuous infusion of D_5W.
    C. Bolus of D_{10}, followed by continuous infusion of 0.45% normal saline.
    D. Continuous IV infusion of Lactated Ringer's.

15. Patients who are undergoing alcohol withdrawal are frequently hypoglycemic. Treatment should include

    A. Bolus of $D_{10}W$, q 2 hour blood glucose monitoring.
    B. TPN with high concentrations of sugars, q 2 hour blood glucose monitoring.
    C. Maintenance fluids of $D_{25}W$ at 125 mL/h peripherally.
    D. Thiamine, then bolus with D_{50}, then infusion of D_5W.

16. Patients who have oral amphetamine overdoses should receive which of the following as part of their treatment regimen?

    A. Ammonium chloride
    B. Ipecac
    C. Caffeine
    D. Theophylline

17. Your patient is undergoing alcohol withdrawal and exhibits diplopia, peripheral neuropathy, confusion, recent memory loss, and hyper-excitability. You suspect that this patient has

    A. Jorn's syndrome.
    B. Leucine deficiency.
    C. Increased caritine levels.
    D. Wernicke–Korsakoff syndrome.

18. Maxine suffered severe respiratory depression following ingestion of a large amount of diazepam. She has now developed atrial fibrillation. Anticipated treatment would include

    A. Amiodarone.
    B. Lidocaine.
    C. Adenosine.
    D. Prostaglandin.

19. Scott is a 44-year-old male who was burned over the anterior chest, both arms, anterior neck, and the lateral aspect of the right leg. He was smoking in bed when the bedcovers caught fire. The burns on his chest and right arm have a white, leather-like appearance, and Scott has no sensation in that area. Which classification of burn in this?
    A. First degree
    B. Second degree, partial thickness
    C. Third degree, full thickness
    D. Fourth degree, full thickness

20. Michael was serving soup at a homeless shelter when one of the other helpers spilled soup on Michael's right hand and arm. The burn on Michael's right arm is pink and blistered. When touched, Michael screams with pain. Which classification of burn is this?
    A. First degree
    B. Second degree, partial thickness
    C. Third degree, full thickness
    D. Fourth degree, full thickness

21. If muscle is burned, which classification of burn is involved?
    A. First degree
    B. Second degree, partial thickness
    C. Third degree, full thickness
    D. Fourth degree, full thickness

22. Your patient has burns on the right arm that are circumferential (all the way around the arm). What is a potential risk with this type of burn?
    A. Infection into the bone
    B. Difficulty removing dead tissue
    C. Compartment syndrome
    D. Escharotomy

23. Sustained compartment pressures of _____ are usually suggestive of compartment syndrome.
    A. 15 mm Hg
    B. 30 mm Hg
    C. 40 mm Hg
    D. 50 mm Hg

24. Initially, the burned area is estimated by the rule of nines, or using the palm as 1% of the body surface area. There are many ways to calculate the body surface area involved. If your patient was burned over 30% of his body and weighs 70 kg, calculate the total fluid requirements during the first 24 hours using the Parkland formula.
    A. 2,100 mL
    B. 6,300 mL
    C. 4,500 mL
    D. 8,400 mL

25. **Calculate the fluid requirements (first 24 hours) for a patient who weighs 65 kg and is burned over 45% of his body using the Parkland formula.**
    A. 29,250 mL
    B. 11,700 mL
    C. 26,000 mL
    D. 10,300 mL

26. **When using the Parkland formula, the preferred fluid for burn resuscitation is**
    A. Normal saline.
    B. D_5/Isolyte M.
    C. Lactated Ringer's.
    D. D_5W.

27. **To minimize inflammation in burns, which of the following therapies may be used?**
    A. Vitamin C
    B. Hyperbaric therapy
    C. Prednisone
    D. Leaving burns open to the air

28. **Carla was admitted to the PCU with recurrent *Pneumocystis carinii* pneumonia. She is currently on protease inhibitors and non-nucleoside reverse transcriptase inhibitors. Which of the following herbals may be contributing to her recurrent *P. carinii* infection?**
    A. St. John's wort
    B. Ginseng
    C. Ginkgo biloba
    D. Thyme

29. **The brown recluse spider is also known as the**
    A. Hobo spider.
    B. Violet spider.
    C. Fiddleback spider.
    D. Huntsman spider.

30. **People often believe that they have been bitten by a brown recluse spider. If they are able to capture the spider and bring it with them, which of the following would confirm a recluse identification?**
    A. Six (6) eyes
    B. The legs are a darker brown than the body.
    C. The legs have thick spines.
    D. The web is obvious and may be found between two trees or in bushes.

31. **Jay, a 68-year-old retiree, was cleaning out an old basement yesterday. He developed a raised area that initially looked like a mosquito bite but is now red, pus-filled, and inflamed. Jay is admitted to the unit with a necrotizing wound. He may also exhibit all of the following signs and symptoms of a brown recluse spider bite except**
    A. Nausea and vomiting.
    B. Dyspnea.
    C. DIC.
    D. Hemolysis and thrombocytopenia.

32. Which spider bite is most often blamed or misdiagnosed for actual MRSA and *Streptococcus* infections, ulcerations, or insect bites?
    A. Black widow
    B. Huntsman
    C. Brown recluse
    D. Daddy long-legs

33. Jay, a 68-year-old victim of a brown recluse spider bite, is leaving your unit. As part of his discharge teaching, you include ways to prevent future bites. Recommendations should include all of the following except:
    A. Shake out all clothing prior to getting dressed
    B. Always wear gloves when touching wood products or rocks and when working in basements or attics
    C. Change all storage boxes to cardboard
    D. Install yellow or sodium vapor light bulbs outdoors

34. Black widow spider venom is how many times more potent than a cobra or coral snake venom?
    A. 2 times
    B. 5 times
    C. 15 times
    D. 20 times

35. All of the following are found in black widow venom except
    A. Thiamine.
    B. Adenosine.
    C. Inosine.
    D. Latrotoxins.

36. Frank is a 25-year-old gardener who is brought to your unit after collapsing at home this evening with a high fever, severe headache, dizziness, tremors, and severe muscle cramping. He is tachycardic, tachypneic, hypertensive, and restless. You note a rash with erythema, edema, and piloerection and two puncture sites on his anterior left ankle. When questioned, Frank reports that he had been bit by something that morning, but didn't know what. You suspect he was bitten by a
    A. Mosquito.
    B. Bee.
    C. Huntsman spider.
    D. Black widow spider.

37. Tyler, a victim of a black widow spider bite, becomes obtunded, bradycardic, apneic, and hypotensive. You should
    A. Administer morphine 2 mg IV.
    B. Administer antivenin.
    C. Tie a tourniquet around the patient's leg.
    D. Prepare to intubate.

38. Frank is preparing to go home after treatment with antivenin for a black widow spider bite. Which of the following discharge instructions is correct?

A. You may experience muscle spasms for only a few days.

B. You may experience tingling and weakness for five years or longer.

C. It is normal to have a rash or fever in the next three days.

D. Contact your physician immediately if you have joint or abdominal pain or begin to have trouble breathing.

39. **Logan, a 24-year-old hiker, was bitten by a rattlesnake 60 minutes ago while hiking with his wife and friends. He was bitten on the left forearm when he reached down in some grass to pick up a hat that had blown loose. Logan's hand and arm are red and swelling. The puncture sites are bleeding, and he complains of pain and blurred vision. His physician wanted Logan to be admitted directly to your unit and the physician will arrive shortly. There is no available antivenin within 100 miles. Which of the following steps should be taken immediately?**

    A. Contact the patient's insurance company to verify coverage

    B. Place a tourniquet around the patient's arm

    C. Remove any rings or watches

    D. Lift the patient's arm above his heart and wrap it in ice

40. **Continuing with the scenario from Question 39, Logan's friends bring in the dead snake that bit him to verify the type of snake. You should tell them**

    A. That they are crazy for hunting down a snake after it has already bitten once.

    B. To be careful with the head because the snake could bite again even when dead.

    C. To get the snake out of the unit as soon as possible.

    D. That you don't need the snake for verification because all snake bites are the same.

41. **All of the following are poisonous snakes except**

    A. Rattlesnakes.

    B. Coral snakes.

    C. Cottonmouths.

    D. Rat snakes.

42. **Helen was bitten and envenomated by a baby rattlesnake 40 minutes ago. In caring for Helen, you know which of the following facts will influence your treatment?**

    A. Baby rattlesnakes bite but do not inject venom.

    B. Baby rattlesnake venom is mostly hemolytic.

    C. Baby rattlesnake venom is mostly neurotoxic.

    D. Baby rattlesnake venom is less concentrated than adult snakes.

43. **Many people today add "exotic herbs" and supplements into their food and diets. Many of these herbs may be very harmful and interact with medicines the patient is on or may result in serious or deadly complications of existing diseases. Aria is a 20-year-old student who is experimenting with flavorings. She made a roast with Scotch broom on it for her parents to try. After ingesting the roast, her father began to feel light-headed and have palpitations and weakness. She is being treated in your unit post cardiac arrest in the emergency room. If not already done in the ER, your priority would be to**

    A. Insert a nasogastric tube and provide gastric lavage with activated charcoal.

    B. Insert a Foley catheter.

    C. Continue quinidine medications taken at home.

    D. Continue the amiodarone infusion.

44. You have been caring for April in the PCCU for terminal breast cancer. She has stopped eating due to nausea and vomiting. Her son asks if he can bring in her favorite dessert to tempt her to eat. After it is cleared with the physician, he brings in "special" brownies only for his mother. Within a few hours after they leave, April is eating, but is noted to be shaking, anxious, and is no longer oriented to time and place. You suspect

   A. April is exhibiting signs of brain metastasis.
   B. April is having a stroke.
   C. April has ingested marijuana and is exhibiting side effects.
   D. April is hypoglycemic and should continue eating.

45. You are discussing herbal remedies at work when you are approached by a family member of your patient who has Alzheimer's disease and has been admitted for pneumonia. She asks if her mother would benefit from drinking ginkgo biloba at home once discharged because she had heard that this herb can decrease symptoms in early Alzheimer's disease. You tell her:

   A. "There is a lot of research, but nothing really supports its use."
   B. "Sure, there are no interactions with other drugs, so she should be fine."
   C. "Her doctor doesn't approve of any natural remedies, so don't tell him if you are using it."
   D. "There could be very dangerous side effects if ginkgo biloba is taken without consulting her physician. I will have him speak with you when he comes in."

46. You are treating Sid, a patient with long QT syndrome. Which of the following herbs should he avoid?

   A. Ginseng
   B. Ginkgo biloba
   C. Marijuana
   D. Oregano

47. Your patient has been receiving nitroprusside. When giving this medication, it is necessary to monitor for

   A. Tachycardia.
   B. Cyanide toxicity.
   C. Retinal changes.
   D. Ataxia.

48. Ted was admitted to your unit after experiencing abdominal cramping, nausea, and severe diarrhea. His EKG shows sinus tachycardia with frequent PVCs. He is currently on an amiodarone infusion. The only significant history was that Ted ate at a seafood restaurant three days ago. Ted is probably suffering from

   A. Irritable bowel syndrome.
   B. Hypokalemia.
   C. Shellfish poisoning.
   D. Celiac disease.

49. **Diana works in the fashion industry and is a cutter in the wool sweater section of her company. This morning, a fire broke out in her section. Diana did not suffer any burns, but she did inhale large quantities of smoke. What would be the most potent toxin she might have inhaled?**
    A. Carbon monoxide
    B. Smoke
    C. Nitrates
    D. Cyanide

50. **Your patient lives in the country and is self-sufficient. As part of his diet, he eats deer and fish. He was admitted for respiratory distress, weight loss, vomiting, and numbness around the mouth. He is also suffering from mouth sores and drools constantly. His probable diagnosis will be**
    A. Botulism.
    B. *Chlamydia* infection.
    C. *Clostridium difficile* infection.
    D. Mercury poisoning.

51. **Your 28-year-old male patient has been prescribed ergotamine. This drug was probably prescribed for**
    A. Erectile dysfunction.
    B. Headaches.
    C. Pruritis.
    D. Nausea.

52. **Patients who are stung by bees numerous times are in danger of developing**
    A. Kidney failure.
    B. Anemia.
    C. Long QT interval.
    D. Hydrocephalus.

53. **A possible side effect of cocaine is**
    A. Malignant hyperthermia.
    B. Cherry red skin.
    C. Paralytic ileus.
    D. Constricted pupils.

54. **Seymour is a 62-year-old who has become septic following a TURP one week ago. During his course of treatment he is prescribed naloxone. The purpose of the naloxone is**
    A. To block prostaglandins.
    B. To stabilize the cell membrane.
    C. To block endorphins.
    D. To block histamine.

55. Continuing with the scenario from Question 54, Seymour is also receiving activated protein C. The actions of this drug include
    A. Blockade of angiotensin II.
    B. Antimicrobial activity.
    C. Antiviral activity.
    D. Profibrinolytic activity.

56. Which of the following drugs may promote anaphylaxis in a patient receiving treatment for status asthmaticus?
    A. Oxygen
    B. Acetylcysteine
    C. Codeine
    D. Guaifenesin

57. Your patient was very anxious prior to undergoing a bronchoscopy. He received an IM injection of 0.20 mg/kg of Versed. His blood pressure dropped from 142/88 to 80/56, and he became bradycardic. To counter this reaction, he should be given
    A. Xanax.
    B. Ativan.
    C. Valium.
    D. Romazicon.

58. Which of the following vasodilators should not be mixed with Lactated Ringer's?
    A. Nesiritide
    B. Captopril
    C. Cardene
    D. Epinephrine

59. If your patient was in the early stage of septic shock, you would expect which of the following hemodynamic parameters?
    A. SVR elevated, CO decreased
    B. CO decreased, CVP elevated
    C. CVP elevated, SVR decreased
    D. CO increased, SVR decreased

60. Today, you had to float to the fast-track side of the ED. A bunch of teenagers carry in their friend who they call "Jonathan" and they leave him in a chair, then speed off in their car. Jonathan was stabbed by a gang member in the right anterior chest. He lost 1,500–1,600 mL of blood. Which of the following signs and symptoms would be expected with this volume of blood loss?
    A. BP decreased, pulse pressure normal, RR 20–30/min
    B. BP normal, RR increased, capillary refill normal
    C. RR increased, BP normal, pulse pressure normal
    D. BP decreased, RR increased, CO decreased

61. Hoss is a ranch foreman. Yesterday he complained of a stiff neck and was very lethargic. Last night he was found unconscious and had apparently vomited and possibly aspirated. Hoss probably has
    A. Pneumonia.
    B. West Nile virus infection.
    C. Western equine encephalitis.
    D. A brain tumor.

62. Helen is a 40-year-old secretary being treated for MRSA. She has been receiving vancomycin, and this morning her trough level result was > 20 mcg/mL. This level
    A. May cause ototoxicity.
    B. May cause nephrotoxicity.
    C. Is therapeutic.
    D. Indicates the current dosage is too low.

63. Marge is a 28-year-old female who gave birth two months ago to a healthy baby boy. She has been suffering from postpartum depression. Marge was admitted with hallucinations, agitation, ventricular arrhythmias, and a possible seizure (witnessed by her husband). She has probably been taking tricyclic antidepressants. Which of the following drugs is classified as a tricyclic antidepressant?
    A. Amitriptyline
    B. Gentamycin
    C. Clonidine
    D. Fluvastatin

64. Continuing with the scenario from Question 63, Marge's husband said the last time she took one of the antidepressant doses was last evening. A blood level was drawn and is considered a trough level. Her treatment should include
    A. Hemodialysis.
    B. Syrup of ipecac.
    C. Sodium bicarbonate.
    D. Trazodone.

65. Which of the following conditions would be a contraindication when scheduling a patient for a transesophageal echocardiogram (TEE)?
    A. Cardiac tumors
    B. Dysphagia
    C. Vegetative endocarditis
    D. Mitral valve regurgitation

66. Your patient was stabbed in the chest two weeks ago. The damage done to the heart required a prosthetic mitral valve replacement. The patient is now experiencing transient chest pain and syncopal episodes. A TEE is ordered. You anticipate which of the following actions prior to the procedure?
    A. Hold all medications 8 hours prior to procedure
    B. Allow the patient to keep dentures in
    C. Administer prophylactic antibiotics
    D. Position patient on the right side

67. **Which of the following conditions would present with lab results showing a decreased sedimentation rate?**
    A. Anemia
    B. Colon cancer
    C. Infection
    D. Congestive heart failure

68. **Contraindications for a pulmonary angiogram would include**
    A. Perfusion deficits.
    B. Vascular filling defects.
    C. Pulmonary thromboembolism.
    D. Pregnancy.

69. **Acetaminophen overdose may take as long as 2 weeks to resolve. From 72 to 96 hours after ingestion, the patient's symptoms will include**
    A. Pallor, lethargy, and metabolic acidosis.
    B. Increased renal function.
    C. Right upper quadrant pain and increased serum hepatic enzymes.
    D. Jaundice, confusion, and coagulation disorders.

70. **The activated coagulation time (ACT) is more sensitive to _____ and _____ than whole blood clotting time.**
    A. oxygenation, hemofiltration
    B. factor VIII, heparin
    C. warfarin, leukemia
    D. liver disease, calcium

71. **CVP catheter infections may be best prevented by which of the following actions?**
    A. Using an antibiotic-coated catheter
    B. Removing the catheter within 48–72 hours of its insertion
    C. Using prophylactic antibiotics
    D. Avoiding continuous heparin infusions

72. **Increased protein may occur in cerebrospinal fluid due to spinal anesthetics, measles, and ethyl alcohol.**
    A. True
    B. False

73. **Which of the following statements about cocaine is false?**
    A. Cocaine use, even for just one time, can cause rhabdomyolysis.
    B. Cocaine and tobacco use are associated with spontaneous abortion.
    C. Specimens should be kept on ice.
    D. Cocaine causes the placenta to shrink.

74. **Patient and family teaching for digital subtraction angiography includes:**
    A. The length of the procedure is approximately 90 minutes.
    B. Women who are breastfeeding should substitute formula for breast milk for one or more days after the procedure.
    C. The patient will be able to change position frequently during the procedure.
    D. The patient will be free to move around during the procedure.

75. **An antidote for ethylene glycol toxicity is**
    A. Digoxin.
    B. Anisindione.
    C. Fomepizole.
    D. Narcan.

76. **GHB (Ecstasy) overdoses can lead to amnesia in what percentage of cases?**
    A. 13%
    B. 21%
    C. 24%
    D. 32%

77. **Poisoning by arsenic may produce the following symptoms:**
    A. Pneumonia and renal dysfunction
    B. Tachycardia and hypertension
    C. Paresthesia and cerebral edema
    D. Convulsions

78. **Cadmium accumulates in the lungs, liver, and kidneys following exposure to**
    A. Cigarette smoke.
    B. Asbestos.
    C. Lead paint.
    D. Fungicides.

79. **Your patient was admitted for severe flank pain and hematuria. He is scheduled for a kidney biopsy. Your patient and family teaching should include:**
    A. The patient should report any pain in the flank or abdomen post procedure.
    B. The patient may pass a small kidney stone after the procedure.
    C. The patient will be on bed rest for 24 hours.
    D. No teaching is necessary.

80. **Your patient has a history of cluster migraine headaches and has been treated with lithium. Her lithium level on admission was 1.7 mmol/L. This would correspond with the following symptoms:**
    A. Somnolence and coma.
    B. Ataxia and diarrhea.
    C. Seizures and flattened T wave.
    D. Manic-depressive behavior.

81. **Following a lung scan (V/Q), you should observe your patient for**
    A. Sixty minutes following the study for possible reaction to the nucleotides.
    B. Signs and symptoms of pneumonia.
    C. Twenty-four hours to measure urine output and maintain strict I&O.
    D. No observation is necessary.

82. **When preparing to obtain a wound culture for MRSA, which of the following tasks should not be performed?**
    A. Obtain a sterile, cotton-tipped culturette swab
    B. Transport the sample on ice to the lab
    C. Culture the site using a rotating motion for 10 seconds
    D. Place the swab in a sodium chloride medium

83. **Factors that may affect results of urine morphine levels include all the following except**
    A. Poppy seed ingestion may produce false-positive results.
    B. 10 mg MS IV may be detectable in urine for as long as 84 hours.
    C. Use of a stealth adulterant will cause negative results in a positive sample.
    D. High levels of lymphocytes will mask morphine in urine.

84. **Blood osmolality is decreased in**
    A. Uremia and dehydration.
    B. Alcoholism and burns.
    C. Diabetes insipidus.
    D. Hyponatremia and overhydration.

85. **Phenytoin serum levels may be affected by which of the following:**
    A. Holding tube feedings 30 minutes after oral phenytoin administration.
    B. Peak levels should be drawn 2 hours after oral administration of phenytoin.
    C. After a change of dose, allow 24 hours before drawing a phenytoin peak level.
    D. None of the above.

86. **Your patient has been scheduled for a PET scan. Your patient teaching should include:**
    A. The patient is to remain NPO.
    B. The test will require the patient to change position several times during the test.
    C. The patient should avoid ingesting large quantities of fluids within 2 hours prior to the PET scan.
    D. Lactating women should not breastfeed for at least 48 hours after the scan.

87. **Your patient's prothrombin time has an increased INR. You question the patient and determine the patient had taken one of the following medications that may have affected the INR level:**
    A. Antacids.
    B. Herbs and natural remedies.
    C. Antihistamines.
    D. Diuretics.

88. **Your patient underwent pulmonary function testing. The respiratory therapist tells you the preliminary result is a low peak expiratory flow rate (PEFR). This might indicate**
    A. Asthma.
    B. Pneumothorax.
    C. Pulmonary cysts.
    D. Heart failure.

89. **Your patient is undergoing a renal arteriogram. After the dye is injected, the patient complains of a "salty taste" in his mouth. You know**
    A. This is the first sign of an anaphylactic reaction.
    B. This will result in termination of the arteriogram.
    C. This is expected and should pass after about five minutes.
    D. This is an emergency.

90. **Rocky Mountain spotted fever is caused by**
    A. A parasite.
    B. Fleas.
    C. A rotavirus.
    D. Fungi.

91. **False-positive results for the sickle cell test may be caused by all of the following except**
    A. Polycythemia.
    B. High blood protein levels.
    C. Anemia.
    D. Multiple myelomas.

92. **Your hospital has just received word of a mass casualty incident. You are called on to report to the ED and assist with triage. The preliminary report is that your facility will be receiving as many as 60 patients. The first patient you see is a male, about 30 years old, with multiple lacerations. He is awake and alert and complaining of pain in the right chest and right upper quadrant. There is no rebound tenderness. You confirm that ribs 7–9 are fractured. You would suspect which of the following underlying conditions/injuries?**
    A. Spleen laceration
    B. Liver laceration
    C. Pneumothorax
    D. Mesenteric infarction

93. **Continuing with the scenario from Question 92, the second patient you see is a 20-year-old female who was trapped in her car for almost two hours by the steering column. She complains of left shoulder pain, left upper quadrant rebound tenderness, and she presents with an obviously fractured lower leg that was splinted by paramedics. The paramedics had listed her as stable and stated that she had no rebound tenderness or guarding at the accident scene. She is tachycardic at 116 and has fractures of ribs 9–10. You suspect**
    A. Ruptured pancreas.
    B. Diaphragm rupture.
    C. Spleen injury.
    D. Lacerated liver.

94. **Continuing with the scenario from Questions 92 and 93, the third patient you encounter is a paramedic who was injured on the way to assist with the mass casualties. He is confused, but complains of back pain at the level of L3. He is hypotensive and has swelling at the level of L1–L3. You would suspect which type of injury?**
    A. Splenic rupture
    B. Kidney laceration
    C. Large bowel rupture
    D. Retroperitoneal liver injury

95. Rick is a fanatic golf fan. He was a spectator at a golf tournament when he was struck by lightning. Rick was thrown about 10 feet into a tree. He suffered a fractured left radius, a concussion, and burns on his left arm, chest, and right leg. He has been somewhat confused since the accident. Which of the following statements about lightning injuries is true?
    A. Internal burns are common.
    B. Barotrauma is rare.
    C. Myoglobinuria is rarely seen.
    D. DC current will most likely cause ventricular fibrillation.

96. Binge eating, mutilation, obesity, drug abuse, and alcoholism are all examples of
    A. Self-destructive behaviors.
    B. Psychotic behaviors.
    C. Neurosis.
    D. Immaturity.

97. All of the following may affect an elderly patient's ability to counter psychiatric emergencies except
    A. Altered or reduced problem-solving and coping mechanisms.
    B. Stable health.
    C. Increased loss of or limited support systems.
    D. Greater financial pressures or limited resources.

98. Clint, a 52-year-old father of six, has suffered a heart attack and requires immediate coronary artery bypass graft. His children and wife are present as well as multiple other family members and church family. You overhear his wife and children speaking about complete insurance coverage; they state that Clint's employer has approved significant sick time for his recovery and has offered Clint the chance to work from home if additional home recuperation time is required. You are determining the level of psychiatric distress in this family. Your first priority is to
    A. Administer psychotic medications.
    B. Examine the range and effectiveness of coping mechanisms.
    C. Work with any available family members, friends, or religious support systems.
    D. Determine if there is a crisis.

99. Amy is the lone survivor of a car crash that killed her parents and two siblings. She is recovering from a pneumothorax, hemothorax, and bilateral broken legs. Amy has been extremely depressed and withdrawn. You are discussing medications, psychiatric therapy, and the increased risk of suicide and suicidal behavior with Amy's distant relatives. The family makes each of the following statements. Which of the statements is false?
    A. "If Amy is considering suicide, she will make statements or give warnings of suicide."
    B. "We should trust our instincts if we feel Amy is in danger."
    C. "As she recovers from her depression, Amy is at greater risk of suicide."
    D. "If Amy talks about suicide or asks about pills, then she is just voicing the thought and will not attempt suicide."

100. Continuing with the scenario from Question 99, Amy is the sole survivor of a crash that killed her immediate family. While recovering from massive injuries, her behavior and moods change rapidly. Which of the following behaviors is most concerning to you as the nurse and indicates possible suicidal behavior?
    A. Drug seeking with multiple requests for pain medications and sedatives
    B. Withdrawal from conversation and interaction
    C. Crying and statements of helplessness
    D. Screaming at her distant relatives

101. Brody is a 46-year-old admitted to the PCU after a barroom brawl in which he suffered multiple minor stab wounds. He is angry and verbally assaults the staff. The goal of anger management for this patient is to do all of the following except
    A. Confront Brody directly with whatever made him angry.
    B. Discuss what in the situation made him angry.
    C. Discuss with Brody alternative and positive ways to express his feelings.
    D. Decide on positive ways for Brody to express his feelings when confronted with frustrating situations in the future.

102. Cassandra was admitted to the DOU for severe anxiety. Which of the following medical conditions may present with such symptoms?
    A. Narcolepsy
    B. Asthma
    C. Hyperglycemia and/or hypoglycemia
    D. Hypercaffeination

103. Stephan is an alcoholic admitted to your unit with cirrhosis. Why is thiamine added to his IV fluids?
    A. Thiamine is a sedative and will ease agitation.
    B. Thiamine decreases the symptoms of DTs.
    C. Thiamine is used to prevent the damage to the brain as a result of Wernicke's syndrome.
    D. Thiamine is used to prevent complications of substance abuse.

104. Harold is experiencing delirium tremens. Nursing interventions include keeping his room well lit and minimizing stimulation. Staff members continuously reorient Harold to time, place, and person. Haldol has been given as ordered, and the patient is in four-point restraints. Which of these nursing interventions should be discontinued?
    A. Reorientation
    B. Medication administration
    C. Restraints
    D. Controlling stimulation

105. You are assisting with triaging of patients after an earthquake. Which of the following steps is your first priority?
    A. Establishing physical conditions
    B. Addressing the media
    C. Getting social services
    D. Reconnecting family members

106. Your patient had a three-vessel CABG procedure and sustained a small stroke during the procedure. The stroke left some residual numbness in the left arm. The family is quite agitated and does not agree with the patient's advance directives. The family informs you that they want everything done for the patient and to ignore the patient's request for no resuscitative measures. Which of the following nursing interventions would be appropriate at this time?
    A. Inform the family that the physician will meet with them to discuss treatment options
    B. Tell the patient about the family's concerns
    C. Notify the physician that all orders are to come from the family
    D. Inform the family that the patient is fully capable of making decisions

107. Your patient is scheduled for implantation of a VAD. About 20 minutes prior to the scheduled start of the procedure, she informs you that she has concerns about side effects and the procedure itself. Your best nursing intervention would be to
    A. See if the patient signed the consent form for the procedure.
    B. Notify the physician that the patient does not have a full understanding of the procedure.
    C. Cancel the procedure.
    D. Answer the patient's questions yourself.

108. A car carrying four teenagers went off a bridge and killed all but one of the teens. Today, a second EEG was done and brain death was confirmed for the fourth teen. The family was approached about organ donation. They requested that the patient remain in the PCU for at least 7–8 days until the older sister can return from a war zone. The appropriate nursing response would be to
    A. Tell the family patients are waiting for the bed.
    B. Notify the physician to tell the family organ donation must be made within 24 hours.
    C. Notify social services and arrange for emergency compassionate leave for the sister.
    D. Wait until the family leaves to procure the organs.

109. A woman who is eight months pregnant was severely injured in an automobile accident. Her condition has been declining over the past week. The husband has been informed of the probable demise of his wife. The patient was made a "Do not resuscitate" and moved to the PCU because she requires more care than the staff on the orthopedic unit can provide. In addition, the physician suspects fetal demise and has notified the husband of this possibility. The husband wants to bring their only other child, an 8-year-old boy, into the PCU to visit his mother. The PCU has a policy that children must be 12 years old to visit. What is an appropriate nursing action at this time?
    A. Sneak the child in during night shift
    B. Take a picture of the mother for the child
    C. Arrange a patient care conference for the next day to discuss options
    D. Inform the husband that the visiting policy is strictly enforced

110. Shawn works sorting mail at the local post office. She finds an envelope that is torn and has white powder falling out of the tear. Shawn is sent to the hospital and admitted to the intensive care unit for possible inhalation anthrax. What is the treatment of choice for Shawn?

A. Penicillin G 2 million units intravenously every 6 hours

B. Ciprofloxacin 400 mg intravenously every 12 hours

C. Doxycycline 500 mg intravenously every 12 hours

D. Augmentin 875/125 mg intravenously every 12 hours

111. **What is the incubation period for inhalation anthrax?**
    A. 7–10 days
    B. 5–7 days
    C. 7–60 days
    D. 20–30 days

112. **What are the initial symptoms of inhalation anthrax?**
    A. Mild, flu-like symptoms
    B. Severe dyspnea and productive cough
    C. High fever, cough, and stridor
    D. Cutaneous lesions, cough, and high fever

113. **4. How long is antibiotic therapy continued for inhalation anthrax?**
    A. 10 days of intravenous antibiotics
    B. 14 days of intravenous antibiotics, then oral antibiotics
    C. 30 days of intravenous antibiotics, then oral antibiotics
    D. 60 days of combined intravenous and oral antibiotics

114. **Which form of isolation should be used for a patient with inhalation anthrax?**
    A. Full isolation with laminar air flow
    B. Droplet precautions
    C. Standard contact precautions
    D. Reverse isolation

115. **Kathy is a 50-year-old female who lives on a farm. She home-cans meat and vegetables every year. Kathy is admitted to the intensive care unit with profound weakness, double vision, slurred speech, and dysphagia. Her initial diagnosis is Guillain-Barré syndrome. While you are interviewing her family, you learn that a few days ago Kathy ingested some home-canned green beans that were several years old. No other family members ate the beans because the color was odd. What do you do with this information?**
    A. Do nothing, it is of no consequence
    B. Notify the physician immediately, Kathy may have botulism
    C. Tell the physician tomorrow during rounds
    D. Continue the interview

116. **What is the causative organism in botulism?**
    A. *Clostridium difficile*
    B. *Clostridium botulinum*
    C. *Clostridium avium*
    D. *Botulinum botulinum*

117. Your hospital is put on an external disaster notice after a ricin poisoning at a local train station. Your progressive care unit prepares to accept casualties. What makes ricin so toxic to humans?
    A. It causes respiratory failure.
    B. It causes renal failure.
    C. It inhibits protein synthesis leading to cell death.
    D. It destroys the mitochondria in the cell, causing cell death.

118. As the charge nurse for a busy telemetry unit, you note an increased frequency of patients with underlying mental disorders being admitted. You overhear some negative comments from other nurses about assignment to these patients. You ask the nurses to complete a self-awareness survey regarding their beliefs and understanding of mental health issues. You will use this information to
    A. Determine which nurses should never care for patients with mental health issues.
    B. Change nursing assignments immediately.
    C. Determine which nurses should be written up and counseled.
    D. Create an education program for the nurses that will increase understanding of mental health issues and explain how to access resources.

119. You are discussing post-discharge psychiatric resources with a patient's family. You note that they are using the terms "psychiatric emergency" and "crisis" interchangeably. To clarify this issue, you tell them that
    A. A crisis is an immediate danger to someone else, and an emergency is a suicide attempt.
    B. A crisis develops over time as a result of a psychological stressor, and an emergency is an immediate situation that, if not corrected, will result in violence.
    C. A crisis occurs when no intervention will be effective, and an emergency is when interventions have the greatest impact.
    D. A crisis is sudden and precedes an emergency when lives may be threatened.

120. While passing the room of your terminally ill patient, you see his wife of 40 years crying at the bedside while she pats the patient's hand. She is unkempt, tired, and unable to focus during conversations. You believe that she is in the middle of a situational crisis. Your best action is to
    A. Call the social worker to speak with her.
    B. Call the appropriate spiritual advisor for this patient.
    C. Call her primary doctor for a prescription for Xanax or Paxil.
    D. Call your charge nurse to cover your other patients while you initiate a conversation with her to identify stressors and develop a list of resources.

121. Which of the following individuals is at highest risk for a psychological emergency?
    A. An 80-year-old home-bound male whose wife has just died and who has no children or living family
    B. A married 20-year-old female who delivered a 35-week gestational infant
    C. A married 56-year-old male who was just laid off from his job of 10 years
    D. A married 36-year-old female newly diagnosed with systemic lupus

122. Your unit has just completed a code lasting two hours for an 18-year-old rape and trauma victim. The patient had seemingly been doing fine the past 3 days while in your unit. Due to overwhelming unknown factors, the patient does not survive. Chaplain services are called in to assist with a nursing staff debriefing. Of all emotions encountered, staff members experiencing which of the following emotions are at highest risk for psychological stress?
    A. Anger
    B. Fear
    C. Anxiety
    D. Denial

123. You are talking to your 24-year-old patient about his newly diagnosed Type II diabetes. He states that he is fine with the diagnosis and knows that he will need to make some changes. His speech is rapid and pressured, and he is making frequent jokes; he also talks about playing football with the guys when he is discharged. You would still be concerned about this patient's psychological health because of his
    A. Rapid, pressured speech.
    B. Frequent jokes.
    C. Talk of social activities.
    D. Failure to identify specific lifestyle changes that will need to be made.

124. Zack, a chronic alcoholic with cirrhosis, has returned again to the DOU after failing rehabilitation that you assisted him in obtaining. Although you previously had a friendly and open relationship, the patient will not look at you and gives only minimal answers to your questions. You tell him:
    A. "I can't believe you wasted the opportunity to get sober at the rehabilitation center."
    B. "I know you want to stay sober, but maybe you need more time."
    C. "I am proud of how long you stayed sober. Let's try again."
    D. "Why don't we work together to find new resources for you to utilize when you are tempted to drink."

125. Adam, a 24-year-old football player, suffered a spinal injury in a motor vehicle accident while intoxicated. He is now a paraplegic without family and financial resources. During wound care, he states, "You shouldn't bother with that—no one cares if I live or die. My life is over. I can't play football, and no one wants a cripple around. If I disappear, no one would even notice." Your best response to his statements is to say:
    A. "Don't talk like that—you are still alive and many paraplegics are active and happy."
    B. "Why would you say that? You had visitors yesterday."
    C. "I understand that your injuries are devastating to you, but I cannot allow you to harm yourself."
    D. "Let's just get through the dressing change, and then I'll have the doctor prescribe something for you."

126. Alicia, the 44-year-old estranged daughter of your patient with myocardial infarction, is overheard in the waiting room telling another family member, "The nurses aren't doing enough for her. If they let her die, I'll make sure they suffer." When Alicia comes in to visit, you note that she is glaring at the staff, her posture is tense, and her movements are quick and forceful. She is pacing the room, will not acknowledge staff members, and uses inappropriate language at the bedside. Your priority is to
    A. Call security to assist in removing Alicia from the unit to a secluded area.
    B. Ignore Alicia's behavior and continue to care for the patient.
    C. Call the police and forbid Alicia from returning.
    D. Make jokes and shame Alicia into behaving.

127. You are caring for a 68-year-old woman who was in a motor vehicle accident in which a child was killed. She is combative and restless, hyperventilating, tachycardic, and has an elevated blood pressure. The patient states, "I've got to leave here. They'll arrest me and they'll lock me up. I can't believe this. There is no way out." You should tell her:
    A. "Just relax. They can't arrest you while you are in the hospital."
    B. "Calm down. It wasn't your fault if the child darted into traffic."
    C. "Stop it. You are working yourself up. Look at me and focus on what I am telling you to do."
    D. "They should arrest you, you killed a child."

128. You are caring for Mr. B., a 34-year-old male who suffered a gunshot wound during a casino bar fight 18 hours ago. He was restrained after being verbally and physically abusive to the staff. You see Mr. B. thrashing around in the bed and he is suddenly awake when you enter the room. He is shaking, has vomited, is tachycardic with an elevated blood pressure, and is talking to people who are not in the room. You suspect Mr. B. is
    A. Experiencing delirium tremens.
    B. Experiencing drug withdrawal.
    C. Experiencing sepsis.
    D. Exhibiting signs of paranoid schizophrenia.

129. Risk assessment for pressure ulcers should be done on admission using
    A. Harrelson's scale.
    B. Cush's anagram.
    C. Ordon's anagram.
    D. Braden scale.

This concludes the Multisystem Questions section.

ANSWERS

1. **Correct Answer: A**
"Body packer" is a term used for people who transport narcotics in their body cavities. In this case, it is probable that a packet has ruptured. More doses of naloxone may be necessary, along with supportive treatment for opioid overdose. Be alert for bradycardia, hypotension, respiratory depression, and hypothermia.

2. **Correct Answer: C**
MODS is usually the result of a direct injury to an organ. A kidney stone or appendicitis should present with pain and tenderness. SIRS is a systemic infection that can present in the elderly with hypothermia and even a WBC of < 4,000 or > 12,000.

3. **Correct Answer: B**
Gentamycin is an aminoglycoside, as are tobramycin and amikacin. These medications are used for gram-negative bacterial infections; however, they must be used with caution because they can cause nephrotoxicity.

4. **Correct Answer: D**
When a sudden flame-up comes near the face, the first instinct is to gasp. This inhalation of superheated air will cause swelling of the tissues in the air passages. This patient was probably very near the flame as his facial hair was burned off, and he is at great risk of a compromised airway and may need intubation. Ideally, Sam should have gone to a dedicated burn unit or to an ICU in case he needed intubation. Potential respiratory issues can be easily overlooked.

5. **Correct Answer: C**
Because of the immediate danger of airway closure, intubation should be done as soon as possible on a prophylactic basis. Once the airway begins to close, intubation may be impossible. At times, even a tracheostomy is extremely difficult.

6. **Correct Answer: C**
Sam is likely suffering from under-resuscitation. Burn patients require large amounts of fluid. Later in this section, you will learn a formula for fluid resuscitation.

7. **Correct Answer: A**
Hypertonic solutions minimize wound edema.

8. **Correct Answer: A**
Aspirin is an acid and causes a profound acidosis. Tinnitus may also be present.

9. **Correct Answer: B**
This question describes an emergency. The pressure must be relieved via an escharotomy, an incision through multiple layers of tissue. Any circumferential burn of the body may lead to impaired function and necessitate escharotomy.

10. **Correct Answer: C**
Lactated Ringer's is used for burn patients because it is part of many of the formulas for burn resuscitation. This solution is preferred for large-volume resuscitation because LR contains 130 mEq/L of sodium compared to normal saline that has 154 mEq/L of sodium. LR also has a higher pH (6.5) compared to normal saline (5.0). The pH of the

LR is close to a normal pH for the body. The patient will be in metabolic acidosis, so the metabolized lactate will buffer the acidosis. LR is also an isotonic crystalloid.

11. **Correct Answer: D**
Electrical burns are insidious and follow the path of least resistance. Muscle tissue breaks down and causes rhabdomyolysis when myoglobin is released into the circulation.

12. **Correct Answer: B**
Ludwig's angina is a submaxillary infection. It is a cellulitis of the neck and floor of the mouth that usually occurs with, or after, dental disease.

13. **Correct Answer: A**
In addition, TNF stimulates increased capillary permeability and promotes the release of IL-1, IL-6, and IL-8.

14. **Correct Answer: B**
Hypoglycemia occurs because of the hepatotoxic effects of acetaminophen. Infusions must also be based on blood glucose results.

15. **Correct Answer: D**
Administer thiamine, then give a D_{50} bolus, and then start an infusion of D_5W.

16. **Correct Answer: A**
Ammonium chloride can convert to ammonia and HCl in the liver. This conversion will indirectly correct metabolic alkalosis, but the ammonia that is generated can produce encephalopathy.

17. **Correct Answer: D**
Wernicke–Korsakoff syndrome is a thiamine deficiency and a metabolic encephalopathy.

18. **Correct Answer: A**
Amiodarone is useful in treatment of atrial fibrillation because the drug decreases sinus rate, increases PD and QT intervals, and results in the development of U waves.

19. **Correct Answer: C**
Full-thickness burns destroy nerve endings because they extend into subcutaneous tissue. The tissue may have a whitish color and will be somewhat firm, with a leather-like appearance. Sometimes you can see clotted vessels through the eschar.

20. **Correct Answer: B**
This type of burn may be superficial or a deep partial-thickness burn. The nerve endings are still intact and this burn is very painful. Sometimes burns can be deceptive. A reddened area can be diagnosed as a first-degree burn, yet may be overlooked when staff calculate the patient's requirements for fluid and nutrient resuscitation. After a few hours, these areas can develop blisters and only then may be recognized as dermal burns. A new way of assessing burn levels uses a laser Doppler during the first week of treatment.

Assessing a burn depth can be tricky. The first step is determine which factors caused the burn (chemical, electrical, thermal), how long the causative mechanism was in contact with the area, blood flow, and where the burn is located. Another thing to consider is the thickness of the skin at the site. Elderly people and children have thinner skin, so burns in those populations tend to be more severe. Burns on the eyelids and genital area are approximately 1 mm thick, whereas burns on the palms and soles of the feet are on areas approximately 5 mm thick. Although the thicker skin offers a bit more thermal protection, the palms and soles of the feet become infected more easily.

21. **Correct Answer: D**

    Not many people are familiar with this classification. This kind of burn not only involves muscle, but also extends through muscle and bone.

22. **Correct Answer: C**

    Escharotomy is a procedure, not a direct risk. The highest risk at this time is compartment syndrome. As a nurse, you must constantly assess the patient for quality of pulses. Edema may be so great as to completely cut off circulation in a limb and cause a myoglobin-related renal failure. Elevating the limb may help drain fluid and mitigate further edema. If the pulse is lost, compartment syndrome is not necessarily the cause. The lost pulse could be due to failure to replace the lost volume secondary to the burn.

23. **Correct Answer: B**

    This level of sustained pressure requires that the physician perform a procedure to release the pressure. If the compartment pressure reaches 40 mm Hg, it requires an immediate escharotomy or fasciotomy. In most burn units, there is some sort of electrocautery device at the bedside or close by. Before performing this procedure, the patient should be sedated and medicated for pain if hemodynamically stable. If the patient experiences a lot of pain, it could be that the elevated pressure resulted from a fluid deficit. When assessing a burned patient, if a weak pulse is present, it is probably due to under-resuscitation.

24. **Correct Answer: D**

    The Parkland formula was developed by Dr. Charles Baxter at Parkland Hospital in Dallas, Texas, in the 1960s and is still utilized today as a standard for fluid resuscitation. Many other formulas are in use as well, but this one is widely known and will probably be on the CCRN examination. The Parkland formula is

    4 mL fluid × patient's weight (in kg) × % of body surface area burned

    In this case, the patient requires $4 \times 70 \times 30 = 8{,}400$ mL fluid for the first 24 hours. Half the calculated volume is given in the first 8 hours, then the remaining volume is given over the next 16 hours.

25. **Correct Answer: B**

    The formula is $4 \times 65 \times 45 = 11{,}700$ mL.

26. **Correct Answer: C**

    Lactated Ringer's is used for burn patients because it is part of many of the formulas for burn resuscitation. This solution is preferred for large-volume resuscitation because LR contains 130 mEq/L of sodium; by comparison, normal saline contains 154 mEq/L of sodium. LR also has a higher pH (6.5) compared to normal saline (5.0). The pH of the LR is close to a normal pH for the body. The patient will be in metabolic acidosis, so the metabolized lactate will buffer the acidosis. LR is also an isotonic crystalloid.

27. **Correct Answer: A**

This question will probably not be on the PCCN exam, but it may show up as a question within the next year or so. Vitamin C is an antioxidant that is used to counter oxidant-mediated effects on the inflammatory cascade. Studies with animals have shown that if vitamin C is given within six hours of a burn, as much as 50% of the fluid needed for resuscitation can be eliminated.

Always remember that with a burn patient you should start at least two large-bore IVs.

Another new treatment involves the use of subatmospheric pressure dressings. These dressings may aid in removing excess fluid and help save areas that would otherwise have to be grafted or removed.

28. **Correct Answer: A**

St. John's wort is contraindicated in patients with HIV/AIDS. This herb interferes with the metabolism of protease inhibitors and non-nucleoside reverse transcriptase inhibitors.

29. **Correct Answer: C**

Depending on the region in which the spider is found, the brown recluse spider may also be called the violin spider or the fiddleback. Although it is normally found in the South, reports have noted this spider's presence from California to Virginia and as far north as Ohio and Michigan. In the United States, there are 13 varieties of recluse spiders.

30. **Correct Answer: A**

The brown recluse spider is just that—a recluse; it will generally avoid humans whenever possible. Because of its reclusive nature, the brown recluse spider's web will be difficult to see or find. These spiders have six eyes instead of the eight eyes seen on most spiders. A dark, violin-shaped mark appears on the part of the body where the legs are attached, with the neck of the "violin" pointing toward the body of the spider. The legs have fine hairs and no spines. The brown recluse spider is no larger than 0.5 inch in body length.

31. **Correct Answer: B**

Patients presenting with recluse spider bites may not initially know that they were bitten and will seek medical help 12–36 hours after the initial bite. Because treatment is so often delayed, symptoms may be difficult to treat. The majority of patients will present with flu-like symptoms. DIC, hemolysis, and thrombocytopenia are severe symptoms. Treatment includes applying ice to control inflammation, keeping the area clean and protected, and treating symptoms. No specific treatment has been proven to be 100% effective. Dapsone has limited support for preventing necrosis. Nitroglycerin patches counter the vasoconstrictive properties of the venom and lead to hemodilution in the bloodstream and increased bleeding at the site to wash the venom out.

32. **Correct Answer: C**

The brown recluse spider is often blamed for necrotic wounds that are actually caused by MRSA, *Streptococcus* infection, ulcerations, and bites from other insects. This spider is generally an isolative spider and will avoid humans whenever possible. Because bites are often not felt at the time of their occurrence, capture and identification of the actual spider that caused the bite is difficult and extremely rare. If the brown recluse is the cause of a bite, if the bite occurs over fatty or soft tissue, the venom may cause necrosis and take months to heal. Necrosis is thought to be caused by the vasoconstrictive properties of the venom.

33. **Correct Answer: C**

    It is recommended that all cardboard be removed from houses and populated areas as soon as possible. Because cardboard is made of wood fibers, when it decays it is similar to a rotting tree stump, a popular haven for the brown recluse. The spider may hide or nest in folds and between layers of cardboard. Sealed plastic containers and bags provide some barriers to habitation. Gloves protect hands from exposure when handling woods and rocks or when working in storage areas such as basements and attics. Yellow or sodium light bulbs do not prevent the spider from nesting, but will limit food availability (lights repel other insects) and make the area less inviting.

34. **Correct Answer: C**

    Black widow venom is 15 times more potent than cobra or coral snake venom. What is fortunate is that black widow spiders are not large and their punctures are at most 1 mm deep (the length of a female's chelicerae or pincher). Males are smaller than the females with smaller chelicerae and, therefore, inject less venom. The high incidence of deaths worldwide caused by black widow spider bites is mostly reflective of the high number and wide distribution of this spider.

35. **Correct Answer: A**

    Thiamine, also known as vitamin B_1, is not found in the black widow venom. Adenosine has two effects in the body: It inhibits the central nervous system and it acts as an anti-inflammatory agent. Adenosine is also broken down into inosine within the bloodstream. Inosine is part of the cascade that leads to muscle movement. Latrotoxin is the main active neurotoxin most responsible for symptoms felt by victims of black widow spider bites. Low-molecular-weight components within the venom are thought to facilitate higher-molecular-weight toxins in permeating cell membranes. The neurotoxin causes cell death by causing a rapid influx of calcium into cells.

36. **Correct Answer: D**

    Black widow spider venom causes massive muscle contractions as the venom circulates throughout the body via blood and the lymphatic system. Symptoms are most often seen in the first 24 hours after a bite. The neurotoxins cause an influx of calcium into cells, resulting in cellular death. In addition to muscle cramping, other symptoms include joint pain, anxiety, insomnia, diaphoresis, severe abdominal cramping and pain, and lacrimation. If the patient has a compromised immunity or co-morbidities, the effects of the toxins could be more deadly. Extreme cases and complications include priapism, acute renal failure, myocarditis, rhabdomyolysis, and paralysis. If untreated, shock, coma, and death may occur.

37. **Correct Answer: D**

    The patient is apneic and bradycardic. Priorities are to maintain the airway to provide ventilation and oxygen therapy. The next step is to administer antivenin as soon as it is available. Morphine may help with pain, but will worsen the bradycardia and hypotension. It is a myth that tying a tourniquet around the affected limb will stop the venom from reaching the bloodstream or lymphatic system. At this point, the venom already has systemic distribution. In minor cases involving healthy adults, symptoms may be managed with pain control, muscle relaxants, and comfort measures. Symptoms should dissipate during the first 3 days after exposure.

38. **Correct Answer: D**

    Joint and abdominal pain (pain related to splenomegaly) as well as dyspnea may be signs of anaphylaxis or serum sickness that occur as long as 2–4 weeks after antivenin administration. If these symptoms arise, patients should be taught to contact their physicians immediately so early treatment can be initiated to prevent complications. Administration of corticosteroids and antihistamines will aid in combating the inflammatory response to the animal proteins in the antivenin. The neurotoxin may cause residual muscle spasms, tingling, weakness, and nervousness for weeks to months after the exposure to the venom. Patients may need to slowly increase activity during their recovery.

39. **Correct Answer: C**

    As swelling continues in the affected limb, it is important to remove any restrictive jewelry or clothing while you are still able to do so without damaging the limb. Do not place a tourniquet or ice on the bite, as this will decrease blood flow to the surrounding tissues. A light bandage on the site will absorb the blood; do not bind the site tightly. Do not raise the site of the bite above the patient's heart, as gravity will increase venom flow back toward the heart. It is best to keep the limb dependent and stabilized. Keep the patient calm, prevent unnecessary movement, and treat shock symptoms if present.

40. **Correct Answer: B**

    A snake may strike again within one hour after death due to reflexes. A snake should never be captured after a strike unless done by experienced personnel. The snake may strike again in fear, leading to a second victim. All bites are not the same. You may be able to identify the snake if dead and present; otherwise, blood tests can determine which venom is present in the blood.

41. **Correct Answer: D**

    Rattlesnakes, coral snakes, and cottonmouths are all venomous (poisonous). Immediate medical attention should be sought for any bite victim. The rat snake is found mostly on the East Coast from Canada to Florida and as far west as Texas and Minnesota. Often mistaken for a cottonmouth, the rat snake has a narrower body.

42. **Correct Answer: C**

    The venom of baby rattlesnakes is more potent than the venom of adult snakes and contains more neurotoxins; hence, symptoms will be more neurologic in presentation. Careful attention should be given to respiratory effort, blood pressure, and muscular control. Baby snakes can bite and inject venom rapidly if threatened or cornered. Their venom may be more neurotoxic, which helps to paralyze a predator so that the baby can escape. In contrast, the adult rattlesnake uses the more hemolytic venom for hunting and consumption. Generally, a snake will not strike an animal that it cannot consume unless threatened or cornered.

43. **Correct Answer: A**

    Scotch broom contains sparteine, which has very powerful cardiovascular effects. Arrhythmias, blood pressure changes (increased or decreased), coagulation changes, and vision changes are possible side effects of this herb. The best action listed would be to lavage the stomach to remove any undigested or partially digested Scotch broom. You will need to insert a Foley catheter, because Scotch broom does have diuretic properties; this step is not a priority, however. Quinidine and amiodarone should be stopped immediately because they will interact with the Scotch broom to cause further cardiovascular collapse by increasing the toxicity of the herb.

44. **Correct Answer: C**

Based on the history presented, it is suspicious that April's behavior toward food and her psychomotor skills would be altered so closely after ingesting a homemade meal. The brownies should be tested for marijuana. Additional side effects of marijuana ingestion may include paranoia, sleeplessness, short-term memory impairment, nausea, respiratory depression, and headaches.

Each state has specific regulations regarding marijuana use for medicinal purposes. Regardless, the staff should have a family conference with the patient to determine the best course of treatment regarding April's symptoms. Self- or family-prescribing should not be permitted during hospitalization. If use of medicinal marijuana is illegal in your state, local law enforcement officials may need to be contacted.

45. **Correct Answer: D**

Although natural, if herbal supplements and herbal use are not regulated, these products can have varying strengths and resultant side effects. Regardless of their personal beliefs, it is vital that the treating staff be aware of any herbal supplements taken separately or in drinks or foods. Although some research has favored ginkgo biloba's use in increasing cerebral blood flow, there have also been documented cases of severe bleeding, seizures, glucose instability, and allergic reactions. Extreme caution should be used with these products for patients on anticoagulation therapy, antiplatelet therapy, anti-inflammatory drugs, diabetic regimen, MAO inhibitors, antipsychotic drugs, and antiseizure medications.

46. **Correct Answer: A**

Ginseng has been known to increase the QT interval, which would put this patient at greater risk for cardiac rhythm complications. Advise patients to carefully read the label before consuming any sports or high-energy drink, as many of these drinks now contain various herbs and high levels of caffeine. Ginseng may also cause breast tissue enlargement in men, erectile dysfunction, increased menstrual bleeding, and hormone imbalances in those with breast cancer, uterine cancer, and endometriosis. These effects may occur because ginseng has effects similar to those associated with estrogen. Ginseng may also cause complications or interactions with anticoagulation therapy, calcium-channel blockers, diabetes management, and it increases the potency of some sedatives.

47. **Correct Answer: B**

Sodium nitroprusside, when used in high doses (10 mcg/kg/min) or over a period of days, can raise blood concentrations of cyanide to toxic levels. Patients who are malnourished or are stressed from surgery may have low thiosulfate reserves. These patients are at increased risk for developing symptoms, even with therapeutic dosing. They may become agitated and combative and these symptoms may be mistaken for ICU psychosis. If patients are given hydroxocobalamin or sodium thiosulfate along with the nitroprusside, the symptoms may be prevented or at least mitigated.

48. **Correct Answer: C**

Shellfish poisoning can cause an individual to exhibit symptoms days after ingestion of the shellfish. The toxin contained in shellfish (e.g., clams and oysters) is called saxotoxin and is not affected by steaming or cooking. It inhibits sodium channels of membranes, thereby blocking propagation of nerve and muscle action potentials. If the nerves are involved, the person may experience paresthesias of the lips, tongue, gums, and face. The paresthesias may spread to the trunk and lead to paralysis and respiratory arrest. There is no definitive treatment for shellfish poisoning, so care is driven by treating symptoms and psychological support.

49. **Correct Answer: D**
Wool and silk give off cyanide gas. Nitriles, like those found in the gloves nurses wear, will burn and give off cyanide. Household plastics like melamine dishes, plastic cups, polyurethane foam in furniture cushions, and many other synthetic materials may produce lethal concentrations of cyanide when burned under certain circumstances. Cyanide inhibits cellular respiration, even when the person has adequate oxygen stores. Cellular metabolism changes from aerobic to anaerobic, and produces lactic acid. The organs with the highest oxygen requirements are the ones most dramatically affected by cyanide inhalation.

50. **Correct Answer: D**
Fish can contain large amounts of mercury. The concentration of mercury can be more than 1,000 times greater in the fish than in the surrounding water. People who eat fish as a main component of their diet may be at risk.
   Organic mercury compounds are very toxic. They may be taken into the body by ingestion, inhalation, skin, and eye contact. The mercury compounds can attack all body systems, causing nausea, lack of appetite, abdominal pain, kidney failure, swollen gums and mouth sores, tremors, seizures, and numbness and tingling in the lips, mouth, tongue, hands, and feet. Patients can become very uncoordinated and feel disconnected from their surroundings. They may lose part or all of their vision and hearing. Additional neurological issues may include memory loss, personality changes, and headache. Organic mercury can pass to a baby via breast milk. Methyl mercury may cause serious birth defects.

51. **Correct Answer: B**
Ergotamine (Ergot) is used as a treatment for migraine headaches. In females, it may be used to promote uterine contraction in childbirth. Because ergotamine promotes contraction of smooth muscles, it can be used to control bleeding.
   In large doses, ergotamine paralyzes the motor nerve endings of the sympathetic nervous system. It can cause disorientation, confusion, convulsions, seizures, severe muscle cramping, and dry gangrene of the extremities. LSD (lysergic acid diethylamide), is chemically related to ergotamine.

52. **Correct Answer: A**
Bee stings deliver proteins in the venom that act as enzymes. The enzymes lyse the cells and the cellular debris accumulates very quickly and actually clogs the kidneys. The patient then dies from kidney failure. Any patient who has been stung multiple times needs to be monitored for at least two weeks following the incident.

53. **Correct Answer: A**
The antidote is Dantrolene. Malignant hyperthermia is usually seen in patients receiving anesthetics. This patient may also require ice packs and a hypothermia blanket. On occasion, bowel irrigations with cold water and cold NG tube irrigations have been necessary. Cherry red skin is a possible effect with carbon monoxide poisoning.

54. **Correct Answer: C**

Excess endorphins need to be mediated. Prostaglandin is blocked by ibuprofen. Corticosteroids are used to stabilize the cell membrane by modifying mediators.

55. **Correct Answer: D**

Activated protein C (Xigris) inhibits factors Va and VIIIa. It also inhibits human tumor necrosis factor production by monocytes and limits thrombin-induced inflammatory responses.

56. **Correct Answer: B**

Mucomyst may actually cause bronchospasm, so it must be used with a bronchodilator. Usually, Mucomyst is contraindicated in status asthmaticus. Codeine is generally not used in status asthmaticus. Guaifenesin is Robitussin, a mild cough syrup.

57. **Correct Answer: D**

Xanax, Valium and Ativan are also benzodiazepines. Flumazenil (Romazicon) is a benzodiazepine antagonist.

58. **Correct Answer: C**

Cardene cannot be mixed with Lactated Ringer's or sodium bicarbonate infusions. According to studies, although the combination does not cause a precipitate, the Lactated Ringer's inactivates 15% to 42% of the drug.

59. **Correct Answer: D**

The patient may have a mild fever and will be in a hyperdynamic state. The endotoxins that are circulating will have vasodilatory effects, so CVP and blood pressure are decreased. The increase in CO is compensatory.

60. **Correct Answer: D**

This patient is in hypovolemic shock. The normal blood volume in an adult is about 5,000 mL. A loss of 1,500 mL of blood would be equal to about one third of the total blood volume. You would expect the heart rate to increase to 120–150, blood pressure to decrease, pulse pressure to narrow, respiratory rate to increase to 25–40, and delayed capillary refill. The skin would be cool and clammy, and there may be neurological issues such as restlessness, anxiety, and confusion.

61. **Correct Answer: C**

Western equine encephalitis is caused by an arbovirus (togovirus). An arbovirus is carried by arthropods. A horse or small mammal was probably infected, and the virus was transferred by a mosquito. This type of encephalopathy is not directly transmitted from human to human. This patient is at high risk for aspiration pneumonia and ARDS.

62. **Correct Answer: B**

A trough level of more than 20 μg/mL is actually a panic level and, if not addressed, will cause nephrotoxicity. Ototoxicity usually occurs if levels are prolonged at > than 30 μg/mL. Vancomycin may cause hypertension, thrombocytopenia, tubular necrosis, colitis, and deafness. The patient may require hemodialysis, hemofiltration, or peritoneal dialysis. Note that charcoal hemofiltration does not remove vancomycin.

63. **Correct Answer: A**

Tricyclic antidepressants act by blocking norepinephrine and serotonin uptake in the central nervous system. These drugs also have anticholinergic properties. The really interesting thing about this group of drugs is that they metabolize in the liver to one of the other tricyclics. You must test for levels of all the tricyclics because the one you are testing for may have metabolized and added to the effects.

64. **Correct Answer: C**

You can give hypertonic saline for hypotension. The ABG results should guide the amount to be given. Hemodialysis will not remove amitriptyline from the patient's system.

65. **Correct Answer: B**

In a TEE, the patient is sedated and the gag reflex reduced by an oral numbing spray. A gastroscope is advanced, which the patient should swallow. The tube is positioned directly behind the heart and allows for sound waves to be reflected off the heart chambers and valves. The left mainstem bronchus can interfere with the view. Some of these types of scopes can generate a three-dimensional picture.

There is a risk with this procedure for the patient to experience reflex bradycardia, esophageal perforation, transient hypoxia, drug-initiated tachycardia, or oversedation. Additional contraindications would include stenosis and obstruction of the esophagus, penetrating chest injuries, and central nervous system depression (no sedatives). An inability to lie flat is another contraindication.

66. **Correct Answer: C**

The patient should receive prophylactic antibiotics to mitigate possible endocarditis, which may be the cause of his symptoms.

67. **Correct Answer: D**

The sed rate may also be decreased in patients with poikilocytosis. Other causes of a low sed rate include cortisone, lecithin, and corticotrophin.

68. **Correct Answer: D**

Pulmonary angiogram requires iodine-based radiographic contrast dye to be injected into the antecubital or femoral vein via catheter to the pulmonary artery. The pulmonary vasculature can then be visualized. The radioactive iodine crosses the blood–placental barrier, which is why this procedure is contraindicated in pregnancy. Other contraindications include allergy to shellfish, iodine, radiographic dye, and renal insufficiency.

69. **Correct Answer: D**

Renal function is possibly decreased, and the patient may have increased ALT and AST. The symptoms will abate in 4 days to 2 weeks.

70. **Correct Answer: B**

The activated coagulation time (ACT) test is easy to do and is reliable. The ACT measures the ability of the blood to clot. Fresh, whole blood is added to a test tube that contains an activator. The activator can consist of glass particles, kayolin, or diatomaceous earth. The result will be the time it takes for a clot to form.

71. **Correct Answer: B**

A major complication with use of CVP catheters is infection. Studies have shown that the initial source of the infection is usually from an initial colonization of skin bacteria that migrate down the catheter. The point of insertion (subclavian or jugular) also has been found to have no bearing on the risk of infection. Heparin may keep the catheter from clotting, but does not have any bearing on potential infections. Prophylactic antibiotics will not prevent catheter infections and may lead to more antibiotic-resistant strains colonizing the catheter. If the catheter remains in place more than 72 hours, there is a significant risk of infection.

72. **Correct Answer: A**
We decided to throw you a curve and put in a true/false question. Protein can show up in the cerebrospinal fluid as a result of more than 30 conditions. Some of these conditions include brain abscess, brain tumor, diabetic neuropathy, encephalitis, heavy-metal poisoning, meningitis, mumps, myxedema, and phenytoin, to name a few.

73. **Correct Answer: D**
Cocaine is classified as a Schedule II central nervous system stimulant. It is also used as a local anesthetic, a bronchodilator, and a vasoconstrictor. Cocaine compromises the heart's antioxidant defense system, and an overdose can cause an MI. Cocaine can also cause aortic dissection, stroke, intestinal ischemia, hallucinations, and adverse effects on fetuses.

74. **Correct Answer: B**
Digital subtraction angiography can be done to diagnose aneurysms, aortic valve stenosis, carotid stenosis, pulmonary emboli, ulcerative plaques, hepatocellular carcinomas, and many other conditions. The procedure carries some risks, including allergic reactions to the contrast dye, anaphylaxis, aphasia, hemiplegia, paresthesia, hemorrhage, infection, renal toxicity, and thromboemboli.

75. **Correct Answer: C**
Ethylene glycol is a compound found in antifreeze. After ingestion, it is converted to oxalic acid, which is excreted by the kidneys. This causes crystals in the urine, acidosis, tetany, and renal failure. Hemodialysis and peritoneal dialysis will remove ethylene glycol from the body.

76. **Correct Answer: A**
Ecstasy use can also cause ataxia, central nervous system depression, coma, bradycardias, hypothermia, hypotension, respiratory depression, and respiratory acidosis.

77. **Correct Answer: D**
Arsenic is found in all human tissues as a trace element, but these levels may become elevated with exposure to additional sources. Approximately 60% of ingested arsenic is excreted in the urine. Arsenic may be found in well water, pesticides, paints, cosmetics, treated wood, and coal. Chronic exposure can lead to various types of cancers.

78. **Correct Answer: A**
Cadmium is a heavy metal with a half-life of 15–20 years. This respiratory irritant can produce pulmonary edema, interstitial pneumonia, and cardiovascular collapse if inhaled. Cadmium is used in the manufacture of storage batteries, alloys, and in electroplating. If cadmium is ingested, the individual will experience severe gastrointestinal symptoms within 30 minutes. Most cadmium collects in erythrocytes and kidney tissues. It is not metabolized in the body.

79. **Correct Answer: A**

     The biopsy may cause bleeding from highly vascular tissue. Flank pain may be the first sign.

80. **Correct Answer: B**

     Lithium is an alkali, a metal salt used mostly in the treatment of bipolar disorder and cluster migraine headaches. In bipolar disorder and alcohol withdrawal, lithium works by altering sodium transport in nerves and muscles, which helps to stabilize mood.

81. **Correct Answer: A**

     An additional consideration is that when you are discarding urine, you should wear gloves when dealing with patients for 24 hours after the test. You must also wash the gloves with soap and water before removing the gloves; then, wash your hands again. Many nurses have needlessly exposed themselves because in their haste to empty fluids for I&Os at shift change, they forget to wear gloves.

82. **Correct Answer: B**

     Wound cultures for MRSA do not have to be placed on ice for transport. They may be kept as long as 8 hours at room temperature.

83. **Correct Answer: D**

     The stealth adulterant will mask morphine in the urine. When heroin is taken, it breaks down into morphine. As little as 10 mg of morphine is detectable in urine for 84 hours; it can even be measured in corpses for about a week.

84. **Correct Answer: D**

     Answers A, B, and C are all causes of increases in blood osmolality.

85. **Correct Answer: D**

     Phenytoin is metabolized in the liver and excreted in bile and urine. It is used as an anticonvulsant and antidysrhythmic agent. Tube feedings should be held before the test for two hours. Peak levels should be drawn 3–9 hours after oral use. As much as five days must be allowed to pass before a change in dose will change results.

86. **Correct Answer: C**

     Patients may eat prior to the PET scan, but they should not drink large quantities of fluid within two hours of the scan unless the patient has, or will have, an indwelling catheter. Caffeinated drinks should be avoided within two hours of the test. It is important to inform lactating women to not breastfeed for at least 20 hours after the scan.

87. **Correct Answer: B**

     Many herbs and natural remedies will affect the INR because they are oral anticoagulants. These products include dan shen, dang gui, dong quai, gingko biloba, garlic, ginseng, and ginger.

88. **Correct Answer: A**

     Because of air trapping, a person with asthma has a low peak flow rate during expiration.

89. **Correct Answer: C**

     The salty taste is normal and the patient may be slightly nauseous, feel the need to cough, or feel flushed. This sensation will pass in about five minutes.

90. **Correct Answer: C**

    Rocky Mountain spotted fever is spread by ticks. Symptoms include a sudden-onset fever for 2–3 weeks and a rash that may cover the entire body. Treatment must include both chloramphenicol and tetracycline.

91. **Correct Answer: C**

    False-positive results may be caused by polycythemia. False-negative results may be due to anemia or the fact that less than 7 mL of blood was drawn for the test.

92. **Correct Answer: B**

    The liver may be lacerated by either blunt or penetrating trauma. In blunt trauma, there will often be fractures of ribs 7–9, overlying the liver. In this case, there is no history of the mechanism of injury. Right upper quadrant tenderness will be present with a liver laceration. Rebound sensitivity and guarding will not be present because blood has not been in the abdomen at least two hours (long enough to cause peritoneal irritation). Suspect liver laceration when penetrating trauma involves the right lower chest or right upper abdomen, or when right upper quadrant tenderness accompanies blunt trauma. The patient needs a CT.

93. **Correct Answer: C**

    Suspect splenic injury when ribs 9–10 on the left side are fractured, or when left upper quadrant tenderness and tachycardia are present. This patient has not complained of pain in the left shoulder, but it is a common complaint with splenic injury. Peritoneal signs such as rebound sensitivity and guarding are delayed until the blood has had time to cause local irritation of the peritoneum. This patient was trapped in her car for almost two hours. Hypotension is a sign of an active bleed.

94. **Correct Answer: B**

    The kidneys are in the retroperitoneal space at the level of T12 to L3. They can be damaged by shearing or compression forces, which can cause laceration or contusion. Suspect renal injuries with fractures to the posterior ribs or lumbar vertebrae. Rupture of the renal artery with a deceleration injury from a crash may cause hypovolemia. There is little collateral circulation to the kidney, so damage to the renal artery may lead to acute tubular necrosis and intrarenal failure. Sometimes, the signs of a kidney injury may be confused with a pancreatic injury. However, you do not generally have hematuria with a pancreatic injury. You will see common signs such as Grey–Turner's sign (flank ecchymosis), Cullen's sign (peri-umbilical bruising), and flank pain. This patient also is exhibiting confusion, which could be caused by anything from a simple concussion to an acute brain injury. The patient needs immediate evaluation.

95. **Correct Answer: C**

    AC current usually causes ventricular fibrillation, whereas DC current usually causes asystole. In some cases, arrhythmias may be delayed for up to 12 hours after the lightning strike.

    The mechanism of lightning strikes is quite complex, and lightning can injure a person in several different ways. In this case, a side splash from another object is probably the cause of this patient's injuries. The lightning may have hit something like a tree, and then bounced off. A direct strike may also have occurred. Another type of strike can occur when the person touches an object that is struck. Ground current effect occurs when energy spreads out across the surface of the earth.

Lightning has two strokes, upward and downward. If they do not meet, energy can be directed outward. Internal burns are rare with lightning-related injuries, and myoglobinuria rarely occurs. Generally, lightning will cause cardiac and respiratory arrest, burns from metals touching the victim (watches, necklaces, golf shoe cleats), and neurological damage.

96. **Correct Answer: A**
Self-destructive behaviors are those that, over time, will shorten or threaten the person's length and quality of life.

97. **Correct Answer: B**
Often elderly persons have unstable health that contributes to psychiatric crisis and emergency. Many elderly individuals have limited support systems as time and circumstances may result in loss of loved ones by death or distance. Limited ability to work, health or disabilities, or limited funds may also lead to greater emotional and psychiatric distress because of financial issues.

98. **Correct Answer: D**
In any potential psychiatric emergency or crisis, it is important to determine if one actually exists. In this scenario, the patient has an extensive and involved support system, financial stability, and effective coping mechanisms, so a psychiatric crisis is not likely to develop. It is still important to carefully monitor for any change in status.

99. **Correct Answer: D**
Careful consideration and observation should be given to any person voicing any thought or plan regarding suicide. Many individuals will provide warnings about their suicidal thoughts, thereby providing those in the family or in proximity the opportunity to intervene. Such warnings are often cries for help and intervention. Family members should pay close attention to any impression or instinct that the person is considering suicide. As individuals enter and exit depression, they are at greatest risk for suicide as they have sufficient mental focus to form a plan and energy or motivation to carry it out.

100. **Correct Answer: C**
Feelings of helplessness or hopelessness indicate psychotic emergencies. Extreme anxiety or ability to recognize options should alert staff and family that the person is at greater risk of suicide, because suicide may be seen by the patient or individual as the only option. The other answers indicate depression and/or levels of grief and emotional expression.

101. **Correct Answer: A**
Direct confrontation with the object of anger may further exacerbate the situation and limit the person's ability to deal positively with the situation. Instead, engage the person in a conversation regarding the stressor and assist him in identifying feelings and options.

102. **Correct Answer: A**
Alterations in chemical or electrolytes may lead to anxiety and agitation that could be misdiagnosed as a psychiatric emergency.

103. **Correct Answer: C**

Wernicke's syndrome is a result of thiamine deficiency. It will result in brain damage if not treated immediately.

104. **Correct Answer: C**

Restraints should be used only if alternative methods for behavioral correction are ineffective. There is no indication that this patient is violent or has caused any threat to staff or self. Restraints should be used only as a last resort to prevent injury to self and staff. Reorientation, medications, and controlling external stimulation are all effective methods for controlling behavior.

105. **Correct Answer: A**

Physical needs must come before psychological needs in any disaster or crisis. According to Maslow's hierarchy of needs, the physical needs must be met first before other needs can be considered. Once the physical needs have been satisfied, then you can focus on locating family, providing social services, and disseminating information to the media.

106. **Correct Answer: D**

Sometimes family members do not have enough education to make proper decisions. In this case, the family needs to know that the patient is still capable of making decisions and that his wishes will be honored.

107. **Correct Answer: B**

Even if the patient signed a consent form, she does not appear to be certain about the procedure or is not fully informed. The nurse must act as advocate and notify the physician.

108. **Correct Answer: C**

Sometimes, the bed is actually emergently needed. In the best possible world, the military could arrange for compassionate leave for the military service member. Hospital personnel certainly should not simply go ahead and try to procure organs as soon as the family leaves.

109. **Correct Answer: C**

This is the best nursing response because it ensures that all members of the healthcare team can join in the decision. Visiting policies vary, but are primarily designed to protect children from disease and from being overwhelmed by equipment and the PCU milieu. Under the circumstances, you would probably want to sneak the kid in on night shift, but many factors should be weighed here. This visit could produce the child's last memory of his mother. The conference will weigh the child's maturity and coping ability. He and the father will probably lose the mother and the sibling. There is no simple answer.

110. **Correct Answer: B**

Ciprofloxacin, a fluroquinolone antibiotic, is the drug of choice for inhalation anthrax. Doxycycline, a tetracycline derivative, may also be utilized but the dosage in this question is incorrect. Penicillin G is not an option because the bacterium, *Bacillus anthracis*, becomes beta lactamase positive, making penicillin ineffective. Augmentin would not be used for this situation and it is only given orally.

111. **Correct Answer: C**

Inhalation anthrax has an incubation period ranging from 7 days to as long as 60 days after exposure. Symptoms are initially vague and flu-like, such as malaise, low-grade fever, and nausea. These symptoms quickly progress to profound diaphoresis, chest discomfort, and rhonchi. The mild symptoms occur in the first 5 days of the illness, followed by a brief rally. The patient then experiences an abrupt onset of high fever and severe respiratory distress. Death occurs as early as 24–36 hours after symptoms begin.

112. **Correct Answer: A**

Inhalation anthrax starts with mild, nonspecific symptoms such as malaise, low-grade fever, fatigue, and cough. If it is left untreated, death occurs within 24–36 hours from respiratory failure.

113. **Correct Answer: D**

Antibiotics for inhalation anthrax are continued for 60 days after exposure, even if exposure is merely suspected. Treatment is initially intravenous, but then changes to oral dosing for the remaining time. The two antibiotics most commonly given are ciprofloxacin and doxycycline.

114. **Correct Answer: C**

According to CDC guidelines, contact precautions are all that is required for inhalation anthrax. Standard precautions may include the use of a face mask if the patient has a productive cough.

115. **Correct Answer: B**

Kathy has botulism from the old green beans she consumed. Because this patient ate the contaminated food a few days ago, it is too late to give her the antitoxin. If she survives the acute phase, she may have lasting fatigue and dyspnea for years, requiring long-term therapy.

Many foods that are home-canned may contain botulism spores. Those foods include beans, fermented fish, tomatoes, chili peppers, asparagus, corn, beets, improperly handled baked potatoes, and garlic or herbs in olive oil. All of these items have a low acid content, which encourages the survival of *Clostridium botulinum* spores. Proper sterilization of home-canning equipment and storage containers can reduce the risk to those consuming these foods. Boiling the foods for at least 10 minutes will also kill the *C. botulinum* spores.

116. **Correct Answer: B**

Clostridium botulinum is a rod-shaped bacterium that is the causative organism of botulism. Only 25% of all U.S. cases of botulism are from food products, and most of these involve home-canned foods. The majority of cases consist of infant botulism, which accounts for more than 70% of all cases of botulism in the United States. The third type of botulism is seen in wounds contaminated by soil containing the botulism spores. Babies younger than 1 year old should not consume honey, especially raw or home-grown honey, because it may contain botulism spores.

117. **Correct Answer: C**

Ricin, which is made from castor beans, is one of the most toxic substances known. It interferes with protein synthesis and causes cell death. Chewing castor beans may cause some symptoms, but the most lethal form of ricin is inhaled. The toxin is not spread by casual contact. The most likely victims in a bioterrorism event would be seen in enclosed areas such as subway trains, buses, or small rooms. For distribution purposes, ricin is usually aerosolized with a liquid such as water or a weak acid.

118. **Correct Answer: D**

Surveys can be used to anonymously identify staff perceptions and determine educational opportunities. Mental health issues impact every person at some point in their lives. Whether the patient's problem arises due to a catastrophic event or ongoing psychological issues, it is important that nurses understand their own biases regarding mental health and be able to identify resources when caring for this population. If the nurses believe the survey will be used punitively, then data may be skewed to reflect what the staff believe the surveyor is looking for, not the truth. Instead of changing assignments immediately, it is best to use the opportunity for education and professional growth.

119. **Correct Answer: B**

A psychological crisis may precede an emergency, though that is not always the case. Although there is no specific definition for either term, accepted criteria for a crisis is that it is a less immediate situation that has developed over time in the presence of a psychological situation. Coping mechanisms may be partially effective, but do not address the situation directly to lead to a conclusion of the problem. A crisis may develop into an emergency if coping mechanisms fail or additional stressors appear. A psychological emergency has multiple elements, including a sense of urgency that if the situation is not resolved, the anxiety may become intolerable and lead to feelings of being overwhelmed. If coping skills have completely failed, the patient may recognize the need for help in alleviating the stressors. Suicide calls, notes, and messages meet these criteria.

120. **Correct Answer: D**

The wife may need time to open up to you, so the nurse will need to ensure that his or her other patients are cared for while this conversation takes place. Even though the social worker and spiritual advisor may need to be called, it is important not to overwhelm the wife until the stressor and situation have been identified. It is not appropriate for the nurse to contact the wife's physician. The wife may need prescriptions during this time, but that decision should be made by her physician upon direct assessment.

121. **Correct Answer: A**

Although each of these situations can be classified as a crisis, the 80-year-old homebound male without family resources is at greatest risk for emergency. Because he is confined to his home, it will be more challenging to get resources to him. Public assistance, friends, and seniors groups may be effective resources to ensure appropriate coping.

122. **Correct Answer: C**

Anger, fear, and denial are all normal emotions in this situation. Staff members who feel anxiety may be at greater risk, even though anxiety is frequently a response in psychological emergencies. Anxiety involves uncertainty about the unknown and may limit the person's ability to identify resources or initiate appropriate coping mechanisms. Debriefings after codes, successful and unsuccessful, are therapeutic and allow staff to verbalize emotions in a safe and stable environment. As a team, the staff may identify ways to support families and one another during crisis and emergency situations.

123. **Correct Answer: A**

Rapid, pressured speech is a sign of tension and indicates that the patient still needs support and assistance in coping with his diagnosis. Humor and social activities can be positive coping techniques as long as they are not used to avoid the stressful situation. This patient will need assistance and education regarding his diagnosis to effectively identify positive lifestyle changes.

124. **Correct Answer: D**

The patient may feel as if he has failed the nurse by not remaining sober and that assistance may be withdrawn. This statement in answer D does not judge the patient, but rather shows the patient that help is still available by initiating communication and encouraging the patient to talk about his struggles with maintaining sobriety. Answer A is judgmental and demeaning. Answer B limits support and indicates to the patient that he unable to succeed. Answer C focuses on the nurse's feelings, rather than those of the patient.

125. **Correct Answer: C**

This response acknowledges the patient's situation without allowing him to manipulate the nurse and indicates that the nurse takes his warning of suicidal talk seriously. This patient should be placed on suicide precautions and moved to a room where he is under direct supervision at all times. The doctor and psychological services will need to be notified immediately. The patient will need continued physical and psychological support during his recovery. Careful monitoring for depression and suicidal thoughts and attempts should be initiated. At this point, the patient is unable to see options or acknowledge positive facts of being alive. Visitors may be seen as pitying and not supportive by the patient. Medication may be necessary, but not until the situation has been fully assessed.

126. **Correct Answer: A**

Safety is your highest priority. By removing the disruptive family member from the unit, her behavior and anger can be managed more safely. It is important to address her directly, acknowledge her anger, and avoid trapping her physically in any corner. Use quiet and even tones that will not escalate her emotions. Ignoring the behavior and making jokes may further anger the daughter and may lead to physical acts of violence. Calling the police may elevate the situation if the daughter has not directly made or acted on threats. If security is unable to assist in diffusing the situation, then hospital personnel may need to call the police.

127. **Correct Answer: C**

The goal at this point is to regulate the patient's breathing and stabilize her vital signs. Using a firm and quiet voice and using simple sentences can help the severely anxious patient focus and diffuse the anxiety. Severely anxious individuals are less able to see options and cope at this stage. Goals should include decreasing unnecessary stress and remaining available to the patient for communication. The other answers speak to facts not in the nurse's knowledge and may increase fear or lead to false hope.

128. **Correct Answer: A**
     The timing of the symptoms is consistent with alcohol withdrawal or delirium tremens (DTs). DTs usually are seen 12–24 hours after last ingestion of alcohol, appearing as blood alcohol levels drop. Effects may peak up to 15 days after DTs begin. Fluids, vitamins, nutrition, and short-term pharmacological treatments are appropriate treatments. The severity of symptoms is affected by the amount and duration of alcohol ingestion as well as the patient's underlying physical health, combination of other drugs taken, and existing psychological status. There are no indications at this time that the patient is septic or has schizophrenia. There may be underlying drug withdrawal symptoms, but the patient history does not provide an indication of this problem.

129. **Correct Answer: D**
     The Braden scale is a validated assessment tool for determining an individual's risk for developing pressure ulcers. Because prevention is the most effective treatment for pressure ulcers, early identification of at-risk patients is critical.

BIBLIOGRAPHY

Ahmed, I., & Beckingham, I. G. (2007). Liver trauma. *Trauma, 9*(3), 171–180.

Ahrens, T. (2006). *Critical care nursing certification.* Columbus, OH: McGraw-Hill.

American Association of Critical-Care Nurses. (2006). *Core curriculum for critical care nursing* (6th ed.). Philadelphia: Saunders.

American Association of Critical-Care Nurses. (2007). *AACN certification and core review for high acuity and critical care* (6th ed.). Philadelphia: Saunders.

American Heart Association. (2007). *Guidelines 2005 for cardiopulmonary resuscitation and emergency cardiovascular care.* Retrieved July 24, 2008 from http://circ.ahajournals.org/content/vol112/24_suppl

Antunez, C., Martin, E., Cornejo-Garcia, J. A., et al. (2006). Immediate hypersensitivity reactions to penicillins and other betalactams. *Current Pharmaceutical Design, 12*(26), 3327–3333.

Atlas, R. M. (2002). Bioterrorism: From threat to reality. *Annual Review of Microbiology, 56,* 167–185. Retrieved March 1, 2008, from Research Library database.

Audi, J., Belson, M., Patel, M., Schier, J., & Osterloh, J. (2005). Ricin poisoning: A comprehensive review. *Journal of the American Medical Association, 294*(18), 2342–2351.

Benson, A., Dickson, W. A., & Boyce, D. E. (2006). ABC of wound healing: Burns. *British Medical Journal, 332*(7542), 649–652.

Benson, L. S., Edwards, S. L., Schiff, A. P., Williams, C. S., & Visotsky, J. L. (2006). Dog and cat bites to the hand: Treatment and cost assessment. *Journal of Hand Surgery, 31*(3), 468–473.

Bergmann, J. F., & Kher, A. (2005). Venous thromboembolism in the medically ill patient: A call to action. *International Journal of Clinical Practice, 59*(5), 555+.

Bistrian, B. (2007). Systemic response to inflammation. *Nutrition Reviews, 65*(12), S170–S172.

Borgel, D., Bornstain, C., Reitsma, P. H., Lerolle, N., Gandrille, S., Dali-Ali, F., et al. (2007). A comparative study of the protein C pathway in septic and nonseptic patients with organ failure. *American Journal of Respiratory and Critical Care Medicine, 176*(9), 878–885.

Bresolin, N. L., Carvalho, F. C., Goes, J. C., Fernandes, V., & Barotto, A. M. (2002). Acute renal failure following massive attack by Africanized bee stings. *Pediatric Nephrology, 17*(8), 625–627.

Bulger, E. M., Jurkovich, G. J., Nathens, A. V., Copass, M. K., Hanson, S., Cooper, C., et al. (2008). Hypertonic resuscitation of hypovolemic shock after blunt trauma. *Archives of Surgery, 143*(2), 139.

Burd, A., & Noronha, F. V. (2005). Theme symposium: What's new in burns trauma? *Surgical Practice, 9*(4), 126–136.

Burns, S. M. (Ed.). (2007). *American Association of Critical-Care Nurses (AACN): AACN protocols for practice: Healing environments* (2nd ed.). Sudbury, MA: Jones and Bartlett.

Cai, S., Singh, B. R., & Sharma, S. (2007). Botulism diagnostics: From clinical symptoms to in vitro assays. *Critical Reviews in Microbiology, 33*(2), 109–125. Retrieved March 1, 2008, from ProQuest Health and Medical Complete database.

Carter, C. (2005). Evaluation and treatment of brown recluse spider bites. *American Family Physician, 72*(7), 1372, 1376.

Cauwels, A. (2007). Nitric oxide in shock. *Kidney International, 72*(5), 557–565.

Centers for Disease Control and Prevention. (2006). *Fast facts: Anthrax information for health care providers.* Retrieved March 3, 2008, from http://emergency.cdc.gov/agent/anthrax/anthrax-hcp-factsheet.asp

Centers for Disease Control and Prevention. (2006). *Ricin: Epidemiology overview for clinicians.* Retrieved March 3, 2008, from http://emergency.cdc.gov.agent/ricin/clinicians/epidemiology.asp

Chauhan, D., Chari, P., Khuller, G., & Singh, D. (2004). Correlation of renal complications with extent and progression of tissue damage in electrical burns. *Indian Journal of Plastic Surgery, 37*(2), 99–104.

Co-Minh, H. B., Demoly, P., Guillot, B., & Raison-Peyron, N. (2007). Allergy Net: Anaphylactic shock after oral intake and contact urticaria due to polyethylene glycols. *Allergy, 62*(1), 92–93.

Conover, M. B. (2003). *Understanding electrocardiography* (8th ed.). St. Louis, MO: Mosby/Elsevier.

Copstead, L., & Banasik, J. L. (2000). *Pathophysiology: Biological and behavioral perspectives* (2nd ed.). Philadelphia: Saunders/Elsevier.

Cosgrove, S. E., Perl, T. M., Song, S., & Sisson, S. D. (2005). Ability of physicians to diagnose and manage illness due to category A bioterrorism agents. *Archives of Internal Medicine, 165*(17), 2002–2006. Retrieved March 3, 2008, from Research Library database.

Curley, M. A. Q. (1998). Patient–nurse synergy: Optimizing patients' outcomes. *American Journal of Critical Care, 7,* 64–72.

De Waele, J. J. (2008). Abdominal compartment syndrome in severe acute pancreatitis: When to decompress? *European Journal of Trauma and Emergency Surgery, 34*(1), 11–16.

Diaz, J. H., & Leblanc, K. E. (2007). Common spider bites. *American Family Physician, 75*(6), 869–873.

Dossey, B. M., Keegan, L., & Guzzetta, C. (2003). *Holistic nursing: A handbook for practice* (3rd ed.). Sudbury, MA: Jones and Bartlett.

Edwards, D. F. (1999). The Synergy Model: Linking patient needs to nurse competencies. *Critical Care Nurse, 19*(1), 88–98.

Emergency Nurses Association & Newberry, L. (2003). *Sheehy's emergency nursing: Principles and practice* (5th ed.). St. Louis, MO: Mosby/Elsevier.

Finkelmeier, B. A. (2000). *Cardiothoracic surgical nursing* (2nd ed.). Philadelphia: Lippincott, Williams & Wilkins.

Garretson, S., & Malberti, S. (2007). Understanding hypovolaemic, cardiogenic and septic shock. *Nursing Standard, 21*(50), 46–55; quiz 58.

Gaspardone, A., & Versaci, F. (2005). Coronary stenting and inflammation. *American Journal of Cardiology, 96*(12A), L65–L70.

Gasparis Vonfrolio, L., & Noone, J. (1999). *Critical care examination review* (3rd ed. revised). Staten Island, NY: Power Publications.

Glapa, M., Kourie, J. F., Doll, D., & Degiannis, E. (2007). Early management of gunshot injuries to the face in civilian practice. *World Journal of Surgery, 31*(11), 2104–2110.

Gonzalez, N. C., Allen, J., Blanco, V. G., Schmidt, E. J., van Rooijen, N., & Wood, J. G. (2007). Alveolar macrophages are necessary for the systemic inflammation of acute alveolar hypoxia. *Journal of Applied Physiology, 103*(4), 1386.

Gueant, J. L., Gueant-Rodriguez, R. M., Viola, M., Valluzzi, R. L., & Romano, A. (2006). IgE-mediated hypersensitivity to cephalosporins. *Current Pharmaceutical Design, 12*(26), 3335–3345.

Hardin, S. R., & Kaplow, R. (Eds.). (2004). *Synergy for clinical excellence: The AACN Synergy Model for Patient Care.* Sudbury, MA: Jones and Bartlett.

Harman, K. R., & Herndon, T. M. (2006). Case management study: Cold-water immersion in a 22-year-old service member. *Military Medicine, 171*(5), 459–462.

Harries, M. (2003). ABC of resuscitation: Near drowning. *British Medical Journal, 327*(7427), 1336–1338.

Hickey, J. V. (2002). *The clinical practice of neurological and neurosurgical nursing* (5th ed.). Philadelphia: Lippincott, Williams & Wilkins.

Holgate, S. T., & Polosa, R. (2008). Treatment strategies for allergy and asthma. *Nature Reviews. Immunology, 8*(3), 218–230.

Howell, J. M., Mayer, T. A., Hanfling, D., & Morrison, A. (2004). Screening for inhalational anthrax due to bioterrorism: Evaluating proposed screening protocols. *Clinical Infectious Diseases, 39*(12), 1842–1847. Retrieved March 1, 2008, from Research Library database.

Hurst, J. R., Perera, W. R., Wilkinson, T. M. A., Donaldson, G. C., & Wedzicha, J. A. (2006). Systemic and upper and lower airway inflammation at exacerbation of chronic obstructive pulmonary disease. *American Journal of Respiratory and Critical Care Medicine, 173*(1), 71–78.

Index case of fatal inhalation anthrax due to bioterrorism in the United States. (2002). *Journal of Cutaneous Medicine and Surgery, 6*(4), 379. Retrieved March 3, 2008, from ProQuest Health and Medical Complete database.

Inhalation anthrax. (2001). *Morbidity and Mortality Weekly Report.* Retrieved March 3, 2008, from http://www.cdc.gov/mmwr/preview/mmwrhtml/mm5043al.htm

Joulin, O., Petillot, P., Labalette, M., Lancel, S., & Neviere, R. (2007). Cytokine profile of human septic shock serum inducing cardiomyocyte contractile dysfunction. *Physiological Research, 56*(3), 291–297.

Kandil, E., Burack, J., Sawas, A., Bibawy, H., Schwartzman, A., Zenilman, M. E., et al. (2008). B-type natriuretic peptide. *Archives of Surgery, 143*(3), 242.

Karmy-Jones, R., Carter, Y., & Stern, E. (2002). The impact of positive pressure ventilation on the diagnosis of traumatic diaphragmatic injury. *American Surgeon, 68*(2), 167–172.

Keel, M., Eid, K., Labler, L., Seifert, B., Trentz, O., & Ertel, W. (2006). Influence of injury pattern on incidence and severity of posttraumatic inflammatory complications in severely injured patients. *European Journal of Trauma, 32*(4), 387–395.

Kemerer, J. J., Reitz, M., & Diaz, J. H. (2007). Diagnosis of brown recluse spider bites is overused/ In reply. *American Family Physician, 76*(7), 943–944; author reply 944, 947.

Kozieras, J., Thuemer, O., & Sakka, S. G. (2007). Influence of an acute increase in systemic vascular resistance on transpulmonary thermodilution-derived parameters in critically ill patients. *Intensive Care Medicine, 33*(9), 1619–1623.

Kury Hughs, S., Nilsson, D. E., Boyer, R. S., Bolte, R. G., Hoffman, R. O., Lewine, J. D., et al. (2002). Neurodevelopmental outcome for extended cold water drowning: A longitudinal case study. *Journal of the International Neuropsychological Society, 8*(4), 588–595.

Legeza, V. I., Galenko-Yaroshevskii, V. P., Zinov'ev, E. V., Paramonov, B. A., Kreichman, G. S., Turkovskii, I. I., et al. (2004). Effects of new wound dressings on healing of thermal burns of the skin in acute radiation disease. *Bulletin of Experimental Biology and Medicine, 138*(3), 311–315.

Leibovici, L., Gafter-Gvili, A., Paul, M., Paramonov, B. A., Kreichman, G. S., Turkovskii, I. I., et al. (2007). Relative tachycardia in patients with sepsis: An independent risk factor for mortality. *QJM, 100*(10), 629–634.

Lipson, J. G., Dibble, S. L., & Minarik, P. A. (Eds.). (1996). *Culture and nursing care: A pocket guide.* San Francisco, CA: UCSF Nursing Press.

McNally, P. (2001). *GI/liver secrets* (2nd ed.). Philadelphia: Hanley & Belfus/Elsevier.

McQuillan, K. A., Von Rueden, K. T., Hartsock, R. L., Flynn, M. B., & Whalen, E. (Eds.). (2002). *Trauma nursing: From resuscitation through rehabilitation* (3rd ed.). Philadelphia: Saunders/ Elsevier.

Medina, J., & Puntillo, K. (2006). *AACN protocols for practice: Palliative care and end-of-life issues in critical care.* Sudbury, MA: Jones and Bartlett.

Merchant, R. C., Zabbo, C. P., Mayer, K. H., & Becker, B. M. (2007). Factors associated with delay to emergency department presentation, antibiotic usage and admission for human bite injuries. *Journal of the Canadian Association of Emergency Physicians, 9*(6), 441–448.

Mitchell, J. W., & Danska, J. (2007). Escharotic lesion after a "brown recluse spider bite." *American Family Physician, 75*(12), 1841–1842.

Modell, J. H., Idris, A. H., Pineda, J. A., & Silverstein, J. H. (2004). Survival after prolonged submersion in freshwater in Florida. *Chest, 125*(5), 1948–1951.

Monneuse, O., Al-Ahmadi, K., & Ahmed, N. (2006). The case of a migrating bullet. *Lancet, 368*(9544), 1392.

Moore, E. E., Cheng, A. M., Moore, H. B., Masuno, T., & Johnson, J. L. (2006). Hemoglobin-based oxygen carriers in trauma care: Scientific rationale for the US multicenter prehospital trial. *World Journal of Surgery, 30*(7), 1247–1257.

Norris, R. L., Wilkerson, J. A., & Feldman, J. (2007). Syncope, massive aspiration, and sudden death following rattlesnake bite. *Wilderness & Environmental Medicine, 18*(3), 206–208. Retrieved March 29, 2008, from Research Library database (Document ID: 1363946451).

O'Brien, J. M., Ali, N. A., Aberegg, S. K., & Abraham, E. (2007). Sepsis. *American Journal of Medicine, 120*(12), 1012.

O'Brien, K. K., Higdon, M. L., & Halverson, J. J. (2003). Recognition and management of bioterrorism infections. *American Family Physician, 67*(9), 1927–1934.

Pagana, K. D., & Pagana, J. (2005). *Mosby's manual of diagnostic and laboratory tests* (3rd ed.). St. Louis, MO: Mosby/Elsevier.

Petroianu, A. (2007). Arterial embolization for hemorrhage caused by hepatic arterial injury. *Digestive Diseases and Sciences, 52*(10), 2478–2481.

Prodan Lange, S., & Shank, S. L. (2008). *Managing the psychiatric crisis homestudy.* Catalog 50 JDE. Lakeway, TX: National Center for Continuing Education.

Ranasinghe, A. M., Hyde, J. A. J., & Graham, T. R. (2002). Management of flail chest, trauma 3. *Trauma, 4*(3), 146.

Regueira, T., Hasbun, P., Rebolledo, R., Galindo, J., Aguirre, M., Romero, C., et al. (2007). Intra-abdominal hypertension in patients with septic shock. *American Surgeon, 73*(9), 865–870.

Rhoads, J. (2007). Epidemiology of the brown recluse spider bite. *Journal of the American Academy of Nurse Practitioners, 19*(2), 79–85.

Richardson, J. D., Franklin, G. A., Heffley, S., & Seligson, D. (2007). Operative fixation of chest wall fractures: An underused procedure? *American Surgeon, 73*(6), 591–596; discussion, 596–597.

Robin-Lersundi, A., Trancho, F. H., Gastardi, J. C., Martinez, A. G., García, A. T., & Balibrea Cantero, J. L. (2003). Penetrating chest gunshot wounds: Conservative treatment. *Surgical Endoscopy, 17*(10), 1677.

Rubin, A. E., Wang, K., & Liu, M. L. (2003). Tracheobronchial stenosis from acid aspiration presenting as asthma. *Chest, 123*(2), 643–646.

Seamon, M. J., Fisher, C. A., Gaughan, J. P., Kulp, H., Dempsey, D. T., & Goldberg, A. J. (2008). Emergency department thoracotomy: Survival of the least expected. *World Journal of Surgery, 32*(4), 604–612.

Seiler, J. G., & Shaw, B. A. (2003). Rattlesnake bite with associated compartment syndrome: What is the best treatment? *Journal of Bone and Joint Surgery, 85*(6), 1163.

Seth, R., Chester, D., & Moiemen, N. (2007). A review of chemical burns. *Trauma, 9*(2), 81–94.

Sharma, O. P., Oswanski, M. F., Singer, D., Raj, S. S., & Daoud, Y. A. H. (2005). Assessment of nonoperative management of blunt spleen and liver trauma. *American Surgeon, 71*(5), 379–386.

Shaw, B. A., & Hosalkar, H. S. (2002). Rattlesnake bites in children: Antivenin treatment and surgical indications. *Journal of Bone and Joint Surgery, 84*(9), 1624–1629.

Skidmore-Roth, L. (2004). *Mosby's 2004 nursing drug reference.* St. Louis, MO: Mosby/Elsevier.

Smeltzer, S., & Bare, B. G. (2003). *Brunner and Suddarth's textbook of medical–surgical nursing* (10th ed.). Philadelphia: Lippincott, Williams & Wilkins.

Sole, M. L., Hartshorn, J., & Lamborne, M. L. (2001). *Introduction to critical care nursing* (3rd ed.). Philadelphia: Saunders/Elsevier.

Spaniolas, K., Velmahos, G. C., Wicky, S., Nussbaumer, K., Petrovick, L., Gervasini, L., et al. (2008). Is upper extremity deep venous thrombosis underdiagnosed in trauma patients? *American Surgeon, 74*(2), 124–128.

Spencer, R. C. (2003). *Bacillus anthracis. Journal of Clinical Pathology, 56*(3), 182–187. Retrieved March 3, 2008, from ProQuest Health and Medical Complete database.

Spies, C., & Trohman, R. G. (2006). Narrative review: Electrocution and life-threatening electrical injuries. *Annals of Internal Medicine, 145*(7), 531–537.

Swanson, D. L., & Vetter, R. S. (2005). Medical progress: Bites of brown recluse spiders and suspected necrotic arachnidism. *New England Journal of Medicine, 352*(7), 700–707.

Taplitz, R. A. (2004). Managing bite wounds. *Postgraduate Medicine, 116*(2), 49.

Turk, T., Vural, H., Ata, Y., Eris, C., & Yavuz, C. (2007). Acute aortic insufficiency after blunt chest trauma: A case report. *Journal of Cardiovascular Surgery, 48*(3), 359–361.

Tzortzaki, E. G., Lambiri, I., Vlachaki, E., & Siafakas, N. M. (2007). Biomarkers in COPD. *Current Medicinal Chemistry, 14*(9), 1037–1048.

Urden, L. D., Stacy, K. M., & Lough, M. E. (2007). *Thelan's critical care nursing: Diagnosis and management* (5th ed.). St. Louis, MO: Mosby.

van Haren, F. M. P., Sleigh, J. W., Pickkers, P., & van der Hoeven, J. G. (2007). Gastrointestinal perfusion in septic shock. *Anaesthesia and Intensive Care, 35*(5), 679–694.

Vassilakopoulos, T., & Hussain, S. N. A. (2007). Ventilatory muscle activation and inflammation: Cytokines, reactive oxygen species, and nitric oxide. *Journal of Applied Physiology, 102*(4), 1687.

Vécsei, V., Arbes, S., Aldrian, S., & Nau, T. (2005). Chest injuries in polytrauma. *European Journal of Trauma, 31*(3), 239–243.

Warwick, A. M., Goonewardene, K., Burton, P. R., Usatoff, V., & Evans, P. M. (2007). HP38P: Management of the traumatic pancreatic injury. *ANZ Journal of Surgery, 77*(s1), A48.

Weber-Carstens, S., Deja, M., Bercker, S., Dimroth, A., Ahlers, O., Kaisers, U., et al. (2007). Impact of bolus application of low-dose hydrocortisone on glycemic control in septic shock patients. *Intensive Care Medicine, 33*(4), 730–733.

Wiegand, D. J. L., & Carlson, K. K. (Eds.). (2005). *AACN procedure manual for critical care* (5th ed.). Philadelphia: Elsevier.

Woltmann, A., Beisse, R., Eckardt, H., Potulski, M., & Bühren, V. (2007). Combined abdominal and spine injuries after high energy flexion–distraction trauma. *European Journal of Trauma and Emergency Surgery, 33*(5), 482–488.

Woods, S., Sivarajan Froelicher, E. S., & Motzer, S. U. (2000). *Cardiac nursing* (4th ed.). Philadelphia: Lippincott, Williams & Wilkins.

Zeller, J. L. (2007). Evaluation of white blood cell count, neutrophil percentage, and elevated temperature as predictors of bloodstream infection in burn patients. *Journal of the American Medical Association, 298*(9), 968.

PCCN Practice Examinations

These practice exams contain some of the same information that is found on the enclosed CD. The questions on the CD are in random order. Allow yourself 2½ hours to complete each of these practice exams. The answers and rationale are at the end of each exam. Keep practicing until you can score at least 80%.

PCCN PRACTICE EXAM 1

1. **Samuel is a 16-year-old tennis player who was admitted to your unit last night with a fractured right tibia and fibula. He is very concerned about how soon he will be able to resume playing tennis. Your reply is guided by the time it normally takes fractures to heal and your knowledge about the stages of healing. The correct order of fracture healing is**
   A. Remodeling, ossification, granulation tissue, fracture hematoma.
   B. Bone union, granulation, consolidation, osteoblast formation.
   C. Fracture hematoma, granulation tissue, callus formation, ossification.
   D. Granulation tissue, consolidation, bone union, ossification.

2. **The most common infection in patients with a ventricular assist device (VAD) is**
   A. Septicemia.
   B. Pericarditis.
   C. Pneumonia.
   D. Pericardial effusion.

3. **BiPAP is somewhat useful in acute respiratory distress syndrome (ARDS) because:**
   A. BiPAP decreases cardiac output.
   B. BiPAP decreases venous return so the lungs drain more effectively.
   C. BiPAP prevents barotrauma.
   D. BiPAP can open collapsed alveoli.

4. **Adin is a 30-year-old male who was thrown from a horse onto a fence; he suffered abdominal trauma with a splenic rupture. While awaiting surgery in the telemetry unit, because the operating rooms were full, he received 12 units of PRBCs. As a telemetry nurse, you know that Adin should also receive**
   A. Potassium.
   B. Whole blood.
   C. Platelets.
   D. Heparin.

5. **Rheumatoid arthritis differs from osteoarthritis in that**
    A. Osteoarthritis affects small joints first.
    B. Osteoarthritis is a localized disease.
    C. Osteoarthritis shows narrowing joint space and subluxation on X-ray.
    D. Stiffness occurs on rising and subsides after 30 minutes.

6. **During a cardiopulmonary arrest, you note that the patient is being forcefully ventilated by the respiratory therapist using a bag-valve mask device. You know this patient is at risk for**
    A. Alveolar collapse.
    B. Barotrauma.
    C. Cardiac tamponade.
    D. Hemothorax.

7. **An aneurysm that is dissecting upward (ascending) produces pain**
    A. In the chest and midscapular area.
    B. In the back of the neck and left shoulder.
    C. From the umbilical area to the shoulder.
    D. In the left shoulder and midsternal area.

8. **Ted was ill 4 days ago with a slight cold. Now he is experiencing ascending weakness in both legs. This symptom is suggestive of which of the following illnesses?**
    A. Guillain-Barré syndrome
    B. Chronic fatigue syndrome
    C. Tetanus
    D. *Clostridium botulinum* infection

9. **Bernard lost his home to a fire this morning. He was burned on the chest and neck while trying to put out the fire. He is dyspneic and has soot on his face, and his eyebrows and nares are singed. The priority of treatment is to**
    A. Maintain cardiac output.
    B. Maintain airway patency.
    C. Treat burned areas.
    D. Obtain ABGs and a carboxyhemoglobin level.

10. **George was initially admitted for pneumonia. He is two years post heart transplant. When you place the EKG monitoring leads, you note sinus tachycardia with PVCs and a 2 mm ST elevation. The patient denies pain. This finding is**
    A. Impossible.
    B. Normal.
    C. Indicative of an RBBB.
    D. Indicative of an inferior MI.

11. **Miriam, a 56-year-old office manager, suffered burns to 30% of her body when a propane tank exploded while she was barbecuing. Prolonged hypoxemia due to complications obtaining and maintaining a patent airway and hypovolemia have led Miriam to develop an ischemic ulcer. An ischemic ulcer that develops following a burn injury is often called a**

    A. Blaze ulcer.

    B. Wave ulcer.

    C. Curling ulcer.

    D. Pyrolonic ulcer.

12. Pulse oximetry readings are considered unreliable when oxygen saturation falls below

    A. 60%.

    B. 90%.

    C. 55%.

    D. 70%.

13. The patient who is status post heart transplant may have significant bradycardia. The drug of choice to treat this condition is

    A. Atropine.

    B. Isuproterenol.

    C. Apresoline.

    D. Adenosine.

14. Analyze the following arterial blood gas result. Use the provided space to the right side to assist in interpretation by writing acidosis, alkalosis, compensated or uncompensated.

    pH 7.38

    CO_2 27

    HCO_3 16

    A. Normal

    B. Compensated respiratory acidosis

    C. Compensated metabolic acidosis

    D. Uncompensated respiratory alkalosis

15. Your patient is 36 hours status post right femoral bypass graft. The patient complains of pain with even slight movement of the limb. You suspect

    A. An arterial obstruction.

    B. A DVT.

    C. A venous obstruction.

    D. A leg cramp from prolonged bed rest.

16. If the function of the Brunner's gland is inhibited in your patient, which condition may occur?

    A. The patient cannot control peristalsis.

    B. The patient may develop a duodenal ulcer.

    C. The patient will suffer recurrent vomiting.

    D. The patient will not feel hungry.

17. Patricia had a renal transplant about one year ago. She was admitted to your unit for severe flu-like symptoms. Which sign or symptom would lead you to suspect that Patricia is having an acute rejection episode?

    A. Pelvic pain

    B. Hypotension

    C. Increased urine output

    D. Decreased urine osmolality

18. Felix has been transferred from the ICU to PCCU after a gunshot wound to his T11–T12 spine. Upon assessment, you find motor paralysis on the same side as the gunshot wound but loss of pain and temperature sensation on the opposite side. This is called
    A. Grey–Turner syndrome.
    B. Cushing syndrome.
    C. Syndrome X.
    D. Brown–Sequard syndrome.

19. Your patient received streptokinase about 30 minutes ago for a lateral wall STEMI. You would expect which of the following events to occur?
    A. Lowered CPK isoenzymes
    B. Reperfusion rhythms
    C. Transient increased chest pain
    D. Mild CHF

20. Sinusitis, hospital-acquired pneumonia (HAP), and ventilator-acquired pneumonia (VAP) pose many challenges for the progressive care nurse. Sometimes the patient will be transferred to your unit with an infection already acquired, and then symptoms will become more pronounced. Which statement is true regarding these conditions?
    A. Good hand washing technique is effective for reducing VAP.
    B. Sinusitis can be prevented by using a smaller-diameter endotracheal tube.
    C. Nasogastric tubes are preferred to orogastric tubes.
    D. Oral tubes are associated with a greater incidence of sinusitis.

21. Heather underwent gastric bypass three days ago. You are continuing her discharge teaching regarding food choices and lifestyle changes. You tell Heather that she will need to limit and eventually stop cigarette use, limit caffeine intake, limit or eliminate alcohol consumption, and participate in stress management or relaxation programs. She demands to know why she has to do each of these things because the "weight is supposed to just fall off." Which of the following statements is correct?
    A. Smoking increases hydrochloric acid production.
    B. Alcohol use delays healing.
    C. Stress decreases peristalsis.
    D. These steps will decrease the risk and complications related to dumping syndrome.

22. Jerri is a quadriplegic with a C6 spinal injury. She is admitted to the step-down unit for a possible myocardial infarction, where she develops severe hypertension and headache. The hospitalist diagnoses autonomic hyperreflexia. What is one cause of autonomic hyperreflexia?
    A. Diarrhea
    B. Suctioning
    C. Constipation
    D. Warm breeze

23. **Seth is a 15-year-old with Down syndrome. He has undergone a graft procedure secondary to a burn on his leg and has not experienced any complications. You are about to teach his mother how to change the leg dressings and the graft-site dressings on the hips. Principles of teaching include**
    A. Teaching all the information at once.
    B. Teaching the information as fast as possible.
    C. Explaining the rationale for the procedure and then demonstrating the procedure.
    D. Speaking slowly so the patient can hear.

24. **A patient with a suspected diagnosis of active tuberculosis has been admitted to your care. The type of protective face mask you should use is the**
    A. N95 respirator.
    B. Particulate mask.
    C. TB face mask.
    D. Hood mask.

25. **Helen developed infective pericarditis after renal failure and sepsis. Her morning labs should show**
    A. Increased WBC, decreased ESR, normal CK-MB.
    B. Normal WBC, decreased ESR, elevated CK-MB.
    C. Increased WBC, increased ESR, elevated CK-MB.
    D. Increased WBC, normal ESR, elevated CK-MB.

26. **Droplet precautions should be taken for a patient with**
    A. Herpes simplex.
    B. Chickenpox.
    C. Mumps.
    D. Wound infection.

27. **High blood viscosity and low oxygen tension are the cause of which of the following types of anemia?**
    A. Pernicious
    B. Aplastic
    C. Sickle cell
    D. Hemolytic

28. **Which of the following conditions mandates the use of pain control?**
    A. Hemothorax
    B. ARDS
    C. Flail chest
    D. Pulmonary contusion

29. **During shift report, you are told that your patient has a 90% occlusion to the circumflex coronary artery. Which type of myocardial infarction is this patient at greatest risk of developing?**
    A. Lateral wall infarction
    B. Anterior wall infarction
    C. Posterior wall infarction
    D. Septal wall infarction

30. Pathologic changes in the lung caused by chronic bronchitis do not include
    A. Destruction of alveolar walls.
    B. An increase in goblet cells.
    C. Disappearance of cilia.
    D. Narrowing of the small airways.

31. Mrs. B., a patient who has a closed head injury, has a Foley catheter. In one hour her urine output increases from 30 mL/h to 1,000 mL/h of very pale, clear urine. The PCCU nurse knows this change is a result of
    A. A volume shift from the third space.
    B. Syndrome of inappropriate antidiuretic hormone.
    C. Diabetes insipidus.
    D. Diuresis from steroids.

32. Mary is a "no code" patient in your PCCU. She has suffered an acute hemorrhagic stroke and is not expected to survive long. You know that her intracranial pressure is rising and she is developing Cushing syndrome. Which signs and symptoms would you expect to see?
    A. Increased systolic blood pressure, widening pulse pressure, bradycardia
    B. Elevated blood pressure, narrowed pulse pressure, tachycardia
    C. Bradycardia, low blood pressure, narrowed pulse pressure
    D. Tachycardia, increased systolic blood pressure, widening pulse pressure

33. Laura suffered a myocardial infarction as a result of 100% occlusion of the left anterior descending and circumflex artery. Although cardiac catheterization returned some blood flow to the left side of her heart, you note a new murmur at the fifth intercostal space, midclavicular line. You suspect
    A. Tricuspid valve stenosis.
    B. Mitral valve regurgitation.
    C. Pulmonic stenosis.
    D. Aortic regurgitation.

34. One factor to be considered when assessing a patient for possible aspiration and chemical/aspiration pneumonitis is
    A. Possibility of using syrup of ipecac.
    B. pH.
    C. Type of infiltrates on CXR.
    D. ABG results.

35. Gina was admitted to the PCU with cough, fever, chills, anorexia, malaise, and headache. She has a pericardial friction rub and a history of rheumatic fever. While examining Gina, you note fine, dark lines in her nail beds and some flat lesions on her palms. These flat lesions are known as
    A. Janeway lesions.
    B. Roth spots.
    C. Osler's nodes.
    D. Pella's sign.

36. **A partial rebreathing mask can deliver what percentage of oxygen?**
    A. 20–40%
    B. 60–80%
    C. 40–60%
    D. > 90%

37. **Which of the following nursing actions would be important in the care of a patient with occlusive disease of the terminal aorta and a nonhealing wound on the left foot?**
    A. Elevate the patient's legs
    B. Place the patient in high Fowler's position
    C. Maintain normothermia
    D. Place the patient on fluid restrictions

38. **Samantha has been suffering with malaise for several weeks. Today, she was admitted for low H and H, epistaxis, and bleeding into the diaphragm. She is bleeding from the gums, even with only the lightest stimulus. Petechiae are noted on her chest and arms. Her platelet count is < 100,000. Samantha's probable diagnosis is**
    A. Aplastic anemia.
    B. ITP.
    C. Hemolytic anemia.
    D. Pernicious anemia.

39. **If your patient's temporary pacemaker is not sensing, your first action should be to**
    A. Place the patient on the right side.
    B. Increase mA output.
    C. Check the sensitivity control for the proper setting.
    D. Immediately turn off the pacer and notify the physician.

40. **You are teaching your patient with COPD about his treatment plan. Which of the following statements would indicate that the patient understands his disease and his treatment plan?**
    A. "I should limit my fluid intake to one liter per day."
    B. "I should use my Serevent inhaler as a rescue inhaler."
    C. "I should elevate and cross my legs while watching television."
    D. "I should avoid drinking or ingesting dairy products."

41. **Lori, a 24-year-old mother of three, has been diagnosed with multiple sclerosis (MS). She was admitted to the telemetry care unit after an acute exacerbation in which she experienced left-side weakness. Multiple sclerosis is which type of disease?**
    A. A motor disorder of the spinal cord
    B. A demyelinating disorder of the brain and spinal cord
    C. A motor disorder of the brain and spinal cord
    D. A demyelinating disease of the spinal cord

42. **Your patient has a potassium level of 2.9 mEq/L. You would expect your patient to exhibit a clinical manifestation of**
    A. Flushed skin, nausea, and constipation.
    B. Cardiac arrhythmias, hypotension, and fatigue.
    C. Weakness, anorexia, and cardiac arrhythmias.
    D. Excessive sweating, seizures, and nausea.

43. **Which of the following are some of the signs and symptoms associated with diabetic ketoacidosis (DKA)?**
    A. Polyuria, polydipsia, polyphagia, dilute urine
    B. Polyuria, polydipsia, polyphagia, fruity breath, dehydration, marked fatigue
    C. Hyperactivity, confusion, nausea, vomiting
    D. Kussmaul's respirations, dilute urine

44. **Bruce is a 17-year-old male who has not been eating correctly for approximately 2 weeks because he is stressed out about asking a girl to the prom. He eats a diet of cereals, pastas, and high-calorie, high-sugar foods. Bruce collapsed at work today after becoming dyspneic. His EKG shows sinus tachycardia without ectopy. He is pale and somewhat irritable, and complains of a headache. His initial diagnosis is folic acid deficiency. Tomorrow Bruce is scheduled for more tests to determine if an underlying disease process is at work. You suspect that he simply has a dietary deficiency and prepare to instruct him about foods that contain high amounts of folic acid. These foods would include**
    A. Green beans.
    B. Fish.
    C. Oranges.
    D. Peanut butter.

45. **Rick is a 30-year-old motorcyclist who lost control of his motorcycle in the rain. He was wearing a helmet and protective gear. Rick suffered a fractured left femur, a fractured rib, a cervical sprain, and road rash on his face and neck. He is admitted with the following vital signs: BP 84/44, HR 100, RR 26 and shallow, T 98.4°F. His 12-lead EKG shows ST elevation in the anterior leads. His CXR shows a normal cardiac silhouette and no infiltrates. His Hgb is 9.0 and his Hct is 32. MB is 18%. Rick is restless and complains of pain in his chest and left leg. What condition would you anticipate?**
    A. Systolic dysfunction
    B. Hypovolemic shock
    C. Pulmonary hypertension
    D. Pulmonary edema

46. **How does hyperglycemic, hyperosmolar, nonketotic syndrome (HHNS) differ from diabetic ketoacidosis (DKA)?**
    A. HHNS has the same onset, higher blood sugars, and more dehydration relative to DKA.
    B. HHNS has a slower onset, lower blood sugars, and less dehydration relative to DKA.
    C. HHNS has a slower onset, much higher blood sugars, and more profound dehydration relative to DKA.
    D. HHNS has the same onset, lower blood sugars, and no dehydration relative to DKA.

47. Examples of colloid solutions would include
    A. Plasma and albumin.
    B. Dextrose and saline.
    C. Plasmanate and dextran.
    D. Saline and Lactated Ringer's.

48. Myron, a 25-year-old marathon runner, is admitted to the progressive care unit after being struck by a car while running. He experienced blunt force trauma to the left side of his head. Nursing management of this patient includes frequent assessments. Which of the following parameters is the most sensitive indicator of Myron's status?
    A. Vital signs
    B. Glasgow Coma Scale score
    C. Level of consciousness
    D. Intracranial pressure

49. Which labs would you anticipate for a patient with hyperglycemic, hyperosmolar, nonketotic syndrome (HHNS)?
    A. Glucose 550, positive ketones, serum osmolality 280 mOsm/L
    B. Glucose 1,258, negative ketones, serum osmolality 375 mOsm/L
    C. Glucose 700, negative ketones, serum osmolality 270 mOsm/L
    D. Glucose 600, positive ketones, serum osmolality 240 mOsm/L

50. Barry has Wolf-Parkinson-White syndrome. He is having increasing bouts of tachycardia. It has been decided to utilize overdrive pacing. How do you explain this type of pacemaker to a new orientee?
    A. The pacemaker is set at a constant rate of 70 bpm and is synchronized.
    B. The pacemaker or AICD is set on demand mode and is asynchronous.
    C. The pacemaker or AICD is set on demand mode and is synchronous.
    D. The pacemaker or AICD is set on inhibit mode and is synchronous.

51. Mrs. T., a 36-year-old housewife, is transferred to DOU after recovering from a subarachnoid hemorrhage due to a ruptured anterior communicating artery aneurysm. Cerebral aneurysms are most often found in which of the following anatomical areas?
    A. Internal carotid arteries
    B. Bifurcations of the anterior–posterior circle of Willis
    C. Temporal artery
    D. Vertebral arteries

52. Kyle is a 22-year-old male who underwent a renal transplant one year ago. The physician suspects that the organ is being rejected. You know that a renal transplant that results from humoral rejection or acute cellular rejection may be definitively diagnosed only via
    A. Ultrasound.
    B. Nuclear scan.
    C. Doppler scan.
    D. Renal biopsy.

53. You have to administer amphotericin B to your patient. To avoid incompatibility, you should give the medication in
    A. Lactated Ringer's.
    B. D_5W.
    C. D_5 Isolyte M.
    D. D_5/0.45 NS.

54. Which physical symptoms do you expect with Cushing syndrome?
    A. Moon facies, edema, weight loss
    B. Moon facies, acne, weight loss
    C. Moon facies, purple striae on trunk, buffalo hump
    D. Moon facies, easy bruising, weight loss

55. Septic shock can occur when pelvic inflammatory disease (PID) spreads to the
    A. Liver.
    B. Uterus.
    C. Lungs.
    D. Gastrointestinal tract.

56. Betty is a 50-year-old female who was admitted to the telemetry unit for acute coronary syndrome. She also has myasthenia gravis and is allowed to keep her pyridostigmine at her bedside so she does not miss a dose. Suddenly, her monitor alarms with a severe bradycardia. You suspect an overdose of pyridostigmine. If that is true, Betty's problem is
    A. Cholinergic crisis.
    B. Acetylcholine crisis.
    C. Myasthenia gravis crisis.
    D. Bradycardia related to Betty's acute coronary syndrome, not her myasthenia gravis.

57. Gene had a DDD pacemaker inserted 3 years ago. He has been admitted for pacemaker syndrome. Which symptoms do you expect to see?
    A. Fatigue, agitation, dyspnea
    B. Fatigue, dizziness, confusion
    C. Fatigue, agitation, forgetfulness
    D. Fatigue, dizziness, syncope

58. John had a thyroidectomy yesterday for thyroid cancer. Today he is delirious, vomiting, hyperthermic, and tachycardic. It is imperative to notify the physician stat because
    A. John has a postoperative infection.
    B. John may have had a cerebrovascular accident.
    C. John may be having a thyrotoxic crisis.
    D. John is hypoxic and needs a tracheostomy.

59. Your patient has just undergone a laparoscopic cholecystectomy and is complaining of pain in the right shoulder. To help alleviate the discomfort, you could
    A. Raise the head of the bed to 45 degrees.
    B. Place the patient in Sim's position.
    C. Place the patient supine.
    D. Give anticholinergics to decrease the patient's secretions and pain.

60. **Which of the following lead changes will identify a lateral MI?**
    A. II, III, aVF
    B. V_1–V_4
    C. V_2–V_6
    D. I, aVL, V_5, V_6

61. **Bettina is 28 years old and was admitted because of increasing malaise and night sweats. She had various blood tests done to try to determine if her systemic lupus erythematosus caused her allergic nephritis. Allergic nephritis may also be caused by**
    A. Inadequate protein consumption.
    B. Weight loss.
    C. Cimetidine.
    D. Water intoxication.

62. **Your patient just underwent a laminectomy. He reports that he feels some numbness and tingling, and says the feelings are new to him. Your response should be to**
    A. Reassure the patient and tell him that the sensations will subside in a few hours.
    B. Logroll the patient to the nonoperative side.
    C. Medicate the patient for anxiety and pain.
    D. Assess the neurological status and report the findings to the physician.

63. **Maria is 60 years old and was alert and active last evening, but was found this morning sitting in her kitchen, hardly able to move. At first, it was thought she had suffered a stroke. Maria was admitted because her EKG showed large R waves in leads V_1 and V_2. Physical parameters include the following:**
    EKG: SR at 92, no ectopy
    Manual cuff BP: 94/62
    Skin: pale, cool, clammy
    RR 18, breath sounds clear, slightly diminished LLL
    O_2 2 L/min via NC
    Moderate jugular venous distention, no bruits
    CVP 18
    Mentation: lethargic

    An expected diagnosis for Maria would be
    A. Aortic insufficiency.
    B. LV hypertrophy.
    C. RV infarction.
    D. Pericarditis.

64. **Glenda, a 49-year-old female with Type II diabetes, is admitted to the progressive care unit for acute coronary syndrome (ACS). She is NPO for angiography. She calls you to her room and tells you she feels "funny." You note that Glenda is pale, diaphoretic, anxious, and restless. What is your next step in evaluating this patient?**
    A. Check vital signs and temperature
    B. Check vital signs, repeat cardiac enzymes, obtain a stat EKG
    C. Check vital signs and blood sugar
    D. Check vital signs, obtain a pulse oximetry reading

65. Lee, a 67-year-old retiree, is being admitted to your unit for chest pain after collapsing at home while trying to fix his roof. He is arguing with his wife that he should not be admitted because he just "overdid it" in the yard. She states to you that his chest pain is more frequent, severe, and prolonged than before. You anticipate which diagnosis?
    A. Exertional angina
    B. Unstable angina
    C. Variant angina
    D. Anginal equivalent

66. Your patient must have an arterial blood gas sample drawn. The respiratory therapist says he is out of prepared syringes and obtains a syringe into which he places heparin. What effect will too much heparin have on the sample, if any?
    A. Decrease the bicarbonate value
    B. No effect
    C. Increase the $PaCO_2$
    D. Totally prevent clotting

67. Rodney is a 40-year-old plumber with chest pain who waited for 16 hours before coming to the hospital. He has a right bundle branch block and a left anterior fascicular block. What is the significance of his condition?
    A. Rodney has extensive myocardial damage.
    B. Rodney needs a pacemaker as soon as possible.
    C. Rodney needs to be transferred to a facility that can do a heart transplant.
    D. This problem will resolve itself over the next few weeks.

68. The cells responsible for forming a barrier for alveoli are
    A. Macrophages.
    B. Type II alveolar epithelial cells.
    C. Type I alveolar epithelial cells.
    D. Cilia.

69. Mort, a 45-year-old stockbroker, was admitted to the progressive care unit for an acute myocardial infarction. He has a schizoaffective disorder for which he has taken lithium for 15 years. You note he has a very high urine output—about 800 cc/h—and an SpG of 1.001. What is wrong?
    A. Mort is experiencing the diuretic effect of a low-sodium diet.
    B. Mort has diabetes insipidus from long-term lithium use.
    C. Mort has excessive oral fluid intake.
    D. Mort has neurogenic diabetes insipidus.

70. Your patient was admitted for malaise, severe dyspnea and he had a syncopal episode at work. The patient states he has a midline burning sensation in his chest that worsens when he is supine. You suspect
    A. A pleural effusion.
    B. Pericardial tamponade.
    C. GERD.
    D. Myocarditis.

71. **What is the primary acid–base disturbance exhibited by patients with AKI?**
    A. Metabolic acidosis
    B. Respiratory acidosis
    C. Metabolic alkalosis
    D. Respiratory alkalosis

72. **Mary Margaret has had an inferior wall MI. Where do you expect to see changes on her 12-lead EKG?**
    A. II, III, AVF
    B. I, II, AVL
    C. I, III, AVF
    D. V_1, V_2

73. **Increases in lung compliance occur with**
    A. Pulmonary edema.
    B. Pleural effusions.
    C. Obesity.
    D. Emphysema.

74. **Beck's triad is a combination of symptoms useful in diagnosing tamponade. The symptoms include:**
    A. Pericardial friction rub, hypertension, RV failure.
    B. Increased pulse pressure, increased JVD, tachycardia.
    C. Tachycardia, hypertension, LV failure.
    D. Distended neck veins, muffled heart sounds, hypotension.

75. **The daughters of your patient with severe biliary obstruction notice that their father has multiple scratches and excoriations over his skin. They are concerned that their father is being abused. You explain:**
    A. "Do not panic, we are not abusing him."
    B. "I understand you are concerned. Because of his high bilirubin levels, he scratches unconsciously."
    C. "He must have gotten out of the restraints."
    D. "He did it to himself as a result of PCCU psychosis."

76. **Your patient has had an anteroseptal MI. Where do you expect to see changes on the 12-lead EKG?**
    A. V_1, V_2, V_3, V_4
    B. V_2, V_3, V_4, V_5, V_6
    C. V_1, V_2, II, III, AVF
    D. V_1, V_2, I, AVL

77. **Bryce suffered a crush injury when a ditch he was digging collapsed on him. You would expect to see which of the following results on his electrolyte panels?**
    A. Hyperphosphatemia
    B. Hypomagnesemia
    C. Hypocalemia
    D. Hyperkalemia

78. Millie is a 78-year-old patient admitted postoperatively 2 days ago after a colon resection for cancer. She has a nasogastric tube through which she is receiving routine doses of antacids. Her morning labs include the following values: WBCs 15.6, neutrophils 9,800. Her chest X-ray is inconclusive. What is Millie's problem?
    A. Pulmonary embolism
    B. Hospital-acquired pneumonia
    C. Congestive heart failure
    D. Atelectasis

79. Your 19-year-old patient was involved in a motor vehicle accident in which he experienced blunt abdominal trauma related to the seat belt placement. He begins complaining of severe abdominal pain around the epigastric area that is knife-like and twisting. You also note that he has a low-grade fever with diaphoresis, abdominal distention, decreased bowel tones, and rebound tenderness. You suspect
    A. Pancreatitis.
    B. Acute liver failure.
    C. Gastrointestinal bleeding.
    D. Abdominal bruising.

80. If the inferior wall of the heart is infarcted, the leads that will most directly reflect the injury are
    A. II, II, and aVF.
    B. I and aVL.
    C. V_1–V_2.
    D. V_5–V_6.

81. Mannie is a 15-year-old victim of a gunshot wound to his left chest. As a result of his injury, he has developed a pneumo-hemothorax. Mannie has been stable all day, with minimal chest tube drainage. Over the past four hours, his O_2 saturation has been decreasing. The physician orders mixed venous gases, and the results show an SVO_2 of 64%. What does this information tell you about the patient's condition?
    A. The amount of shunting that is occurring
    B. CO_2 levels
    C. HCO_3 levels
    D. PO_2 level

82. To determine if your patient has a genetic predisposition for malignant hyperthermia, which of the following drugs might be used?
    A. Halothane
    B. Caffeine
    C. Accolate
    D. Singulair

83. Mr. Ingram, a non-alcohol-abusing patient, was diagnosed with portal hypertension with direct variceal bleeding. His wedge hepatic venous pressure is less than his portal pressure due to portal vein thrombosis. This difference may be the result of

A. Chronic active hepatitis.

B. Umbilical vein catheterization as a neonate.

C. Metastatic carcinoma.

D. Congestive heart failure.

84. **Mr. B. was admitted to your unit to rule out myocardial infarction two days ago. He has a history of GERD and stomach ulcers. Mr. B. is due to be discharged today on digoxin and oral antacids. You review his A.M. labs prior to beginning your physical assessment. Lab results are as follows:**

WBC 11,000/mm^3	RBC 5.2 × 10/mm^3	PLT 350,000/mm^3
Hgb 13 g/dL	Hct 48 mL/dL	
Potassium 4.5 mEq/L	Total calcium 13.5 mg/dL	Magnesium 1.87 mg/dL
Sodium 140 mEq/L	Chloride 104 mEq/L	

You would probably expect to see which of the following signs and symptoms during your assessment of Mr. B.?

A. Hypotension, prolonged QT interval, junctional tachycardia

B. Bradycardia, confusion, hypertension, decreased grasp strength

C. Muscle spasms, hypertonicity, ventricular tachycardia

D. Second-degree Type 2 heart block, shortened QT interval, hypotension

85. **Grant, a 21-year-old student, had an appendectomy in another state while on spring break one week ago. He is admitted to the DOU with fever, nausea and vomiting, and abdominal pain with a red, swollen surgical incision. You anticipate**

A. Immediate surgery with IV antibiotics.

B. Hydration and antibiotics.

C. Bedside excision of an abscess.

D. Bedside wound debridement.

86. **Acetaminophen overdose may cause hypoglycemia and should be treated with**

A. Continuous IV of D$_5$W at 100 cc/h.

B. Bolus of D$_{50}$, followed by continuous infusion of D$_5$W.

C. Bolus of D$_{10}$, followed by continuous infusion of 0.45% normal saline.

D. Continuous IV infusion of Lactated Ringer's.

87. **Which of the heart valves is most commonly affected by infective endocarditis?**

A. Aortic

B. Pulmonic

C. Mitral

D. Tricuspid valve

88. **The type of cardiomyopathy that is characterized by replacement of normal cells by fatty tissue is known as**

A. Hypertrophic.

B. Dilated.

C. Arrhythmogenic.

D. Restrictive.

89. Gordon, a 74-year-old retired teacher, is being admitted for dehydration and malnutrition after collapsing in his apartment. His daughter reports that he has been eating very bland, soft foods for three weeks due to reflux and difficulty swallowing. You suspect
    A. Partial tongue paralysis.
    B. Esophageal neoplasm.
    C. Tracheal neoplasm.
    D. Gastric cancer.

90. The new-onset dysrhythmia most commonly seen in a patient with pulmonary edema is
    A. Supraventricular tachycardia.
    B. RBBB.
    C. Ventricular tachycardia.
    D. Atrial fibrillation.

91. Erica was diagnosed with pericarditis on admission yesterday to the progressive care unit. She is complaining of intermittent, sharp, knife-like pain in her chest. In which position would you place her to help alleviate some of the pain?
    A. Lay her flat with her feet elevated
    B. Sit her up and lean her forward on a stable bedside table
    C. Place her prone in Trendelenburg
    D. Position her on her right side

92. Which of the following therapies would be appropriate to use in the treatment of acute hypoglycemia (blood sugar less than 50 mg/dL)?
    A. Small, frequent meals, increased carbohydrate consumption
    B. Intravenous D_{50} administration, oral glucose, and treat the cause
    C. Increased carbohydrate diet, intravenous glucose
    D. Treat the cause, increased carbohydrate consumption

93. Your patient will be having an LVAD placed this evening and will be cared for in your unit. Family members are quite anxious to learn more about the device and to participate in the patient's care. An important point when teaching caregivers is to make certain they understand which changes in the patient's condition should be reported immediately to the staff. A complication that should be reported immediately would be
    A. Irritation or redness at the incision.
    B. A temperature of 99.6°F.
    C. Any change in the mentation of the patient.
    D. A rise in blood pressure of more than 10 mm Hg.

94. Georgina, a 20-year-old exchange student from Hungary, is brought in by her roommate after 7 weeks of flu-like symptoms, increasing bruising, headaches, pounding pulses, and fever. Which diagnosis and cause are mostly likely?
    A. DIC related to bacterial infection
    B. Acute liver failure related to unintentional overdose of acetaminophen
    C. Vitamin K deficiency related to poor nutritional intake
    D. Anemia related to Gaucher's disease

95. What does the second "V" in Joanne's "VVI" pacemaker stand for?
    A. Ventricular paced
    B. Ventricular inhibited
    C. Ventricular sensed
    D. Ventricular programmed

96. Your patient is undergoing alcohol withdrawal and exhibits diplopia, peripheral neuropathy, confusion, recent memory loss, and hyperexcitability. You suspect that this patient has
    A. Jorn's syndrome.
    B. Leucine deficiency.
    C. Increased caritine levels.
    D. Wernicke–Korsakoff syndrome.

97. Your patient is a 45-year-old carpenter who was admitted for cardiomyopathy. His initial ejection fraction was 21%, and he has been confused most of the time since admission yesterday. On admission, his EKG showed ST depression in leads V_1–V_4. The patient has become more dyspneic and is getting restless. Current vital signs and parameters are as follows:
    EKG: ST at 116
    Bilateral pretibial and pedal edema; sacral edema also present
    Manual cuff BP: 102/70
    Skin pale, cool
    Temperature: 99°F
    RR 30, breath sounds clear, slightly diminished RLL
    O_2 4 L/min via mask
    Mentation: oriented to self, confused at times
    What condition does this patient appear to be suffering from at this time?
    A. An anterior MI
    B. Inferior wall MI
    C. Biventricular failure
    D. Right ventricular failure

98. Functions of the thyroid gland, adrenal gland, and male and female reproductive glands are regulated by the
    A. Pineal gland of the brain.
    B. Thyroid gland.
    C. Pineal–pituitary axis.
    D. Hypothalamic–pituitary.

99. Joab, a 40-year-old Orthodox Jew, presents with an unintentional weight loss of 20 pounds, fatigue, anorexia, and chronic, watery diarrhea with bloody mucus. He is tachycardic, tachypneic, hyperthermic, with an Hgb of 7 g/dL and an Hct of 21%. You suspect
    A. Colonic diverticulitis.
    B. Ulcerative colitis.
    C. Pancreatitis.
    D. Cholecystitis.

100. Kenneth is a 54-year-old male who was admitted with a non-STEMI inferior wall MI. He is complaining of dyspnea, weakness, bilateral crackles, and demonstrates orthopnea. Kenneth has developed an S_3 heart sound. You suspect he has also developed
   A. A pulmonary embolus.
   B. Pulmonary hypertension.
   C. A fat embolism.
   D. Cardiogenic shock.

101. Gordon was attempting to install his new propane barbeque system when the flame ignited because the regulator had been set too high. The resulting flame burned Gordon's left hand and arm. The burn on his left arm is pink and blistered. When touched, Gordon yells with pain. This classification of burn is
   A. First degree.
   B. Second degree, partial thickness.
   C. Third degree, full thickness.
   D. Fourth degree, full thickness.

102. Your patient has been diagnosed with pulmonary hypertension. Which of the following compensatory mechanisms would be expected if the patient suffered from chronic hypoxia?
   A. Polycythemia
   B. Hypoplasia of the pulmonary vasculature
   C. Thinning of blood vessels in the lungs
   D. Cor pulmonale

103. Ibrahim, a 45-year-old truck driver, was cleaning out his rented storage room yesterday. After doing so, he developed a raised area that initially looked like a mosquito bite but is now red, pus-filled, and inflamed. Ibrahim is admitted to the unit with a necrotizing wound. He may also exhibit all of the following signs and symptoms of a brown recluse spider bite except
   A. Nausea and vomiting.
   B. Dyspnea.
   C. DIC.
   D. Hemolysis and thrombocytopenia.

104. John is a 32-year-old engineer who has been on hemodialysis for three years. He missed his last two treatments. He is lethargic, lacks stamina, and is very edematous. His ABGs show the following results: pH 7.30, $PaCO_2$ 32, HCO_3 17, PaO_2 90. John's results indicate
   A. Metabolic alkalosis.
   B. Respiratory acidosis.
   C. Metabolic acidosis.
   D. Respiratory alkalosis.

105. Which of the following bariatric surgical methods does not result in the suturing or removal of gastrointestinal tissue or organs?
    A. Vertical banding
    B. Gastric banding
    C. Biliopancreatic diversion
    D. Roux-en-Y proximal gastric bypass

106. Francine was admitted three days ago for management of a deep vein thrombosis. During your initial assessment this morning, you found her sitting on the side of the bed and leaning forward. The patient states that this position relieved her newly developed chest pain. She also states that the pain is worse on inspiration. You notify the physician, who orders a CXR and lab work. The results show that the patient's sed rate and WBCs are elevated. Francine most likely has
    A. Pericarditis.
    B. A thoracic aneurysm.
    C. A pulmonary embolus.
    D. Pulmonary edema.

107. Julianna works in the fashion industry and is a cutter in the wool sweater section of her company. This morning, a fire broke out in her section. Julianna did not suffer any burns, but she did inhale large quantities of smoke. What would be the most potent toxin she might have inhaled?
    A. Carbon monoxide
    B. Smoke
    C. Nitrates
    D. Cyanide

108. Seymour is receiving activated protein C. The actions of this drug include
    A. Blockade of angiotensin II.
    B. Antimicrobial activity.
    C. Antiviral activity.
    D. Profibrinolytic activity.

109. Holly is a 20-year-old female who was admitted to your unit with status asthmaticus. She has been taking Accolate, Allegra and has been using a Proventil HFA rescue inhaler at home. Today she was working in her garden and could not catch her breath. Her bronchospasms worsened, so she was transported to the ED. In the ED she received albuterol, oxygen, and epinephrine without significant improvement. On auscultation, inspiratory and expiratory wheezing with a prolonged expiratory phase is heard throughout the lung fields. Holly is using accessory muscles for respiration and is tachycardic and tachypneic. She is placed on 2 L/min O_2 via NC and ABGs are drawn. Blood gas results are as follows: pH 7.56, PaO_2 102 mm Hg, $PaCO_2$ 28 mm Hg, HCO_3 25 mEq/L. These blood gas results show
    A. Uncompensated respiratory acidosis.
    B. Compensated metabolic alkalosis.
    C. Compensated metabolic acidosis.
    D. Uncompensated respiratory alkalosis.

110. Janet was admitted to your progressive care unit with an anaphylactic reaction to a bee sting. Multiple labs were drawn and her calcium level is 11.9 mg/dL. This value may indicate which of the following conditions?
    A. Hypoparathyroidism
    B. Excessive calcium intake
    C. Hyperparathyroidism
    D. Recent fracture of a long bone

111. A patient can be presensitized and is more likely to experience organ rejection if he or she has a history of
    A. Multiple pregnancies.
    B. Small or reduced lumens in the bile ducts.
    C. Destruction of small airways.
    D. Cytomegalovirus (CMV) infections.

112. Monty is a 47-year-old patient with severe bronchitis who has been treated with a non-rebreather mask for five days. He is exhibiting increased distress with chest discomfort, restlessness, a dry hacking cough with dyspnea, and numbness in his extremities. Pulmonary function tests (PFTs) indicate a decreased vital capacity (VC), decreased compliance, and decreased functional residual capacity (FRC). As the nurse caring for this patient, you should
    A. Prepare for intubation with 100% FiO_2 (fraction of inspired oxygen).
    B. Administer Lasix 40 mg IV.
    C. Take the patient for a CT scan and prepare to give tPA.
    D. Check the pulse oximetry correlation with an arterial blood gas sample and decrease the FiO_2.

113. Your patient was stabbed in the chest two weeks ago. The damage done to the heart required a prosthetic mitral valve replacement. The patient is now experiencing transient chest pain and syncopal episodes. A TEE is ordered. You anticipate which of the following actions prior to the procedure?
    A. Hold all medications 8 hours prior to the procedure
    B. Allow the patient to keep dentures in
    C. Administer prophylactic antibiotics
    D. Position the patient on the right side

114. Wellen's syndrome
    A. Is the same as Prinzmetal's angina.
    B. Occurs with proximal stenosis of the LAD.
    C. Is also called crescendo angina.
    D. Is also called variant angina.

115. Mrs. C. was a direct admission to your unit from her physician's office following sudden epistaxis with severe headache. She is now obtunded. During your initial assessment, you note gingival bleeding, generalized ecchymosis, and petechial hemorrhages on both legs. You suspect Mrs. C. may have

    A. DIC.

    B. Pulmonary emboli.

    C. A fat embolism.

    D. ITP.

116. Amanda, a 23-year-old horse trainer, was admitted three days ago with a right fractured femur and fractures of two ribs. She has been on O_2 at 60% since her admission. During your assessment, you note a temperature of 100°F, heart rate of 120, respiratory rate of 32, increased cough, and decreased breath sounds on the right side without tracheal deviation. You suspect Amanda's symptoms are the result of

    A. Pulmonary edema.

    B. Atelectasis.

    C. Pneumothorax.

    D. Sepsis.

117. An antidote for ethylene glycol toxicity is

    A. Digoxin.

    B. Anisindione.

    C. Fomepizole.

    D. Narcan.

118. Your patient was admitted for severe flank pain and hematuria. He is scheduled for a kidney biopsy. Your patient and family teaching should include:

    A. The patient should report any pain in the flank or abdomen post procedure.

    B. The patient may pass a small kidney stone after the procedure.

    C. The patient will be on bed rest for 24 hours.

    D. No teaching is necessary.

119. If the oxyhemoglobin curve shifts to the right, one of the factors that will affect this shift is

    A. A decrease in CO_2.

    B. A decrease in pH.

    C. A decrease in temperature.

    D. A decrease in 2,3-DPG.

120. Your patient has been diagnosed with hemolytic anemia. She has been in the progressive care unit for three days. You believe her condition was caused by

    A. An inappropriate TPN solution.

    B. A folate deficiency.

    C. Bone marrow aspiration.

    D. Intra-aortic balloon counterpulsation (IABP).

121. Binge eating, mutilation, obesity, drug abuse, and alcoholism are all examples of

    A. Self-destructive behaviors.

    B. Psychotic behaviors.

    C. Neurosis.

    D. Immaturity.

122. A patient is at high risk for ventricular septal defect or rupture or even a ventricular aneurysm if an infarct occurs in the
    A. Left anterior descending artery.
    B. Left main coronary artery.
    C. Left circumflex artery.
    D. Right coronary artery.

123. Santos, a 50-year-old father of six, has suffered a heart attack and requires immediate coronary artery bypass grafts. His children and wife are present as well as multiple other family and church members. You overhear his wife and children speaking about the fact that Santos has complete insurance coverage. According to them, his employer has approved significant sick time for recovery and has offered Santos the flexibility to work from home if additional home recuperation time is required. You are determining the level of psychiatric distress in this family. Your first priority is to
    A. Administer psychotic medications.
    B. Examine the range and effectiveness of coping mechanisms.
    C. Work with any available family members, friends, or religious support systems.
    D. Determine if there is a crisis.

124. Your patient had 1,100 mL of pleural effusion removed via thoracentesis and immediately began coughing and was dyspneic. You believe he has developed
    A. A pneumothorax.
    B. Re-expansion pulmonary edema.
    C. Cardiac tamponade.
    D. A hemothorax.

125. Complications associated with ventricular assist devices (VADs) include
    A. Thromboembolism.
    B. Thrombocytopenia.
    C. Dissection of the aorta.
    D. Septicemia.

Congratulations! You have completed PCCN Practice Exam 1. Keep reviewing the questions in the book and learn the rationale for the answers.

PCCN PRACTICE EXAM 1 ANSWERS

1. **Correct Answer: C**
   The correct order of fracture healing is fracture hematoma, granulation tissue, callus formation, and ossification.

2. **Correct Answer: C**
   Pneumonia secondary to immobility is the primary reason for infection with VADs. There may also exist a need for some type of ventilatory support. Just the fact that tubes are placed into the body means that they are a potential source of infection, but this risk is usually minimized by good hand washing and aseptic technique.

3. **Correct Answer: D**
   Answers A, B, and C are complications of BiPAP. BiPAP must be regulated so as not to cause barotrauma, yet still keep alveoli from collapsing during expiration. The patient may have to be mechanically ventilated at some point if the BiPAP is not effective.

4. **Correct Answer: C**
   PRBCs contain no platelets, and platelets must be given to aid in hemostasis.

5. **Correct Answer: B**
   Osteoarthritis (OA) is a localized disease with a variable and progressive development, whereas rheumatoid arthritis (RA) is a systemic disease with exacerbations and remissions. Other differences include:
   - Onset of the disease: OA occurs after age 40; RA occurs in the teens to thirties.
   - Gender: OA affects more females; RA affects more males initially and then more females after age 50.
   - Weight: OA patients are often overweight, RA patients do not experience any weight change or weight loss.
   - Joints impacted: OA affects weight-bearing joints; RA initially affects small joints, but then progresses.

6. **Correct Answer: B**
   The ventilatory pressures caused by excessive force with the BVM can exceed the intrathoracic and intrapleural pressures, causing barotrauma. This excessive pressure can damage several organs in the thorax and even organs in the abdomen. The lungs are susceptible to collapse (pneumothorax). Barotrauma may also damage major blood vessels.

7. **Correct Answer: A**
   Quite often the patient will describe a ripping or tearing sensation and severe pain. Hypotension may be present as the dissection progresses. Warning signs include hypertension, a new murmur (aortic insufficiency), weak peripheral pulses, and possible deterioration of level of consciousness. Aneurysms that dissect downward may radiate pain to the lower abdomen, lower back, and legs.

8. **Correct Answer: A**
   Guillain-Barré syndrome is a demyelinating autoimmune process affecting the spinal and cranial nerves. It is seen after viral infections. The most common form is the ascending variety, which demonstrates bilateral ascending weakness.

9. **Correct Answer: B**
Airway patency is always a priority. Bernard probably inhaled superheated air and toxins. Most of the products found in a home will give off carbon monoxide when burned. These toxins, plus the CO produced by the fire, may cause edema of the air passages.

10. **Correct Answer: B**
Patients with heart transplants do not feel cardiac pain because the heart has been denervated.

11. **Correct Answer: C**
A Curling ulcer is a peptic ulcer that develops after a burn injury in which blood flow to the gastrointestinal system is compromised. Hypoxemia further compounds the ischemia because O_2 requirements of the gastrointestinal tract cannot be met.

12. **Correct Answer: D**
The accuracy of pulse oximetry is affected by patient motion, low perfusion, venous pulsation, light, poor probe positioning, edema, anemia, and carbon monoxide levels. It is important to compare pulse oximetry values against arterial blood gas values to validate values that are less than 70%.

13. **Correct Answer: B**
When the heart is denervated, there is no connection to the autonomic nervous system, so a reflexive response does not occur. A sympathetic stimulant must be used. If no other complications occur, the ventricle will eventually adjust to not receiving autonomic input.

14. **Correct Answer: C**
These findings are characteristic of compensated metabolic acidosis. The pH is between 7.35 and 7.45, so the value is compensated. Because it is closer to 7.35, the value is considered acidotic. To determine whether the acidosis is respiratory or metabolic, find the value that represents acidosis:$HCO_3 < 22$ mEq/L.

15. **Correct Answer: A**
Pain is a cardinal sign of an arterial obstruction. The nurse should check for pallor, another sign of an arterial blockage, sensation, and the quality of pulses. If the obstruction is venous, the limb may exhibit cyanosis.

16. **Correct Answer: B**
Brunner's gland is a mucus-producing gland within the duodenum. If inhibited, it fails to produce sufficient amounts of mucus to protect the duodenum and an ulcer may develop. Sympathetic stimulation will inhibit this gland's function. Chronic sympathetic stimulation of any kind, such as chronic stress, will impact mucus production and increase the risk of ulcer.

17. **Correct Answer: A**
The transplanted kidney is placed in the pelvic area, so pelvic pain is an ominous sign. Patients who have undergone kidney transplants should be educated to notify their physicians immediately if suffering from pelvic pain, as it is a symptom of rejection.

18. **Correct Answer: D**
Brown–Sequard syndrome causes ipsilateral (same-side) motor paralysis and contralateral (opposite-side) loss of pain and temperature sensation. This syndrome occurs because of the way the pyramidal tracts cross in the spinal column.

19. **Correct Answer: B**
Reperfusion rhythms such as ventricular tachycardia, sinus bradycardia, accelerated idioventricular rhythm, and underlying sinus rhythms with ventricular ectopy may occur. The patient should experience less chest pain. The CPK isoenzymes may actually become elevated temporarily as blood flows freely through newly opened arteries. CHF is not a result of this therapy.

20. **Correct Answer: A**
You cannot prevent sinusitis simply by using a smaller-diameter ET. If anything, the smaller tube will make the patient's work of breathing more difficult, though it will not necessarily contribute to an infectious process. Orogastric tubes are preferred over nasogastric tubes whenever possible. Good hand washing technique has been shown to be effective in reducing all types of hospital-acquired infections.

21. **Correct Answer: D**
Dumping syndrome is a common side effect of gastric bypass surgery if the surgery includes a partial gastrectomy. The rapid emptying of the stomach's highly acidic chyme into the duodenum or directly into the jejunum results in burning or digestion of the mucosal lining, causing the pain associated with dumping syndrome. Smoking inhibits normal healing, and it may prolong healing significantly to allow further damage and possible perforation of the mucosal lining. Alcohol and caffeine increase hydrochloric acid production within the stomach, making the chyme more acidic. Stress, especially chronic stress, results in sympathetic stimulation and inhibition of the Brunner's glands, which produce mucus that protects the duodenal lining, resulting in increased risk for ulcers.

22. **Correct Answer: C**
Autonomic hyperreflexia, also known as autonomic dysreflexia, is caused by numerous stimuli, such as bowel or bladder dysfunction, cool breezes, a clogged urinary catheter, and constipation.

23. **Correct Answer: C**
Family members are probably quite used to providing care for this patient. Do not ignore the patient. There is no point in speaking slowly unless the caregiver or the patient has difficulty understanding instructions. Teaching quickly is counterproductive and may be considered rude and unprofessional. Allow time for a return demonstration of skills and allow for questions. Seth may very well understand all that you are trying to communicate.

24. **Correct Answer: A**
The N95 respirator is the primary mask to filter for TB particles and should be test-fit prior to use.

25. **Correct Answer: C**
Renal failure and sepsis may lead to pericarditis, so A.M. labs should show an increased WBC and increased ESR. With cardiac tissue involvement, an elevated CK-MB is expected. An additional lab would include uremia. Assessment findings would also include elevated ST segments, arrhythmias, and pleural effusions on echocardiography.

26. **Correct Answer: C**
Mumps requires droplet precautions or isolation. Droplets have approximately a 3-foot reach while speaking or coughing, so healthcare staff need to wear masks when in close contact with the patient. Herpes simplex, chickenpox, and wound infections may

require contact and/or airborne precautions depending on the disease and the stage of disease process. Your infection control officer and the CDC will maintain updated recommendations regarding multiple infective organisms and are excellent resources.

27. **Correct Answer: C**

   Sickle cell anemia occurs primarily in the African American population. Affected individuals are homozygous for HgS and have more HgS than HgA. This causes some of the cells to form a "sickle" shape—curved with rough edges. A crisis occurs when low oxygen tension (postulated) causes a proliferation of these cells. As these cells travel through the microcirculation, their sharp edges damage capillaries. A simple thing like cold weather can precipitate massive sickling. Other identified risk factors include dehydration, vomiting, diarrhea, high altitude, excessive exercise, and stress. When the sickled cells break apart, they occlude the microcirculation and lower oxygen tension, which initiates more sickling. A crisis is a very painful time for the patient, and oxygen, pain management, and fluids are very important.

28. **Correct Answer: C**

   Flail chest results when two or more adjacent ribs are broken in two or more places, so that the chest wall becomes unstable. During normal inspiration, the chest wall moves outward with an increase in negative intrathoracic pressure. In flail chest, the opposite movement of the chest wall is seen. This is known as a "paradoxical" movement. Eventually the patient will experience atelectasis and alveolar collapse, with possible development of ARDS. To adequately stabilize the fracture, sometimes neuromuscular blockade is used. The patient must be given pain medication and sedation. Also, pain management is a priority because the work of breathing (WOB) needs to be reduced. To appreciate what patients are going through, just think about a time you have had a pain in your side and how difficult it was to take a full breath.

29. **Correct Answer: A**

   The circumflex artery feeds the left atrium and left ventricle. Infarctions as a result of occlusion of this artery result in lateral or left-side heart damage. The left anterior descending artery and the circumflex artery both branch off from the left coronary artery.

30. **Correct Answer: A**

   Chronic bronchitis is diagnosed when the bronchitis lasts for three months within a 12-month period and occurs in 2 consecutive years. Symptoms are a result of hyperplasia of the mucus-secreting glands in the airway, which results in impaired ventilation. Bronchitis does not affect oxygenation function at the alveolar level.

31. **Correct Answer: C**

   Diabetes insipidus (DI) is a serious decrease in antidiuretic hormone (ADH). The most common causes of neurogenic DI are closed head injury and removal of a posterior pituitary tumor. ADH is produced by the posterior pituitary gland. Closed head injury and cerebral edema lead to pressure on the pituitary gland, thereby decreasing ADH production. Other common causes of DI are lung cancer (small or oat-cell carcinoma), leukemia, and lymphoma.

32. **Correct Answer: A**

   Cushing syndrome is also known as Cushing's triad. These symptoms are late indicators of a serious deterioration of neurologic status. This patient is at very high risk for herniation and imminent death.

33. **Correct Answer: B**

   New-onset or acute mitral valve regurgitation is often a result of myocardial infarction of the left anterior descending and circumflex arteries. These arteries feed the papillary muscles supporting mitral valve function. Prolonged ischemia causes the papillary and/or chordae tendinae of the mitral valve to rupture, which prevents full closure of the mitral valve during systole. As the blood flows back into the left atrium, the murmur can be auscultated.

34. **Correct Answer: B**

   The pH of the aspirate is very important. If the aspirate is acidic, pulmonary edema is created almost immediately due to the collapse and breakdown of the alveoli, capillaries, and their interface. Atelectasis, possible intra-alveolar hemorrhage, and some interstitial edema lead to hypoxia. Alkalotic aspirate destroys surfactant, which causes alveolar collapse, leading to hypoxia. Other factors to identify are the type of material aspirated and the amount. Syrup of ipecac is used for some cases involving ingestions. ABGs would be considered more of a diagnostic tool.

35. **Correct Answer: A**

   Gina has endocarditis. Janeway lesions are flat, painless erythematous areas on palms and soles of the feet predominately. Osler's nodes are small, painful nodules associated with endocarditis; they are found on the fingers and toes. Roth spots are seen when examining the retina; these rounded, white areas are also associated with endocarditis. Pella's sign is not a medical term. It is thought that microvascular clots form in the heart and pass through the microcirculation and impede peripheral circulation, sometimes causing necrosis.

36. **Correct Answer: C**

   To reach O_2 levels of 40–60%, the non-rebreather mask should have an intact reservoir and oxygen should be administered at a rate of 6–10 L/min. Humidity cannot be used with the mask effectively, resulting in dry mucus membranes. Nebulizer therapies should not be used with this form of O_2 support.

37. **Correct Answer: C**

   Patients with peripheral vascular disease are often hypothermic because of poor circulation. Healing is slowed because of the decrease in circulation. The nurse should provide proper alignment without impeding circulation and monitor peripheral pulses for their presence and quality. The color and temperature of the extremity should be monitored and the results charted.

38. **Correct Answer: B**

   Idiopathic thrombocytopenia purpura is the result of a low platelet count. Sometimes platelets are destroyed early and systematically, theoretically as part of an autoimmune response. Hemorrhages may occur in the brain, which may lead to stroke and increased intracranial pressure.

39. **Correct Answer: C**

   The first step is to check the sensitivity control. Even though most of these pacemakers have a cover, the dial may have been moved and indicate a fixed rate is set. If the pacemaker continues to fire, it may cause an R-on-T phenomenon and cause ventricular tachycardia or fibrillation. If the patient has an adequate rhythm, you can turn off the pacemaker and notify the physician. If the patient has a nonsustaining rhythm, you can try positioning the patient on the left side to see if the wire will come in contact with the myocardium. You can also try turning up the mA level. Either way, the physician must be notified and vital signs carefully monitored until the physician can reposition the electrodes.

40. **Correct Answer: D**

Dairy products may actually increase bronchospasm and increase the amount of phlegm produced. Fluid intake should be increased to approximately 3 L per day. Serevent is a long-lasting inhaler and can take up to an hour to work.

41. **Correct Answer: B**

Multiple sclerosis is a demyelinating disorder of the white matter of the brain and spinal cord. It can be intermittent, progressive, or relapsing. Multiple sclerosis follows either an acute course or a progressive course. A major cause of disability in young adults age 16–40, it affects more females than males.

42. **Correct Answer: C**

This patient is hypokalemic and will exhibit muscle weakness, anorexia, and cardiac arrhythmias.

43. **Correct Answer: B**

Polyuria, polydipsia, and polyphagia are known as the "three P's." The fruity breath is from ketone production when fatty acids are broken down. Dehydration is due to osmotic diuresis. Fatigue is due to potassium shifting from inside the cells to the intravascular space.

44. **Correct Answer: D**

Other foods that have a high folic acid content include red beans, broccoli, asparagus, liver, and beef.

45. **Correct Answer: A**

The injuries to the chest may have caused a pulmonary artery laceration or a cardiac contusion, which is more likely. The patient's blood pressure is low and the EKG shows ST-segment elevation in the anterior leads. If the myocardium is contused, it will react the same way as if an MI had occurred. The ST-segment elevation may be the result of a physiologic insult to a coronary artery and an area of the myocardium is ischemic. The pumping function of the myocardium is compromised and may need additional support with inotropes. The patient may need to undergo angiography and/or surgery. Volume replacement may be necessary. This patient is probably in the first stage of cardiogenic shock.

46. **Correct Answer: C**

HHNS develops slowly in Type II diabetes. This condition most often occurs in elderly patients or those with undiagnosed diabetes mellitus. The blood sugars are generally more than 600 mg/dL and can exceed 1,500 mg/dL. The other differentiation between HHNS and DKA is the lack of ketones seen with HHNS.

47. **Correct Answer: C**

Plasmanate and dextran are examples of colloids. Other colloids include Hespan and albumin. Plasma is a blood product often seen as fresh frozen plasma (FFP); Plasmanate is a plasma protein fraction (only 5% of the solution is human plasma), with the remaining volume consisting of normal saline and albumin. Dextrose, normal saline, and Lactated Ringer's are examples of crystalloid solutions.

48. **Correct Answer: C**
Level of consciousness is the most sensitive indicator of neurologic status in a patient. Brain tissue is extremely sensitive to even minute changes in oxygen and glucose levels. When cerebral edema occurs, as in a closed head injury, these levels change very quickly, affecting the level of consciousness of a patient.

49. **Correct Answer: B**
Blood sugars of more than 600 mg/dL, negative serum ketones, and serum osmolality greater than 310 mOsm/L are typical findings with hyperglycemic, hyperosmolar, nonketotic syndrome (HHNS). The pH is usually greater than 7.3, and the blood urea nitrogen (BUN) may be elevated. Osmolality is the best predictor of survivability (better than blood sugar levels).

50. **Correct Answer: B**
This patient needs a pacemaker or AICD that can deliver a more powerful impulse. The asynchronous mode will override Barry's internal pacemaker.

51. **Correct Answer: B**
Approximately 85% of cerebral aneurysms are located at the anterior bifurcations of the circle of Willis; the remaining 15% are found at the posterior bifurcations.

52. **Correct Answer: D**
Ultrasound may be difficult to obtain or interpret due to ascites, obesity, or fluid in the retroperitoneal area. Doppler scans measure blood flow and the flow is diminished due to prerenal and intrinsic AKI. Nuclear scans are of limited value because the excretion rates may be slowed by disease. Renal biopsy is the gold standard for diagnosing rejection.

53. **Correct Answer: B**
Reconstitution or administration with any other solution or with a solution that contains a bacteriostatic agent, such as benzyl alcohol, may cause the antibiotic to precipitate. The drug should not be administered if any precipitation or foreign matter is present. Reconstitution should utilize sterile needles and aseptic technique. IV rate should be slow, and a small test infusion should be given prior to a full dose to observe for side effects. IV site rotation and heparin flushes may limit complications of phlebitis.

54. **Correct Answer: C**
Numerous physical changes occur with Cushing syndrome (also known as Cushing disease): thinning hair, acne, moon facies, increased body hair, buffalo hump on the upper back, purple striae on the trunk, truncal obesity with thin extremities, and easy bruising.

55. **Correct Answer: A**
Pelvic inflammatory disease (PID) is an infective disease of the pelvic cavity most often caused by *Neisseria gonorrhoeae* or *Chlamydia trachomatis*. If the infection is left untreated and spreads to the liver, the presenting pain will be in the upper right quadrant. Infection in the liver allows the organism to become systemic via blood flow through the liver; however, liver function tests remain normal.

56. **Correct Answer: A**

Cholinergic crisis is a life-threatening problem with any overdose—accidental or otherwise. It causes bradycardia, severe weakness, cardiac arrest, and occasionally respiratory arrest.

57. **Correct Answer: C**

Pacemaker syndrome is caused by a loss of atrial kick or regurgitation against a closed A-V valve. Gene's atrial lead may have become damaged or failed.

58. **Correct Answer: C**

Thyrotoxic crisis is a rare but serious problem in post-thyroidectomy patients, undertreated hyperthyroidism cardiopulmonary disease, and hemodialysis patients.

59. **Correct Answer: B**

Right shoulder pain following laparoscopic cholecystectomy occurs when CO_2 is not reabsorbed during or after surgery. As CO_2 accumulates within the abdomen, it can aggravate the phrenic nerve and the diaphragm, causing pain and making it difficult to breathe. To relieve the pressure and irritation of CO_2 on the phrenic nerve, place the patient in Sim's position (left side with knees drawn up toward the chest), which moves the CO_2 away from the nerve and eases pain.

60. **Correct Answer: D**

A lateral MI is identified by changes in leads I, aVL, V_5, and V_6.

61. **Correct Answer: C**

Cimetidine interferes with creatinine excretion in the renal tubule. Renal function does not decrease, but the level of creatinine does rise. If diminished renal function exists, an allergic nephritis may develop.

62. **Correct Answer: D**

Laminectomy is a surgical procedure used to gain access to a herniated disk via removal of part of the posterior arch of the vertebra. Because this procedure involves spinal manipulation, any change in or worsening of neurological symptoms from preoperative status must be reported immediately to the physician once the patient's neurological status has been thoroughly assessed. Improvements in neurological status may not be noticed immediately after surgery, but should occur over time.

63. **Correct Answer: C**

Of the choices given here, the problem is in the right ventricle. The high CVP and jugular distention indicate a problem with the right ventricle—it cannot pump effectively. The lethargy may be unrelated and needs to be evaluated because it is a significant change for this patient.

64. **Correct Answer: C**

Glenda is most likely experiencing a hypoglycemic event due to her NPO status. The other options are not wrong but the question asks about a person with diabetes who is NPO.

65. **Correct Answer: B**

The changes in the quality, frequency, and duration of chest pain indicate unstable angina and may foretell an increased risk for a myocardial infarction. This patient should be closely monitored for EKG changes and rhythm disturbances. In addition, extensive teaching should begin with the family and patient on identification of the symptoms of a myocardial infarction and basic CPR should the patient go into a cardiac arrest outside of the hospital.

66. **Correct Answer: A**

The heparin will have dilutional effects and will decrease the bicarbonate and $PaCO_2$ levels.

67. **Correct Answer: B**

Because your patient has lost two of the three main fascicles that innervate the heart, he is at great risk for sudden death. He needs a pacemaker as soon as possible.

68. **Correct Answer: C**

Type I cells line the outside of the alveoli; they are easily inflamed by inhaled toxins or heated air. Type I cells maintain the blood–gas interface. Type II cells produce surfactant.

69. **Correct Answer: B**

This patient has nephrogenic diabetes related to lithium use. Prolonged use of lithium causes insensitivity to vasopressin in the renal tubules, making the tubules incapable of absorbing water. Treatment involves administration of hydrochloro-thiazide or indomethicin.

70. **Correct Answer: D**

Myocarditis can also present with inspiratory pain. Pain when supine is a cardinal sign of myocarditis. Other findings can include symptoms that are consistent with a respiratory infection, and an S_3, S_4, and a pericardial friction rub may be present.

71. **Correct Answer: A**

A patient with AKI cannot excrete ammonium or acid ions in sufficient quantities to aid in the excretion of hydrogen. The buildup of the hydrogen causes the acidosis.

72. **Correct Answer: A**

Leads II, III, and AVF are the ones in which you would identify an inferior wall MI.

73. **Correct Answer: D**

Answers A, B, and C decrease lung compliance. Other factors that decrease compliance are atelectasis, fibrotic changes, abdominal distention, pain (causes splinting), and flail chest (pain and loss of structure).

74. **Correct Answer: D**

With tamponade, tachycardia is an early sign. A narrowed pulse pressure occurs and fluid cannot be ejected from the heart. The muffled heart sounds occur because the fluid in the sac minimizes the transmission of sound waves.

75. **Correct Answer: B**

This answer acknowledges the daughters' concerns and provides education. Elevated bilirubin levels deposited in the skin result in unconscious scratching and excoriations. When a patient has increased PT, PTT, and INR levels, hematomas may also be present. Answer A provides no explanation for the scratches and decreases communication with the family. Restraints are inappropriate for this patient. ICU/PCCU psychosis can lead to abnormal behavior, but it is not the reason for this patient's behavior.

76. **Correct Answer: A**
The anteroseptal MI is seen in leads V_1, V_2, V_3, and V_4. The septal leads are V_1 and V_2. The anterior leads, which overlap, are V_2, V_3, and V_4.

77. **Correct Answer: D**
The patient will become hyperkalemic as potassium from the cells is released into the vasculature as a result of the crush injury.

78. **Correct Answer: B**
Millie's age, time in the hospital, nasogastric tube, and use of antacids are all risk factors for HAP. The fact that her chest X-ray is inconclusive is not unusual with elderly patients, as they often have other underlying diseases that make it difficult to identify pneumonia.

79. **Correct Answer: A**
Acute pancreatitis may occur as a result of seat belt trauma to the pancreatic duct or abdominal ischemia. Acute liver failure is characterized by flu-like symptoms, jaundice, confusion, and enlarged liver. Gastrointestinal bleeding is associated with a history of ulcers and/or esophageal varices with hemodynamic changes, narrowing pulse pressures, hematemesis, and hyperactive bowel tones. Abdominal trauma does not produce the knife-like and twisting pain, and tenderness and a marbled appearance would be noted.

80. **Correct Answer: A**
Leads I and aVL will show damage to the higher areas of the lateral wall. Leads V_1 and V_2 will show septal wall damage. Leads V_5 and V_6 will show damage to the apical area.

81. **Correct Answer: A**
SVO_2 shows shunting. Normally, a 5% physiologic shunt occurs due to blood in the bronchial, pleural, and Thebesian veins. When the patient has infection, trauma, or ARDS, blood is shunted at a higher rate and is seen as a lowered SVO_2.

82. **Correct Answer: B**
In malignant hyperthermia, the use of anesthetic agents such as Halothane causes muscles to contract and the patient to become hypothermic. Caffeine is used diagnostically because it can contract muscles at higher doses without the danger of depolarizing cell membranes. The antidote for malignant hyperthermia is dantrolene.

83. **Correct Answer: B**
Pre-hepatic (pre-sinusoidal) factors lead to hepatic venous pressures less than portal pressures. Umbilical vein catheterizations as a neonate (within the first month of life) due to neonatal illness or prematurity may cause damage to the vessel. Chronic active hepatitis is an intrahepatic (sinusoidal) factor. Wedge hepatic venous pressures are increased or equal to portal pressures. Metastatic carcinoma and cardiac diseases such as CHF can cause portal hypertension and may indirectly cause variceal bleeding.

84. **Correct Answer: B**
Mr. B. would exhibit signs and symptoms of hypercalcemia, as confirmed by his calcium level of 13.5 mg/dL. Signs and symptoms would include smooth-muscle relaxation, lethargy, confusion, shortened QT interval, bradycardia, heart blocks, bundle branch blocks, and hypertension. Symptoms can be further compounded by the effects of digitalis and possible digitalis toxicity.

85. **Correct Answer: A**

    This patient is exhibiting signs and symptoms of an abscess following the surgical intervention for appendicitis. This complication occurs in 5–33% of patients. Surgical debridement of the incision and IV antibiotics are appropriate immediate treatment to prevent sepsis. Hydration and antibiotics alone will not treat the abscess. Bedside excision of the abscess alone may reduce the amount of infected fluid and tissue at the site, but will not prevent further infection. Bedside wound debridement places the patient at high risk of further contamination of the site. In approximately 2% of cases, the abscess may be intra-abdominal and may require surgical intervention under anesthesia as well as continued antibiotic treatment.

86. **Correct Answer: B**

    Hypoglycemia occurs because of the hepatotoxic effects of acetaminophen. Infusions must also be based on blood glucose results.

87. **Correct Answer: C**

    The mitral valve is the most common site at which infective endocarditis develops. The aortic valve is the next most common valve affected. The valve least likely to be affected by infective endocarditis is the pulmonic valve. The tricuspid valve is often involved secondarily as a result of IV drug abuse.

88. **Correct Answer: C**

    "Arrhythmogenic" is a relatively new classification for cardiomyopathy. The normal myocardial cells are replaced by fatty tissue and fibrous tissue. The right ventricle is primarily affected. Conduction cannot occur normally, so the patient will have multiple ventricular arrhythmias and right ventricular failure. Young people with arrhythmogenic cardiomyopathy are at risk for sudden death. The cause of this condition is unknown, but some research has shown a possible link to an autosomal dominant gene.

89. **Correct Answer: B**

    This patient is exhibiting classic progression of a developing esophageal neoplasm. Complications that coincide with this disease process are related to changes in nutritional intake. Narrowing of the esophageal lumen results in increasing difficulties and pain when swallowing, causing the individual to consume an increasingly softer diet, until ultimately the patient can swallow only liquids. A diagnosis of partial tongue paralysis would be supported if the patient also had difficulty speaking, but that symptom is not listed in the question. Gastric cancer is indicated when the patient has indigestion and fullness, not difficulty swallowing. Tracheal neoplasms would be associated with more respiratory distress.

90. **Correct Answer: D**

    Atrial fibrillation is the result of the constant stretching and disruption of normal pathways in the atrium due to increased preload from the pulmonary congestion.

91. **Correct Answer: B**

    Pericarditis results in inflammation of the layers of the pericardial sac. Deep respirations, trunk rotation, and flat positioning allow the parietal and visceral layers of the pericardial sac to rub against each other. Upright and forward positioning pulls the heart away from the diaphragmatic pleura of the lungs and eases the cardiac pain.

92. **Correct Answer: B**
    Administration of D_{50}, oral glucose, and treating the cause are the most effective ways to manage acute hypoglycemia. The other answers include increased carbohydrate consumption, which would be prohibited in acute hypoglycemia. The optimal diet would consist of small, frequent meals and reduced consumption of carbohydrates.

93. **Correct Answer: C**
    The nurse would monitor the patient's vital signs. This family is so eager to help that they would probably have someone at the bedside many hours during the day. Any change in mentation is very significant, and the family can help monitor the patient when the nurse is away from the room. This family will be ready to embrace learning and assume more tasks as time passes if they are positively reinforced for their efforts.

94. **Correct Answer: B**
    Acute liver failure related to acetaminophen overdose would be consistent with this patient's presentation. Individuals without full command of the English language are at risk for overdose when self-medicating if the medication label is not read and understood correctly. The symptoms listed are inconsistent with DIC and vitamin K deficiency. Gaucher's disease is a genetic enzyme deficiency disease that is typically diagnosed in childhood, symptoms are progressive and worsen as glucocerebroside collects in the spleen and liver. This patient would also present with skeletal weakness, neurological complications, swollen lymph nodes, and pain not restricted to just the last 7 weeks.

95. **Correct Answer: C**
    Using ICHD nomenclature, the second "V" indicates the chamber sensed.

96. **Correct Answer: D**
    Wernicke–Korsakoff syndrome is a thiamine deficiency and a metabolic encephalopathy.

97. **Correct Answer: C**
    The heart cannot pump the fluid out and the lungs are congested (dyspnea). Edema is a sign of pump failure. The patient will probably develop ascites and hepatomegaly.

98. **Correct Answer: D**
    The hypothalamic–pituitary axis releases a number of hormones that inhibit or release several other hormones that affect body functions.

99. **Correct Answer: B**
    Based on the presenting symptoms and his ethnicity, Joab likely has ulcerative colitis. He may also have leukocytosis and cachexia. Colonic diverticulitis presents with left upper quadrant pain, hyperthermia, vomiting, chills, diarrhea, and tenderness over the descending colon. Pancreatitis presents with left upper quadrant pain that radiates to the back or chest, hyperthermia, rigidity, rebound abdominal tenderness, nausea and vomiting, jaundice, Cullen's sign, Grey–Turner's sign, abdominal distention, and diminished bowel sounds. Cholecystitis presents with right upper quadrant or epigastric pain, pain that lasts up to six hours after a fatty meal, vomiting, and increased white blood cell counts.

100. **Correct Answer: D**
    The MI has impaired the heart's ability to pump effectively. The cardiac output falls and the body reacts by vasoconstricting the peripheral circulation and increasing the

heart rate. Tachycardia is also the result of catecholamine release, with increased myocardial oxygen consumption. The left ventricle works harder, but has been compromised by the MI. Preload increases because fluid cannot be pumped out of the chambers effectively. The S_3 heart sound is a signal of increased preload. Pulmonary congestion occurs due to increased left heart pressures.

101. **Correct Answer: B**

    This type of burn may be either a superficial or deep partial-thickness burn. The nerve endings are still intact and the burn is very painful. Sometimes burns can be deceptive. A reddened area diagnosed as a first-degree burn may be overlooked when staff calculate the patient's requirements for fluid and nutrient resuscitation. After a few hours, these areas can develop blisters, only then being recognized as dermal burns. A new way of assessing burn levels is by using a laser Doppler during the first week of treatment.

    Assessing burn depth can be tricky. The first step is determine which factors caused the burn (chemical, electrical, thermal), how long the causative mechanism was in contact with the area, blood flow, and where the burn is located. Another issue to consider is the thickness of the skin at the site. Elderly people and children have thinner skin, so burns in those populations tend to be more severe. Burns on the eyelids and genital area are about 1 mm thick, whereas burns on the palms and soles of the feet are on areas about 5 mm thick. Although the thicker skin offers a bit more thermal protection, the palms and soles of the feet become infected more easily.

102. **Correct Answer: A**

    The effects of acute hypoxia are reversible. Chronic hypoxia causes permanent changes in the lungs and pulmonary vasculature (hyperplasia and hypertrophy), which will cause thickening of the blood vessels and narrow their lumens. Polycythemia develops and the blood viscosity increases. An increased number of cells will be available to carry oxygen, but the increased viscosity of the blood will increase pressure in the pulmonary vasculature and force the right ventricle to pump harder to maintain the CO level. The right ventricle will hypertrophy and eventually weaken, so that the patient develops right heart failure (cor pulmonale).

103. **Correct Answer: B**

    Patients who have recluse spider bites may not initially know that they were bitten and often seek medical help 12–36 hours after the initial bite. Because treatment is delayed, symptoms may be difficult to treat. The majority of patients may present with flu-like symptoms. DIC, hemolysis, and thrombocytopenia are severe symptoms. Treatment includes applying ice to control inflammation, keeping the area clean and protected, and treating symptoms. No specific treatment has been proven to be 100% effective. Dapsone has limited support for the prevention of necrosis. Nitroglycerin patches counter the vasoconstrictive properties of the venom, leading to hemodilution in the bloodstream and increased bleeding at the site that washes the venom out.

104. **Correct Answer: C**

    More specifically, this result would indicate an uncompensated metabolic acidosis. The pH is low, as is the $PaCO_2$.

105. **Correct Answer: B**

    In gastric banding, an adjustable band is placed around the upper portion of the stomach to create a small, 1- to 2-ounce area to act as the stomach. Because the size is restricted without suturing of the stomach or removal of any tissue, the procedure may be reversed for medical reasons such as pregnancy. Vertical banding, biliopancreatic diversion, and Roux-en-Y proximal gastric bypass all include some permanent change to the normal gastric pathway.

106. **Correct Answer: A**

The CXR will probably show pericardial effusion. The elevated sed rate and WBC indicate infection. In pericarditis, leaning forward often relieves chest pain, whereas lying supine makes it worse. Pain may worsen on inspiration as the lungs expand and come in contact with the pericardium. The patient will probably have a fever as well. It is necessary to assess the patient for any signs of cardiac tamponade and to make certain use of anticoagulants is discontinued.

107. **Correct Answer: D**

Wool and silk give off cyanide gas. Nitriles, like those found in the gloves nurses wear, will give off cyanide when burned. Household plastics such as melamine dishes, plastic cups, polyurethane foam in furniture cushions, and many other synthetic compounds may produce lethal concentrations of cyanide when burned under certain circumstances. Cyanide inhibits cellular respiration, even when the person has adequate oxygen stores. Cellular metabolism changes from aerobic to anaerobic, and the body produces lactic acid. The organs with the highest oxygen requirements are the ones affected most dramatically by cyanide inhalation.

108. **Correct Answer: D**

Activated protein C (Xigris) inhibits factors Va and VIIIa. It also inhibits human tumor necrosis factor production by monocytes and limits thrombin-induced inflammatory responses.

109. **Correct Answer: D**

The pH is elevated, indicating alkalosis. The HCO_3 level is normal and the $PaCO_2$ is decreased, which indicates respiratory alkalosis.

110. **Correct Answer: C**

Hyperparathyroidism can be either primary or secondary in nature. Primary hyperparathyroidism involves excess secretion of parathyroid hormone (PTH) and may be related to a breakdown of the feedback system to the parathyroid glands or overgrowth of the glands. Secondary hyperparathyroidism is generally related to a chronic disorder such as chronic renal failure or a malabsorption state.

111. **Correct Answer: A**

Other possible causes of organ transplant rejection include transfusions, previous organ transplants, and blood type incompatibilities. Answers B, C, and D are the results of organ rejections, not causes.

112. **Correct Answer: D**

Monty is exhibiting signs and symptoms of oxygen toxicity after 5 days of oxygen therapy at > 50% FiO_2. Non-rebreather masks provide a minimum of 60% FiO_2 at 6 L/min. An arterial blood gas result would show an increased PaO_2 > 100 mm Hg, ruling out respiratory failure (PaO_2 < 60 mm Hg), which would require intubation. The dry, hacking cough rules out pulmonary edema and the need for Lasix. Numbness in the extremities is from the presence of oxygen radicals in the blood, not a neurologic impairment, which would indicate the need for a CT scan with possible tPA administration.

113. **Correct Answer: C**

The patient should receive prophylactic antibiotics to mitigate possible endocarditis, which may be the cause of his symptoms at this time.

114. **Correct Answer: B**

Wellen's syndrome is a type of angina that occurs when the LAD is stenosed proximally. The ST segment is not elevated more than 1 mm in leads V_1–V_3, there is mild T-wave inversion in leads V_2–V_3, and Q waves are not pathologic (greater than 25% of the total length). Because of the location of the stenosis, surgery is required emergently. Variant angina is the same as Prinzmetal's angina; this pain occurs at rest and is associated with vasospasm. Crescendo angina means that over time it takes less to initiate the pain, and the pain lasts longer.

115. **Correct Answer: A**

Disseminated intravascular coagulation is an overstimulation of the clotting cascade. Both the intrinsic and extrinsic pathways are activated at the same time, which causes an acceleration of the clotting process. When the clots lyse, the fibrin split products are anticoagulants. Eventually, all the clotting factors are used up and no further clots can form. Heparin is sometimes used to interrupt the clotting cycle.

116. **Correct Answer: B**

Three days of high FiO_2 has resulted in a nitrogen washout resulting in atelectasis. Nitrogen's high partial pressure is necessary to maintain alveoli inflation. It is important to titrate FiO_2 to maintain saturations within a prescribed range when oxygen therapy is utilized. Pulmonary edema would result in coarse breath sounds. With a unilateral pneumothorax, a tracheal deviation would be noted. Sepsis would not necessarily present with diminished breath sounds, but rather with additional findings of increased purulent secretions, coarse breath sounds, and altered laboratory diagnostic results.

117. **Correct Answer: C**

Ethylene glycol is a compound found in antifreeze. After ingestion, it is converted to oxalic acid, which is excreted by the kidneys. This causes formation of crystals in the urine, acidosis, tetany, and renal failure. Hemodialysis and peritoneal dialysis will remove ethylene glycol from the body.

118. **Correct Answer: A**

The biopsy may cause bleeding from highly vascular tissue. Flank pain may be the first sign.

119. **Correct Answer: B**

A shift to the right means hemoglobin has less affinity for oxygen. 2,3-Diphosphoglyceride (2,3-DPG) is needed to help force O_2 off the hemoglobin molecule. Thus, if the 2,3-DPG level is decreased, hemoglobin will hang on O_2 more tightly. If the temperature is increased, the tissues need more O_2. If the PCO_2 is elevated, the tissues need more oxygen.

120. **Correct Answer: D**

At about the third day following admission, many patients develop anemias. A reduced folate level would lead to megaloblastic anemia. Bone marrow aspiration is a diagnostic procedure, and TPN solutions would not lead to development of anemia. The IABP could, indeed, cause cells to lyse, as could prosthetic heart valves, heart–lung bypass, and bacterial endotoxins.

121. **Correct Answer: A**

Self-destructive behaviors are those that, over time, will shorten or threaten the length and quality of life.

122. **Correct Answer: B**

An infarct in the left main coronary artery is an ominous sign. Sudden death may occur, along with heart blocks and atrial and ventricular dysrhythmias.

123. **Correct Answer: D**

In any potential psychiatric emergency or crisis, the first issue is to determine whether one actually exists. In this scenario, the patient has an extensive and involved support system, financial stability, and effective coping mechanisms, so a psychiatric crisis is not likely to develop. Even so, it is important to carefully monitor for any change in status.

124. **Correct Answer: B**

Removal of large amounts of pleural fluid (> 1,000 mL) increases negative intrapleural pressure. Edema occurs when the lung does not reexpand. In turn, the patient develops a severe cough and dyspnea. If the symptoms occur during a thoracentesis, the procedure should be stopped.

125. **Correct Answer: A**

Answers B, C, and D are complications of an intra-aortic balloon pump (IABP). Other common complications from VADs include infection and bleeding.

PCCN PRACTICE EXAM 1 ANSWER SHEET

Use this sheet to test yourself with the Practice Exam.

1. A B C D	26. A B C D	51. A B C D
2. A B C D	27. A B C D	52. A B C D
3. A B C D	28. A B C D	53. A B C D
4. A B C D	29. A B C D	54. A B C D
5. A B C D	30. A B C D	55. A B C D
6. A B C D	31. A B C D	56. A B C D
7. A B C D	32. A B C D	57. A B C D
8. A B C D	33. A B C D	58. A B C D
9. A B C D	34. A B C D	59. A B C D
10. A B C D	35. A B C D	60. A B C D
11. A B C D	36. A B C D	61. A B C D
12. A B C D	37. A B C D	62. A B C D
13. A B C D	38. A B C D	63. A B C D
14. A B C D	39. A B C D	64. A B C D
15. A B C D	40. A B C D	65. A B C D
16. A B C D	41. A B C D	66. A B C D
17. A B C D	42. A B C D	67. A B C D
18. A B C D	43. A B C D	68. A B C D
19. A B C D	44. A B C D	69. A B C D
20. A B C D	45. A B C D	70. A B C D
21. A B C D	46. A B C D	71. A B C D
22. A B C D	47. A B C D	72. A B C D
23. A B C D	48. A B C D	73. A B C D
24. A B C D	49. A B C D	74. A B C D
25. A B C D	50. A B C D	75. A B C D

(Over for questions 76–150)

76. A B C D	101. A B C D	126. A B C D
77. A B C D	102. A B C D	127. A B C D
78. A B C D	103. A B C D	128. A B C D
79. A B C D	104. A B C D	129. A B C D
80. A B C D	105. A B C D	130. A B C D
81. A B C D	106. A B C D	131. A B C D
82. A B C D	107. A B C D	132. A B C D
83. A B C D	108. A B C D	133. A B C D
84. A B C D	109. A B C D	134. A B C D
85. A B C D	110. A B C D	135. A B C D
86. A B C D	111. A B C D	136. A B C D
87. A B C D	112. A B C D	137. A B C D
88. A B C D	113. A B C D	138. A B C D
89. A B C D	114. A B C D	139. A B C D
90. A B C D	115. A B C D	140. A B C D
91. A B C D	116. A B C D	141. A B C D
92. A B C D	117. A B C D	142. A B C D
93. A B C D	118. A B C D	143. A B C D
94. A B C D	119. A B C D	144. A B C D
95. A B C D	120. A B C D	145. A B C D
96. A B C D	121. A B C D	146. A B C D
97. A B C D	122. A B C D	147. A B C D
98. A B C D	123. A B C D	148. A B C D
99. A B C D	124. A B C D	149. A B C D
100. A B C D	125. A B C D	150. A B C D

PCCN PRACTICE EXAM 2

1. **Stroke volume consists of which of the following factors?**
   A. Blood volume, viscosity, impedance
   B. Cardiac output, heart rate, compliance
   C. Contractility, preload, afterload
   D. Compliance, impedance, heart rate

2. **Ben was just transferred to your progressive care unit. He had been in the ICU two weeks. He was intubated for a time because of his ARDS. On arrival in your unit, you note that he is tachycardic and restless. Ben states, "I can't be here now. What if something like this happens to me again?" The nurse's best response would be:**
   A. "The nurses in our unit can take care of you."
   B. "We are not very far away at the nurses' station."
   C. "Your insurance will not cover another day there."
   D. "You sound concerned about leaving our ICU."

3. **An absolute contraindication for a single-lung, double-lung, or heart–lung transplant would be**
   A. Previous cardiothoracic surgery.
   B. Kidney disease.
   C. Liver disease.
   D. Psychiatric illness.

4. **What is the mean arterial pressure (MAP) for a patient with a blood pressure of 120/70 and a heart rate of 80?**
   A. 82
   B. 2.4
   C. 50
   D. 85

5. **Amy is the lone survivor of a car crash that killed her parents and two siblings. She is recovering from a pneumothorax, hemothorax, and bilateral broken legs. She has been extremely depressed and withdrawn. You are discussing medications, psychiatric therapy, and the increased risk of suicide and suicidal behavior with Amy's distant relatives. The family makes each of the following statements. Which of these statements is false?**
   A. "If Amy is considering suicide, she will make statements or give warnings of suicide."
   B. "We should trust our instincts if we feel Amy is in danger."
   C. "As Amy recovers from her depression, she is at greater risk of suicide."
   D. "If Amy talks about suicide or asks about pills, then she is just voicing the thought and will not attempt suicide."

6. **Which of the following therapies would be appropriate to use in the treatment of acute hypoglycemia (blood sugar less than 50 mg/dL)?**
   A. Small, frequent meals, increased carbohydrate consumption
   B. Intravenous D_{50} administration, oral glucose, and treat the cause
   C. Increased carbohydrate diet, intravenous glucose
   D. Treat the cause, increased carbohydrate consumption

7. SaO$_2$ values account for what percentage of oxygen (O$_2$) carried within the blood-stream?
   A. 2–3%
   B. 10–24%
   C. 97–98%
   D. 100%

8. The resistance against which the right ventricle must use to eject its volume is known as
   A. Resting heart pressure.
   B. Systemic vascular resistance.
   C. Central venous pressure.
   D. Pulmonary vascular resistance.

9. Nursing care for a patient with glaucoma would not include
   A. Applying cool compresses to the patient's forehead.
   B. Darkening the environment.
   C. Providing a quiet and private space.
   D. Encouraging the patient to cough.

10. If you hear faint breath sounds on the left side of the chest and normal sounds on the right side immediately after your patient has been intubated, most likely
    A. The patient has a tumor.
    B. The physician has intubated the esophagus.
    C. The ET is at the carina.
    D. The right mainstem has been intubated.

11. While passing your terminally ill patient's room, you see his wife of 40 years crying at the bedside while she pats his hand. She is unkempt, tired, and unable to focus during conversations. You believe that she is in the middle of a situational crisis. Your best action is to
    A. Call the social worker to speak with her.
    B. Call the appropriate spiritual advisor for this patient.
    C. Call her primary doctor for a prescription for Xanax or Paxil.
    D. Call your charge nurse to cover your other patients while you initiate a conversation with the wife to identify her stressors and develop a list of resources.

12. You ask a fellow nurse to carry a newly drawn ABG specimen to the lab. She does not place the sample on ice. What effect will the lack of icing have on the sample?
    A. None
    B. It will invalidate the sample.
    C. The pH will rise.
    D. The PaO$_2$ will rise.

13. Mr. Ironclaw is from a nearby Indian reservation. He is retired, is on a fixed income, and does not have insurance. He is being discharged today after an overnight observational stay for chest pain. In planning his discharge care, which of the following issues should be considered first to increase compliance with his plan of care once the patient is home?

A. Arrange for home nursing visits every day for 1 week
B. Ask the physician to consider an over-the-counter antiplatelet medication
C. Schedule the patient's follow-up appointment with the cardiologist in 3 months
D. Suggest a gym membership so that the patient can begin exercising

14. **Arthur is a 50-year-old patient with a history of DKA. He currently has a blood glucose level of 460 mg/dL and a potassium level of 6.2. You have started an insulin drip. You know that the insulin drip will**
    A. Draw more potassium from the intracellular space.
    B. Draw more potassium from the extracellular space.
    C. Not change potassium levels.
    D. Move potassium back into the intracellular space.

15. **Assessment of the abdomen should occur in which order?**
    A. Inspection, palpation, auscultation, percussion
    B. Auscultation, inspection, palpation, percussion
    C. Percussion, inspection, palpation, auscultation
    D. Inspection, auscultation, percussion, palpation

16. **Amy is the sole survivor of a crash that killed her immediate family. While recovering from massive injuries, her behavior and moods rapidly change. Which of the following behaviors is most concerning to you as the nurse and indicates possible suicidal behavior?**
    A. Drug seeking with multiple requests for pain medications and sedatives
    B. Withdrawal from conversation and interaction
    C. Crying and statements of helplessness
    D. Screaming at her distant relatives

17. **Potential complications of loop diuretics would include**
    A. Hypercalcemia.
    B. Increased BUN.
    C. Hypokalemia.
    D. Hypertension.

18. **Your patient is in status asthmaticus. Her ABGs indicate uncompensated respiratory alkalosis. The most probable cause of this acid–base imbalance is**
    A. An adverse effect of albuterol.
    B. A side effect of theophylline.
    C. Hyperventilation.
    D. Hypoventilation.

19. **William was diagnosed with unstable angina. He is scheduled for an exercise stress test. William tells you that he has a "bad hip" and an old knee injury that makes it difficult for him to walk or stand for more than 20 minutes. You tell him:**
    A. "You need to walk for only 10 minutes."
    B. "You can ride a bike for 20 minutes instead."
    C. "I will call the physician and ask for the weight-lift test."
    D. "I will call the physician and ask for a stress echocardiography test."

20. Eileen, a 30-year-old female, was admitted 3 days ago with a right fractured femur and fractures of two ribs. She has been on 60% O_2 since admission. During your assessment, you note a temperature of 100°F, heart rate of 120, respiratory rate of 30, increased cough, and decreased breath sounds on the right side without tracheal deviation. You suspect the patient's symptoms are the result of
    A. Pulmonary edema.
    B. Atelectasis.
    C. Pneumothorax.
    D. Sepsis.

21. **Why are hyperglycemia and hyperlipidemia seen concurrently in diabetes mellitus?**
    A. Very-low-density lipoprotein (VLDL) production increases in response to increased insulin production.
    B. Insulin resistance promotes VLDL production.
    C. Lipid breakdown is hindered by hyperinsulinemia.
    D. Glucose increases cause the liver to increase lipid production.

22. **The oxyhemoglobin dissociation curve**
    A. Shows the relationship between dissolved oxygen and the affinity for oxygen by the hemoglobin molecule.
    B. Is a graphic representation of carbon dioxide content versus oxygen content in arterial blood.
    C. Is a measure of methemoglobin.
    D. Is a way to calculate gas transport across the alveoli.

23. **Ethel P. suffered a cardiac arrest at home. The family did not perform CPR, and the paramedics arrived 6 minutes after the arrest began. The patient was found in pulseless V-tach. Defibrillation was performed, and CPR was continuous during transport to the ED. The patient was transferred to the telemetry unit because of a bed shortage in the ICU. The physician initiated hypothermic measures and administered vecuronium. In this case, the medication was used to**
    A. Control ventricular dysrhythmias.
    B. Prevent shivering.
    C. Act as a sedative.
    D. Relieve pain.

24. **After being resuscitated following a cardiac arrest, Myra spent a week recovering in the MICU. This morning she was admitted to your progressive care unit. Because the resuscitation was prolonged, Myra developed acute renal failure. The definition of acute renal failure would be**
    A. Trauma to one or both kidneys.
    B. Decrease in renal perfusion from shock or anaphylaxis.
    C. A sudden or rapid decline in renal filtration function.
    D. An obstruction to passage of urine.

25. **Falsely low readings on a pulse oximeter may be due to**
    A. Electronic interference from hemodialysis.
    B. Fever.
    C. Vascular dyes.
    D. Polycythemia.

26. A definitive diagnosis of myocarditis can be made via
    A. An endomyocardial biopsy.
    B. Transesophageal ultrasound.
    C. Transmural catheterization.
    D. Chest X-ray.

27. Brody is a 46-year-old carpenter admitted to the PCU after a barroom brawl in which he suffered multiple minor stab wounds. He is angry and verbally assaultive with the staff. The goal of anger management for this patient is to do all of the following except
    A. Confront him directly with whatever made him angry.
    B. Discuss what in the situation made him angry.
    C. Discuss with Brody alternative and positive ways to express his feelings.
    D. Decide on positive ways for Brody to express his feelings when confronted with frustrating situations in the future.

28. Hannah was admitted to the ICU with a temperature of 102.3°F, headache, dyspnea, dry cough, and chills. Her lab results indicate a low white blood cell count, low platelets, and elevated C-reactive protein level. Hannah's history includes a recent trip to a remote Chinese village within the past two weeks. You suspect Hannah may have
    A. Pneumonia.
    B. SARS.
    C. Influenza.
    D. Pericarditis.

29. Your patient was admitted for severe dyspnea, dysphagia, palpitations, and an intractable cough. On auscultation, you hear a loud S_1 and a right-sided S_3 and S_4. This patient probably has
    A. Mitral insufficiency.
    B. Myocarditis.
    C. Atrial stenosis.
    D. Mitral stenosis.

30. Your telemetry patient suddenly develops right pupil dilation. What does this change indicate?
    A. Basilar skull fracture
    B. Uncal herniation
    C. Brain stem herniation
    D. Cerebral vascular accident

31. Carbon monoxide has an affinity for hemoglobin thought to be 200–300 times greater than oxygen's affinity for hemoglobin. Elimination of carbon monoxide occurs via the
    A. Kidneys.
    B. Liver.
    C. Spleen.
    D. Lungs.

32. **Regarding stable angina, which of the following statements is true?**
    A. A positive treadmill test will indicate CAD.
    B. A thallium test will not diagnose LV dysfunction.
    C. The treadmill test will miss as much as 20% of single-vessel disease.
    D. CK-MB isoenzymes and troponins will not increase.

33. **Which of the following individuals is at highest risk for a psychological emergency?**
    A. An 80-year-old home-bound male whose wife has just died and who has no children or living family
    B. A married 20-year-old female who is delivering a 35-week gestational infant
    C. A married 56-year-old male who was just laid off from his job of 10 years
    D. A married 36-year-old female who is newly diagnosed with systemic lupus erythematosus

34. **What are the three major problems associated with macrovascular disease that accompanies diabetes mellitus?**
    A. Retinopathy, coronary artery disease, cerebrovascular accident
    B. Peripheral neuropathy, coronary artery disease, cerebrovascular accident
    C. Coronary artery disease, cerebrovascular accident, peripheral vascular disease
    D. Diabetic peripheral neuropathy, peripheral vascular disease, cerebrovascular accident

35. **An anterior wall infarction may be seen in leads**
    A. V_4 and R.
    B. V_5–V_6.
    C. V_7–V_9.
    D. V_2–V_4.

36. **Increases in lung compliance occur with**
    A. Pulmonary edema.
    B. Pleural effusions.
    C. Obesity.
    D. Emphysema.

37. **The wife of your 60-year-old patient with newly diagnosed acute hepatitis A asks if her husband is getting better. His AST, ALT, alkaline phosphate, and GGT levels are returning to normal after being severely high. His PT, INR, and bilirubin levels are still rising. You tell her:**
    A. "Of course. The important labs are improving."
    B. "I can't talk to you. You don't have power of attorney."
    C. "No, but you have to wait for the doctor."
    D. "Although some of the labs are stabilizing, the increasing PT, INR, and bilirubin indicate that your husband is still very ill."

38. **Stimulation of the vasomotor center in the medulla occurs when the partial pressure of oxygen changes. This sequence is initiated by**
    A. Baroreceptors.
    B. Chemoreceptors.
    C. The Purkinje system.
    D. The Bainbridge reflex.

39. **Cassandra was admitted to the DOU for severe anxiety. Which of the following medical conditions is likely to present with severe anxiety?**
    A. Narcolepsy
    B. Asthma
    C. Hyperglycemia and/or hypoglycemia
    D. Hypercaffeination

40. **Devin was admitted for abrupt-onset fever, chills, vomiting, diarrhea, and headache that developed in the past 24 hours. He had recently been on a cruise to Barbados. Devin is probably suffering from**
    A. A *Pseudomonas* infection.
    B. Influenza.
    C. A *Klebsiella* infection.
    D. Legionnaire's disease.

41. **Symptoms of right-sided heart failure include**
    A. Pulmonary edema.
    B. Elevated pulmonary pressures.
    C. Hepatomegaly.
    D. Orthopnea.

42. **Blood gas results you would expect to see with thrombotic emboli are:**
    A. pH 7.42, PaO_2 88, $PaCO_2$ 28, HCO_3 22
    B. pH 7.50, PaO_2 74, $PaCO_2$ 52, HCO_3 24
    C. pH 7.32, PaO_2 86, $PaCO_2$ 29, HCO_3 26
    D. pH 7.32, PaO_2 90, $PaCO_2$ 30, HCO_3 24

43. **Which symptoms are to be expected with thyrotoxic crisis?**
    A. Hypotension, bradycardia
    B. Hyperthermia, bradycardia
    C. Flushing, hypoventilation
    D. Hypertension, hyperthermia

44. **Joe underwent CABG surgery 4 days ago and was transferred to your care yesterday. Today he complains of dull aching around the sternum. You note increased tenderness to touch along the sternal edge and contracted intercostal muscles. You should**
    A. Contact the physician for an order for a 12-lead EKG, cardiac enzymes, and morphine.
    B. Culture swab the wound for bacterial infection.
    C. Do nothing; Joe's pain is normal.
    D. Administer morphine and diazepam as ordered.

45. **When assessing a patient with a chest tube drainage system, which of the following statements would be correct?**
    A. Check for subcutaneous emphysema around the insertion site by auscultation.
    B. If the system uses a Pleur-Evac with auto-transfusion connection, make certain all clamps are open.
    C. The average chest tube size for an adult is 20 Fr.
    D. If using a chest tube drainage system with a one-way valve and suction, water is required to maintain a tight seal.

46. Which of the following types of cells would be considered a nongranular leukocyte?
    A. Eosinophils
    B. Neutrophils
    C. Basophils
    D. Monocytes

47. Your unit has just completed a code lasting two hours for an 18-year-old rape and trauma victim. The patient had seemingly been doing fine the past 3 days while in your unit. Due to overwhelming unknown factors, the patient does not survive. Chaplain services are called in to assist with a nursing staff debriefing. Of the emotions encountered during this debriefing, staff members experiencing which of the following emotions are at highest risk for psychological stress?
    A. Anger
    B. Fear
    C. Anxiety
    D. Denial

48. Central cyanosis is usually seen when the Hgb level is
    A. 2 g/dL.
    B. 5 g/dL.
    C. 8 g/dL.
    D. 10 g/dL.

49. You are using the PQRST method of pain assessment for your patient complaining of chest pain. The "S" in this acronym stands for
    A. Sensitivity.
    B. Severity.
    C. Standard.
    D. Symptoms.

50. Stephan is an alcoholic admitted to your unit with cirrhosis. Why is thiamine added to his IV fluids?
    A. Thiamine is a sedative and will ease agitation.
    B. Thiamine decreases the symptoms of DTs.
    C. Thiamine is used to prevent damage to the brain that results from Wernicke's syndrome.
    D. Thiamine is used to prevent complications of substance abuse.

51. The drug of choice to treat AV nodal and atrioventricular reentrant arrhythmias is
    A. Amiodarone.
    B. Clonidine.
    C. Quinidine.
    D. Adenosine.

52. Oliguria is a urine output of 100–400 mL/d and is usually the result of
    A. Pyelonephritis.
    B. Rhabdomylitis.
    C. Prerenal syndrome.
    D. Acute glomerular nephritis.

53. Henry is a 76-year-old gentleman who was admitted for end-stage mesothelioma. Which of the following occupations would lend itself to a diagnosis of mesothelioma?
    A. Bricklayer
    B. Gardener
    C. Office manager
    D. Shipbuilder

54. You are talking to your 24-year-old patient about his newly diagnosed Type II diabetes. He states that he is fine with the diagnosis and knows that he will need to make some changes. His speech is rapid and pressured, he makes frequent jokes, and he talks about playing football with the guys when he is discharged. You would still be concerned about this patient's psychological health because of his
    A. Rapid, pressured speech.
    B. Frequent jokes.
    C. Talk of social activities.
    D. Failure to identify specific lifestyle changes that will need to be made.

55. An example of a systolic murmur would be
    A. Tricuspid stenosis.
    B. Tricuspid insufficiency.
    C. Mitral stenosis.
    D. Pulmonic insufficiency.

56. Mr. Davis is a 33-year-old businessman who is in town for an important conference. He was brought to the hospital after collapsing following complaints to hotel staff of continuous right upper quadrant pain, nausea, vomiting, and fever. He is complaining to you about his work schedule and not being able to take off work. He asks you which course of treatment will result in less hospital time. You tell him:
    A. "I understand your concern. I will ask the physician to speak to you about treatment options."
    B. "Delaying surgery may increase mortality."
    C. "Fifty percent of patients who delay surgery may require emergency surgery."
    D. "Laparoscopic surgery requires even less hospital time and has a decreased risk of bile duct injury."

57. Your employer asks that you be immunized for hepatitis B. You should expect
    A. One dose, with a booster every 10 years.
    B. Two doses, with the second occurring at 4–8 weeks.
    C. Three doses, with the second occurring at 1–2 months, and the third at 4–6 months.
    D. One dose every 4 years.

58. Erica was diagnosed with pericarditis on admission yesterday to the progressive care unit (PCU). She now complains of intermittent, sharp, knife-like pain in her chest. In which position would you place her to help alleviate some of the pain?
    A. Lay her flat with her feet elevated
    B. Sit her up and lean her forward on a stable bedside table
    C. Place her prone in Trendelenburg
    D. Position her on her right side

59. George B. is a 55-year-old high school teacher with meningitis. Today he is having a lumbar puncture. As his PCCU nurse, you know that cerebrospinal fluid (CSF) should be
    A. Hazy, with a glucose level of 85.
    B. Clear, with RBCs present.
    C. Clear and colorless, with less than 45 mg/dL of protein.
    D. Clear and colorless, with a white blood cell count of more than 150 cells/mm^2.

60. Patrick is a 24-year-old male with cystic fibrosis. Because of his condition, he is at high risk for which of the following electrolyte imbalances?
    A. Hypernatremia
    B. Hypocalcemia
    C. Hyponatremia
    D. Hypercalcemia

61. Brenda was admitted to your unit for observation after falling 10 feet into a ravine. She was diagnosed with systemic lupus erythematosus (SLE) two years ago. She suffered a concussion, three fractured ribs, a fractured radius, and a sprained ankle. She is on a Holter monitor and is receiving IV fluids and antibiotics. Which of the following conditions would be exacerbated by her SLE?
    A. Hypotension
    B. Constipation
    C. Pericarditis
    D. Polycythemia

62. Harold is experiencing delirium tremens. Nursing interventions include keeping the room well lit and minimizing stimulation. Staff members continuously reorient Harold to time, place, and person. Haldol has been given as ordered, and the patient is in four-point restraints. Which of these nursing interventions should be discontinued?
    A. Reorientation
    B. Medication administration
    C. Restraints
    D. Controlling stimulation

63. The normal range for hematocrit in an adult female would be
    A. 20–40%.
    B. 28–35%.
    C. 37–47%.
    D. 42–55%.

64. A drug that will significantly decrease the INR is
    A. Naficillin.
    B. Vitamin K.
    C. High-dose vitamin C.
    D. Cyclosporine.

65. Analyze the following arterial blood gas results. Use the provided space to the right side to assist in interpretation by writing acidosis, alkalosis, compensated, or uncompensated.

    pH 7.46

    CO_2 34

    HCO_3 24

    A. Normal
    B. Compensated respiratory acidosis
    C. Compensated metabolic acidosis
    D. Uncompensated respiratory alkalosis

66. Sara, an 18-year-old model, is a recovering anorexic. You are preparing to transfer her to her home when you note that she has not touched her lunch. You should tell her:

    A. "It's okay. I know that hospital food is not gourmet, but the dinners are more appetizing."
    B. "If you don't eat, we will have to put a feeding tube in you."
    C. "You need to eat to regain strength and prevent complications. We will work with you to find foods that you like."
    D. "Food is not your enemy. Eating this is not going to make you fat."

67. Kenneth is a 54-year-old male who was admitted with a non-STEMI inferior wall MI. He is complaining of dyspnea, weakness, bilateral crackles, and demonstrates orthopnea. He has developed an S_3 heart sound. You suspect Kenneth has also developed

    A. A pulmonary embolus.
    B. Pulmonary hypertension.
    C. A fat embolism.
    D. Cardiogenic shock.

68. What percentage of the body's potassium may be found in the extracellular fluid?

    A. 2%
    B. 5%
    C. 10%
    D. 98%

69. You are assisting with triaging of patients after an earthquake. Which of the following actions is your first priority?

    A. Establishing physical conditions
    B. Addressing the media
    C. Getting social services
    D. Reconnecting family members

70. A probable candidate for a coronary artery bypass graft might have

    A. An ejection fraction of 55% and diabetes.
    B. Right main artery disease.
    C. An ejection fraction of 35% and coronary artery disease.
    D. A previous history of cardiac surgery.

71. **This form of hepatitis is often misdiagnosed as gastroenteritis:**
    A. Hepatitis A.
    B. Hepatitis B.
    C. Hepatitis C.
    D. Hepatitis E.

72. **Zack, a chronic alcoholic with cirrhosis, has returned again to the DOU after failing rehabilitation that you assisted him in obtaining. Although you previously had a friendly and open relationship, now he will not look at you and gives only minimal answers to questions. You tell him:**
    A. "I can't believe you wasted the opportunity to get sober at the rehabilitation center."
    B. "I know you want to stay sober, but maybe you need more time."
    C. "I am proud of how long you stayed sober. Let's try again."
    D. "Why don't we work together to find new resources for you to utilize when you are tempted to drink."

73. **What differentiates a transient ischemic attack (TIA) from a reversible ischemic neurologic deficit (RIND)?**
    A. A TIA lasts less than 24 hours; a RIND lasts more than 24 hours.
    B. A TIA lasts less than 6 hours; a RIND lasts more than 48 hours.
    C. A TIA lasts more than 24 hours; a RIND lasts less than 24 hours.
    D. A TIA lasts less than 24 hours; a RIND lasts less than 6 hours.

74. **A vasodilator used in the treatment of anginal pain is**
    A. Morphine.
    B. Ticlid.
    C. Aspirin.
    D. NTG.

75. **Hypokalemia may cause**
    A. Respiratory alkalosis only.
    B. Metabolic alkalosis only.
    C. Both respiratory and metabolic alkalosis.
    D. Metabolic acidosis only.

76. **Your priority in caring for a patient with a cerebrovascular accident is**
    A. Preventing decubitus ulcers.
    B. Preventing aspiration of food or fluid.
    C. Preventing contractures.
    D. Preventing depression.

77. **Your patient had a three-vessel CABG procedure and sustained a small stroke during the procedure. The stroke left some residual numbness in the patient's left arm. The family is quite agitated and does not agree with the patient's advance directives. The family informs you that they want everything done for the patient and to ignore the patient's request for no resuscitative measures. Which of the following nursing interventions would be appropriate at this time?**
    A. Inform the family that the physician will meet with them to discuss treatment options
    B. Tell the patient about the family's concerns
    C. Notify the physician that all orders are to come from the family
    D. Inform the family that the patient is fully capable of making decisions

78. **A patient is at high risk for ventricular septal defect or rupture or even a ventricular aneurysm if an infarct occurs in the**
    A. Left anterior descending artery.
    B. Left main coronary artery.
    C. Left circumflex artery.
    D. Right coronary artery.

79. **Analyze the following arterial blood gas results. Use the provided space to the right side to assist in interpretation by writing acidosis, alkalosis, compensated, or uncompensated.**
    pH 7.43
    CO_2 31
    HCO_3 20
    A. Uncompensated metabolic alkalosis
    B. Compensated respiratory acidosis
    C. Compensated respiratory alkalosis
    D. Uncompensated respiratory alkalosis

80. **If blood pressure is lower by at least 10–11 mm Hg on inspiration than on expiration, this is known as**
    A. Pulsus alternans.
    B. Pulse pressure.
    C. Pulsus paradoxus.
    D. Pulsus parvus.

81. **During a Whipple procedure, which of the following organs is removed?**
    A. Gallbladder
    B. Esophagus
    C. Ascending colon
    D. Jejunum

82. **Which of the following nursing diagnoses would be the most appropriate for a patient with Guillain-Barré syndrome?**
    A. Impaired motor weakness, impaired respiratory function, acute pain
    B. Impaired respiratory function, impaired nutrition, acute pain
    C. Impaired motor weakness, impaired bowel function, acute pain
    D. Impaired respiratory function, impaired bowel function, acute pain

83. **Rebecca is a Jehovah's Witness who has just undergone a cardiac surgical procedure. Her Hgb and Hct are falling and are now 6.5 and 24, respectively. Her chest tubes have drained 1,750 mL of fluid in the last four hours. The anticipated treatment for this patient would be to administer**
    A. One unit of type-specific whole blood.
    B. 500 cc of albumin.
    C. 250 mL of fresh frozen plasma.
    D. Continuous-circuit auto-transfusion.

84. Adam, a 24-year-old football player, suffered a spinal injury in a motor vehicle accident while intoxicated. He is now a paraplegic without family and financial resources. As you are providing wound care, he states, "You shouldn't bother with that, no one cares if I live or die. My life is over. I can't play football, and no one wants a cripple around. If I disappear, no one would even notice." Your best response to his statements is:
    A. "Don't talk like that, you are still alive, and many paraplegics are active and happy."
    B. "Why would you say that? You had visitors yesterday."
    C. "I understand that your injuries are devastating to you, but I cannot allow you to harm yourself."
    D. "Let's just get through the dressing change, and then I'll have the doctor prescribe something for you."

85. It is recommended that adults consume _____ of potassium daily.
    A. 500 mg
    B. 1,000 mg
    C. 2,000 mg
    D. 3,500 mg

86. Lea is experiencing dumping syndrome post gastric bypass surgery after eating any meal. Which of the following medications should Lea stop immediately?
    A. Nitroglycerin
    B. Insulin
    C. Pepcid
    D. Reglan

87. Your patient is scheduled for implantation of a VAD. About 20 minutes prior to the scheduled start of the procedure, she informs you that she has concerns about side effects and the procedure itself. Your best nursing intervention would be to
    A. See if she signed the consent form for the procedure.
    B. Notify the physician that the patient does not have a full understanding of the procedure.
    C. Cancel the procedure.
    D. Answer the patient's questions yourself.

88. Holly received 4 mg of morphine IV and now is unresponsive. In addition, her respiratory rate and depth are diminished. The antidote for morphine is
    A. Regitine.
    B. Bicarbonate.
    C. Naloxone.
    D. Atropine.

89. Nursing management of a patient with Guillain-Barré syndrome includes which of the following?
    A. Monitoring labs and neurologic signs
    B. Monitoring respiratory status and neurologic signs
    C. Monitoring respiratory status and lab results
    D. Monitoring labs results and urinary output

90. Your patient has just transferred from the ICU to your unit. The patient had an abdominal aortic aneurysm repair two days ago. He is somewhat restless, but his vital signs are stable. He keeps pointing at the lumbar area of his back and saying that he has discomfort in that area. This may indicate
    A. A blister from the surgical ground pad.
    B. A need for repositioning.
    C. Irritation from the dressing.
    D. Retroperitoneal bleeding.

91. Which of the following statements is true regarding the use of laryngeal mask airways (LMA)?
    A. Nurses routinely insert these airways.
    B. There is a low risk of aspiration with an LMA.
    C. An LMA is a temporary airway.
    D. The vocal cords must be visualized when the LMA is inserted.

92. The area most commonly affected by aortic aneurysms is the
    A. Aortic arch.
    B. Abdominal area.
    C. Thoracic area.
    D. Lumbar area.

93. Alicia, the 44-year-old estranged daughter of your patient with myocardial infarction, is overheard in the waiting room telling another family member, "The nurses aren't doing enough for her. If they let her die, I'll make sure they suffer." When she comes in to visit, you note that the daughter is glaring at the staff, her posture is tense, and her movements are quick and forceful. She is pacing the room, will not acknowledge staff members, and uses inappropriate language at the bedside. Your priority is to
    A. Call security to assist in removing the daughter from the unit to a secluded area.
    B. Ignore the daughter's behavior and continue to care for the patient.
    C. Call the police and forbid the daughter from returning.
    D. Make jokes and shame the daughter into behaving.

94. Hilda, a 24-year-old mother of six, is 7 months pregnant when she is admitted to your unit for severe HELLP syndrome. She is also at risk for which of the following conditions?
    A. Intra-abdominal hypertension (IAH) and abdominal compartment syndrome (ACS)
    B. Decreased intracranial pressure (ICP)
    C. Hypocarbia
    D. Increased platelets

95. A car carrying four teenagers went off a bridge and killed all but one of the teens. Today, a second EEG was done and brain death was confirmed for the fourth teen. When the family was approached about organ donation, they requested that the patient remain in the PCU for at least 7–8 days until the older sister could return from a war zone. The appropriate nursing response would be to
    A. Tell the family that patients are waiting for the bed.
    B. Notify the physician to tell the family that organ donation must be made within 24 hours.
    C. Notify social services and arrange for emergency compassionate leave for the sister.
    D. Wait until the family leaves to procure the organs.

96. What is the treatment of choice once a diagnosis of pheochromocytoma is made?
    A. Diet changes
    B. Antihypertensive medications
    C. Surgical removal of the tumor
    D. Diuretics

97. You are discussing EKG interpretation with your nursing orientee. She asks you why there is such a difference in the size of the waves. You would tell her that:
    A. The P wave represents repolarization of the atrium and the QRS wave represents depolarization of the ventricles; the size difference is related to lead placement.
    B. The P wave represents repolarization of the atrium and the QRS wave represents repolarization of the ventricles; the size difference is related to the muscle mass involved in the polarization.
    C. The P wave represents depolarization of the atrium and the QRS wave represents depolarization of the ventricles; the size difference is related to the muscle mass involved in the polarization.
    D. The P wave represents depolarization of the atrium and the QRS wave represents repolarization of the ventricles; the size difference is related to lead placement.

98. Your patient has a confirmed flail chest. Which alteration in acid–base balance would you expect?
    A. Metabolic alkalosis
    B. Metabolic acidosis
    C. Respiratory acidosis
    D. Respiratory alkalosis

99. Ian was diagnosed with Addison's disease. In Addison's disease, what happens to the potassium level?
    A. Hyperkalemia related to the decrease in aldosterone secretion
    B. Hyperkalemia related to the increase in aldosterone secretion
    C. Hypokalemia related to the decrease in aldosterone secretion
    D. Hypokalemia related to the increase in aldosterone secretion

100. Bernard was admitted for pneumonia. He is two years post heart transplant. When you place the EKG monitoring leads, you note sinus tachycardia with PVCs and a 2-mm ST elevation. The patient denies pain. This finding is

A. Impossible.

B. Normal.

C. Indicative of an RBBB.

D. Indicative of an inferior MI.

101. **You are caring for a 68-year-old woman who was in a motor vehicle accident in which a child was killed. She is combative and restless, hyperventilating, tachycardic, and has an elevated blood pressure. She states, "I've got to leave here. They'll arrest me—they'll lock me up. I can't believe this. There is no way out." You should tell her:**

    A. "Just relax. They can't arrest you while you are in the hospital."

    B. "Calm down. It wasn't your fault if she darted into traffic."

    C. "Stop it. You are working yourself up. Look at me and focus on what I am telling you to do."

    D. "They should arrest you, you killed a child."

102. **Your patient is 36 hours status post right femoral bypass graft. The patient complains of pain with even slight movement of the limb. You suspect**

    A. An arterial obstruction.

    B. A DVT.

    C. A venous obstruction.

    D. A leg cramp from prolonged bed rest.

103. **You are teaching your patient with COPD about his treatment plan. Which of the following statements would indicate that the patient understands his disease and his treatment plan?**

    A. "I should limit my fluid intake to one liter per day."

    B. "I should use my Serevent inhaler as a rescue inhaler."

    C. "I should elevate and cross my legs while watching television."

    D. "I should avoid drinking or ingesting dairy products."

104. **A quadriplegic patient has undergone a CABG and has had no complications. You are about to teach his wife how to change the chest dressings and the graft site dressings on the legs. Principles of teaching include**

    A. Teaching all the information at once.

    B. Teaching the information as fast as possible.

    C. Explaining the rationale for the procedure, and then demonstrating it.

    D. Speaking slowly so the patient can hear.

105. **You are caring for Mr. B., a 34-year-old male who received a gunshot wound during a casino bar fight 18 hours ago. He was restrained after being verbally and physically abusive to the staff. You see him thrashing around in the bed and suddenly awakens when you enter the room. The patient is shaking, has vomited, is tachycardic, has an elevated blood pressure, and is talking to people not in the room. You suspect he is**

    A. Experiencing delirium tremens.

    B. Experiencing drug withdrawal.

    C. Experiencing sepsis.

    D. Exhibiting signs of paranoid schizophrenia.

106. **A factor that would decrease lung resistance is**
    A. Endotracheal tube size.
    B. Bronchospasm.
    C. Secretions.
    D. Albuterol administration.

107. **Jenny B. has had a transsphenoidal resection of a pituitary tumor. Her postoperative care should include**
    A. Vital signs, I&O monitoring, and neurologic signs.
    B. Monitoring neurologic signs, urinary output, and moustache dressing changes.
    C. Monitoring I&O, moustache dressing changes, and daily weights.
    D. Changing nasal packing daily, neurologic signs, and daily weights.

108. **Tachyarrhythmias that are refractive to conventional therapies may have to be treated with radio-frequency ablation. This treatment is usually successful on reentry tachyarrhythmias. The radio-frequency destroys myocardial tissue via**
    A. Radiation.
    B. Heat.
    C. Cold.
    D. Overriding the signal to ablate the pacemaker.

109. **A woman who is eight months pregnant was severely injured in an automobile accident. Her condition has been declining over the past week. The husband has been informed of the probable demise of his wife. She was made a "do not resuscitate" and moved to the PCU because she requires more care than the staff on the orthopedic unit can provide. In addition, the physician suspects fetal demise and has notified the husband of this possibility. The husband wants to bring their only other child, an 8-year-old boy, into the PCU to visit his mother. The PCU has a policy that children must be 12 years old to visit. What is an appropriate nursing action at this time?**
    A. Sneak the child in during night shift
    B. Take a picture of the mother for the child
    C. Arrange a patient care conference the next day to discuss the options
    D. Inform the husband that the visiting policy is strictly enforced

110. **You are preparing Bill for a paracentesis. Which of the following actions is the first step in assisting with a paracentesis?**
    A. Have the patient void or insert a Foley catheter
    B. Exam the abdomen for dullness
    C. Order an upright X-ray of the abdomen
    D. Position the patient with the affected side up

111. **The cardinal signs of respiratory failure include all of the following except**
    A. Tachypnea.
    B. Diaphoresis.
    C. Restlessness.
    D. Headache.

112. Helen developed infective pericarditis after renal failure and sepsis. Morning labs should show an
    A. Increased WBC, decreased ESR, normal CK-MB.
    B. Normal WBC, decreased ESR, elevated CK-MB.
    C. Increased WBC, increased ESR, elevated CK-MB.
    D. Increased WBC, normal ESR, elevated CK-MB.

113. Magnesium is required for all of the following physiological functions except
    A. To always act as an antagonist with calcium.
    B. For enzyme activation.
    C. Synthesis of nucleic acid and proteins.
    D. For functioning of the sodium–potassium pump.

114. During shift report, you are told that your patient has a 90% occlusion to the circumflex coronary artery. Which type of myocardial infarction is this patient at greatest risk of developing?
    A. Lateral wall infarction
    B. Anterior wall infarction
    C. Posterior wall infarction
    D. Septal wall infarction

115. John Doe is admitted to the PCCU for seizure activity. The nurse should anticipate which of the following laboratory tests?
    A. CBC, lipid panel, toxicology screen
    B. CBC, toxicology screen, LFTs
    C. CBC, CMP, lipid panel
    D. CBC, CMP, sedimentation rate, CRP, RPR, toxicology screen

116. As the charge nurse for a busy telemetry unit, you note an increased frequency of patients with underlying mental disorders being admitted. You overhear some negative comments from other nurses regarding assignment to these patients. You ask the nurses to complete a self-awareness survey regarding their beliefs and understanding of mental health issues. You will use this information to
    A. Determine which nurses should never care for patients with mental health issues.
    B. Change nursing assignments immediately.
    C. Determine which nurses should be written up and counseled.
    D. Create an education program for the nurses that will increase understanding of mental health issues and ways to access resources.

117. Janet is being treated in the PCU for burns sustained to 15% of her body when she was trapped in her house during a fire. She is at high risk for developing which of the following conditions?
    A. Peptic ulcer
    B. Pancreatitis
    C. Cholecystitis
    D. SRES

118. Richard is a 61-year-old male with a significant history of emphysema. He started smoking when he was five years old and until his current admission continued to smoke as many as five packs of cigarettes per day. In addition, he has uncontrolled diabetes and peripheral vascular disease. Three days ago, Richard had a major stroke when he was walking down the stairs. He suffered a broken pelvis and fractured his left radius. He has been comatose since his admission with a flat-line EEG study. His wife has agreed that "do not resuscitate" (DNR) should be issued for Richard. She has also agreed to discontinue ventilatory support. His physician recommends that he receive morphine as a comfort measure during this process. Richard's wife has been informed that the morphine will make him more comfortable, but may decrease his ability to ventilate and, in fact, may hasten his demise. This type of ethical dilemma is known as a

    A. Null ethical principle.

    B. Double effect.

    C. Slippery slope.

    D. Palliative principle.

119. Gina was admitted to the PCU with cough, fever, chills, anorexia, malaise, and headache. She has a pericardial friction rub and a history of rheumatic fever. While examining Gina, you note fine, dark lines in her nail beds and some flat lesions on her palms. These flat lesions are known as

    A. Janeway lesions.

    B. Roth spots.

    C. Osler's nodes.

    D. Pella's sign.

120. A diastolic murmur will occur as a result of regurgitant blood flow over which of the following valves?

    A. Mitral, aortic

    B. Mitral, tricuspid

    C. Pulmonic, aortic

    D. Tricuspid, pulmonic

121. Your patient was admitted and treated for torsades de pointes. You are now teaching the patient about adding foods that are rich in magnesium to the diet. Your patient asks about each of the following foods. Which of the following is a poor source of magnesium?

    A. Honey

    B. Broccoli

    C. Almonds

    D. Chocolate

122. Which type of device can deliver precise, high flow rates of O_2?

    A. Partial rebreather

    B. Venturi mask

    C. Non-rebreathing mask

    D. Transtracheal catheter

123. **You are discussing postdischarge psychiatric resources with your patient's family. You note that they are using the terms "psychiatric emergency" and "crisis" interchangeably. To clarify this issue, you tell them that**
    A. A crisis is an immediate danger to someone else, whereas an emergency is a suicide attempt.
    B. A crisis develops over time as a result of a psychological stressor, whereas an emergency is an immediate situation that, if not corrected, will result in violence.
    C. A crisis occurs when no intervention will be effective, whereas an emergency is when interventions have the greatest impact.
    D. A crisis is sudden and precedes an emergency, when lives may be threatened.

124. **A nursing action prior to the patient undergoing an MRI is to ascertain if the patient has any _____ that would prevent the test from occurring.**
    A. autograft heart valve
    B. metal dental fillings
    C. unremoved bullets
    D. burn grafts

125. **Matthew has had an AICD for 6 months. He has been admitted to your unit for syncope. You notice his pulse is very irregular, and he complains of getting "zapped" often. On his monitor, the rhythm is sinus bradycardia with numerous pacemaker spikes. What could be wrong?**
    A. Matthew's AICD has a faulty lead.
    B. Matthew has had a myocardial infarction.
    C. The battery in Matthew's AICD is losing power.
    D. Matthew has experienced a generator failure of his AICD.

Congratulations! You have completed PCCN Practice Exam 2. Keep reviewing the questions in the book and learn the rationale for the answers.

PCCN PRACTICE EXAM 2 ANSWERS

1. **Correct Answer: C**
   Answer A gives the components of afterload. Answers B and D give mixed components of cardiac output.

2. **Correct Answer: D**
   Therapeutic communication occurs when the patient's feelings are validated. This response allows for the patient to express the concerns he has about the transfer. The other answers are closed and judgmental and do not allow for any expression of feeling from the patient.

3. **Correct Answer: D**
   Patients with a history of psychiatric illness may be unable to comprehend or follow through a complicated postoperative medication regimen.

4. **Correct Answer: A**
   The mean arterial pressure (MAP) takes into account that the diastolic phase of the cardiac cycle comprises two thirds of the cycle. The calculation for the MAP is MAP = 2(DBP) + (SBP) / 3. If you took the average of the diastolic blood pressure (DBP) and systolic blood pressure (SBP), it would not account for the importance of the diastolic phase. The heart rate does not enter into this calculation. Patients should maintain a MAP of at least 60 to ensure adequate perfusion to the brain and kidneys. This calculation is incredibly simple to do and will provide you with early trending for your patient.

5. **Correct Answer: D**
   Careful consideration and observation should be given to any person voicing any thought or plan regarding suicide. Many individuals will provide warnings about their suicidal thoughts, thereby providing those in the family or in proximity with an opportunity to intervene. Warnings are often cries for help and intervention. Family members should pay close attention to any impression or instinct that the person is considering suicide. As individuals enter and exit depression, they are at greatest risk for suicide because they have sufficient mental focus to form a plan and energy or motivation to carry it out.

6. **Correct Answer: B**
   Once the blood glucose is less than 300 mg/dL, D_5WNS should be added to slow the drop in glucose. Hourly blood glucose levels should be continued. The anion gap should slowly be lowered to less than 20.

7. **Correct Answer: C**
   The percentage of total oxygen carried within the bloodstream attributed to the SaO_2 is 97–98%. SaO_2 is the arterial saturation of hemoglobin. This percentage corresponds to the percentage of hemoglobin on the red blood cells that carries O_2. Typically this percentage is in the range of 93–99%. PaO_2 is the percentage of oxygen within the bloodstream that is free or dissolved in the plasma. A normal value for this parameter (which is documented in mmHg) is in the range of 80–100 mm Hg.

8. **Correct Answer: D**
   Pulmonary vascular resistance represents a mean pressure in the systemic vasculature. The higher the resistance, the harder the heart has to work against it. For example,

cold will cause vasoconstriction, so that the heart has to pump harder to deliver blood through the narrowed vasculature.

9. **Correct Answer: D**

   Glaucoma is characterized by complications of increased intraocular pressure (IOP) and resulting damage to the ocular nerve. Coughing increases intracranial pressure and thus intraocular pressure, resulting in further damage to the optic nerve. Nursing staff should take precautions to avoid any increase in intracranial or intraocular pressure.

10. **Correct Answer: D**

    The right mainstem bronchus is somewhat wider and has less of an angle off the mainstem bronchus, so it is much more readily intubated.

11. **Correct Answer: D**

    The wife may need time to open up to you, so you will need to ensure that your other patients are cared for. Even though the social worker and spiritual advisor may need to be called, it is important not to overwhelm the wife until the stressor and situation has been identified. It is not appropriate for the nurse to contact the wife's physician, although the wife may need prescriptions during this time; that decision should be made by her physician upon direct assessment.

12. **Correct Answer: B**

    The $PaCO_2$ will rise approximately 3–10 mm Hg per hour. The PaO_2 and the pH will decrease.

13. **Correct Answer: B**

    Although the patient may want to be compliant with his plan of care, financial limitations may prohibit expensive treatments, medications, and support services. If the patient is to start an antiplatelet medication, request from the physician that over-the-counter medications be considered in preference to more expensive brand-name drugs if the patient cannot afford to continue drugs started while in the hospital. The patient may be better able to afford and continue a baby aspirin therapy rather than Plavix. If brand-name and generic drugs are required, attempt to contact the drug manufacturer to obtain information about discounts or special programs. Home visits would be paid for by the patient. Follow-up phone calls by the unit staff or case management personnel may prove cost-effective in verifying patient compliance and answering any questions that he has. A cardiology appointment would likely be scheduled earlier than 3 months to ensure that the patient's plan of care is effective and appropriate for his needs. Although exercise is beneficial, the cost of a gym membership might be prohibitive. Instead, suggest starting a walking club with other friends or neighbors so that the patient can slowly increase his level of activity while limiting costs. The companionship will also improve the patient's psychological and social health.

14. **Correct Answer: D**

    Potassium is pulled from the intracellular space as a result of metabolic acidosis. The insulin drip will help correct the metabolic acidosis by allowing potassium to return to normal levels.

15. **Correct Answer: D**

    Assessment of the abdomen proceeds as follows: (1) inspection to determine landmarks and appearance, (2) auscultation to establish location and quality of bowel tones, (3) percussion to note whether tones are different for various internal organs, and (4) palpation to establish wall tone, tenderness, and size of organs. Performing percussion and palpation prior to inspection or auscultation could affect the assessment findings. Although you may think this is too basic a concept to test on the PCCN exam, it is the simple things that are often overlooked and cause you to miss a question on the exam.

16. **Correct Answer: C**
Feelings of helplessness or hopelessness indicate a psychotic emergency. Extreme anxiety or inability to recognize options should alert staff and family that the patient is at greater risk of suicide because suicide may be seen by the patient or individual as the only option; these signs are a warning of suicide. The other options indicate depression and/or levels of grief and emotional expression.

17. **Correct Answer: C**
Because of the high volume of urine excreted, additional complications may include hypocalcemia, dilutional hyponatremia, hyperglycemia, and hypochloremic acidosis.

18. **Correct Answer: C**
The patient is probably very anxious and hyperventilating because she is unable to get enough oxygen due to bronchial constriction. Hypoventilation causes a buildup of CO_2, leading to respiratory acidosis. This patient has not received theophylline. Albuterol may cause tachycardia, but not an acid–base imbalance.

19. **Correct Answer: D**
The exercise stress test requires the patient to walk on a treadmill or ride a stationary bike for at least 30–60 minutes. For this patient, that level of exertion would be difficult or even impossible because of his decreased mobility and pain. The best choice is to first inform the physician of the patient's stated limitations and request an alternate test. The stress echocardiography uses dobutamine to stress the cardiac tissues without requiring the patient to walk or ride. The weight-lift test does not exist.

20. **Correct Answer: B**
Three days of high FiO_2 has resulted in a nitrogen washout resulting in atelectasis. Nitrogen's high partial pressure is necessary to maintain alveoli inflation. It is important to titrate FiO_2 to maintain saturations within a prescribed range when oxygen therapy is utilized. Pulmonary edema would result in coarse breath sounds. A unilateral pneumothorax is associated with tracheal deviation. Sepsis would not necessarily present with diminished breath sounds, but rather with additional findings of increased purulent secretions, coarse breath sounds, and altered laboratory diagnostic results.

21. **Correct Answer: B**
Insulin resistance predisposes the patient to elevated blood glucose and increased insulin production. Very-low-density lipoprotein (VLDL) production increases with hyperinsulinemia.

22. **Correct Answer: A**
The oxyhemoglobin dissociation curve reflects the patient's physiological circumstances and their effect on hemoglobin's affinity for oxygen.

23. **Correct Answer: B**
Vecuronium is a paralytic and will prevent shivering. If the patient shivers, her temperature will rise.

24. **Correct Answer: C**

   Acute renal failure is now known as acute renal injury (AKI). It can be classified as pre-renal, intrinsic, or postrenal. Because material covered on the PCCN exam reflects practice up to two years ago, we thought that the new terminology should be acknowledged here. Some item writers may use this new terminology on the exam.

25. **Correct Answer: C**

   Some dyes interfere with the sensor's ability to conduct red and infrared light—namely, methylene blue, fluroscein, indocyanine green, and indigo carmine.

26. **Correct Answer: A**

   Endomyocardial biopsy is the only definitive way to diagnose myocarditis.

27. **Correct Answer: A**

   Direct confrontation with the object of anger may further exacerbate the situation and limit the person's ability to deal positively with the situation. Instead, engage the patient in a conversation regarding the stressor and assist in identifying feelings and options.

28. **Correct Answer: B**

   Severe acute respiratory syndrome (SARS) is a type of community-acquired pneumonia caused by the SARS-associated coronavirus. Incubation is usually 2–14 days, and is spread via droplets. SARS is usually acquired in underdeveloped areas. There is no cure; instead, symptoms are treated as they appear. It is incumbent on the nurse to make certain the patient is in a negative-pressure isolation room, and an N-95 respirator mask must be used.

29. **Correct Answer: D**

   This could be caused by mitral stenosis, an ischemic left ventricle, or failure of a left ventricle. The S_3 and S_4 sounds suggest both a fluid problem and a pressure problem.

30. **Correct Answer: B**

   Ipsilateral (same-side) pupil dilation is the symptom seen with uncal herniation across the tentorium. The tentorium is a fold of dura mater that supports the temporal and occipital lobes. This herniation puts pressure directly on CN III, causing pupil dilation.

31. **Correct Answer: D**

   In cases of severe carbon monoxide (CO) poisoning, hyperbaric therapy must be utilized to force the CO molecule off the hemoglobin. The CO is then eliminated by the lungs.

32. **Correct Answer: D**

   Treadmill stress testing may miss as much as 40% of single-vessel disease. LV dysfunction may be diagnosed via a thallium test (myocardial scintigraphy). A positive treadmill test may not be positive for CAD.

33. **Correct Answer: A**

   Although each of these patients can be classified as being in crisis, the 80-year-old home-bound male without family resources is at greatest risk for emergency. Because he is home-bound, it will be more challenging to get resources to him. Public assistance, friends, and seniors groups may be effective resources to ensure appropriate coping.

34. **Correct Answer: C**

   Coronary artery disease, cerebrovascular accident, and peripheral vascular disease are the three major problems associated with macrovascular disease and are often seen in

Type II diabetes mellitus. Mortality or morbidity in these patients typically relates to the macrovascular changes. Diabetes leads to early atherosclerosis and atherosclerotic heart disease. The other problems listed (retinopathy and peripheral neuropathy and diabetic nephropathy) are microvascular diseases.

35. **Correct Answer: D**

Leads V_4 and R indicate right ventricular damage. Leads V_5 and V_6 indicate apical injury. Leads V_7–V_9 are specific to the posterior wall.

36. **Correct Answer: D**

Answers A, B, and C decrease lung compliance. Other factors that decrease compliance are atelectasis, fibrotic changes, abdominal distention, pain (causes splinting), and flail chest (pain and loss of structure).

37. **Correct Answer: D**

The lab changes indicate near-complete hepatocellular necrosis. Answer D indicates a still-critical condition without diagnosing a condition. Answer A ignores the serious indicators of impending complete hepatocellular necrosis and gives rise to false hope. Answer B ignores the fact that the patient's wife has privilege to the information as next of kin. Answer C does answer the question, but fails to provide appropriate information.

38. **Correct Answer: B**

Even minute changes in the partial pressure of oxygen, pH, and the partial pressure of carbon dioxide will result in changes in the heart and respiratory rates. These changes are initiated by the chemoreceptors located in the carotid and aortic bodies.

39. **Correct Answer: A**

Alterations in chemical or electrolytes may lead to anxiety and agitation, which might potentially be misdiagnosed as a psychiatric emergency.

40. **Correct Answer: D**

Devin has the classic symptoms of Legionnaire's disease. If left untreated, this infection may lead to hypotension, acute kidney injury, shock, respiratory failure, and death.

41. **Correct Answer: C**

Answers A, B, and D are symptoms of left-sided heart failure. When the right side of the heart fails, that failure is often due to left-sided failure. The right ventricle cannot adequately pump blood out, so filling pressures rise and the blood backs up, resulting in hepatomegaly. As a consequence, the CVP pressure is elevated. Additional symptoms may include splenomegaly, ascites, abdominal pain, S_3 and S_4 heart sounds, and weight gain.

42. **Correct Answer: B**

The blood gas results show respiratory acidosis with hypoxemia.

43. **Correct Answer: D**

Symptoms of thyrotoxic crisis include hypertension, hyperthermia, flushing, tachycardia (especially atrial tachyarrhythmia), high-output heart failure, nausea and vomiting, psychosis, and delirium. Treatment includes supportive care and medications to block catecholamine effects.

44. **Correct Answer: D**

    Joe is presenting with chest wall pain, most likely as the result of his open heart surgery. Although the pain is expected, to support his recovery and achieve the best possible outcome, the nurse will need to address the patient's pain and discomfort. If the pain is left untreated, Joe may not perform deep breathing exercises or participate fully in physical therapy, thereby placing him at risk for other postoperative complications. Morphine and diazepam will treat both pain and muscle spasms. There is no indication of infection to the wound site, and the pain described by the patient is not consistent with another infarction. EKG changes would most likely be seen. The physician should be contacted if the pain and spasms do not resolve with morphine and diazepam administration or if the pain should present differently with EKG changes.

45. **Correct Answer: B**

    When using an auto-transfusion drainage system, make sure to connect the system per manufacturer's recommendations. Most connections will be color-coded for easy setup. Clamps must remain open to allow for blood collection and prevent increases in intrathoracic pressures. Subcutaneous air should be checked by palpation and borders marked for further monitoring. The average adult-size catheter is 28 or 36 Fr. If a one-way valve system and suction are used, water is not required to maintain a seal because the valve performs this function.

46. **Correct Answer: D**

    Monocytes and lymphocytes are classified as agranulocytes. Monocytes are the largest leukocytes, but they account for only a small portion of the total cell count for WBCs. When monocytes mature, they become tissue macrophages and work as phagocytes. When a phagocyte is found in the liver, it is called a Kupffer cell. When it is found in the lungs, it is called an alveolar macrophage. When it is found in the connective tissues, it is called a histiocyte.

    Macrophages contain lysosomal enzymes and chemicals that can destroy bacteria. If a macrophage is activated by an antigen, it will secrete monokines, which control communication between all the cells involved in an immune response.

47. **Correct Answer: C**

    Anger, fear, and denial are normal emotions in this situation. Nevertheless, for those staff members who feel anxiety, they are at greater risk. Anxiety is an emotion commonly encountered in psychological emergencies. It reflects uncertainty of the unknown and may limit the person's ability to identify resources or initiate appropriate coping mechanisms. Debriefings after codes, successful and unsuccessful, are therapeutic and allow staff to verbalize their emotions in a safe and stable environment. As a team, the staff may identify ways to support families and one another during crisis and emergency situations.

48. **Correct Answer: B**

    Usually, central cyanosis is seen when the level of deoxygenated Hgb reaches 5 g/dL. The cyanosis can be seen on the lips and possibly on the mucous membranes. It can be an early sign of hypoxemia in patients with polycythemia. These patients will be cyanotic when 5 g/dL is desaturated. Sometimes these patients are called "blue bloaters." In anemic patients, central cyanosis is a late sign and they will not necessarily be cyanotic.

49. **Correct Answer: B**

    The PQRST pain assessment method is used to collect assessment data regarding chest pain in a logical manner that ensures complete assessment data is gathered.
    - P stands for *provokes*. Does any activity specifically provoke the pain?
    - Q represents the *quality* of the pain. Typical adjectives used include sharp, stabbing, squeezing, pressure, tightness, dull, indigestion-like, and pulsating.
    - R is *radiation,* the starting location to the ending location of the pain. For example, pain may radiate from the chest to the jaw, a specific arm, the back, and/or the abdomen.
    - S is for *severity* of the pain. Some patients may have altered pain sensation from other disease processes such as diabetes, neuropathies, and multiple sclerosis; as a consequence, they may not present with typical symptoms for a myocardial infarction.
    - T stands for *time.* Time is important when considering use of antithrombolytics as treatment, as these medications are highly time sensitive and any delay in administering them will affect the effectiveness of the treatment.

50. **Correct Answer: C**

    Wernicke's syndrome is a result of thiamine deficiency. It will result in brain damage if not treated immediately.

51. **Correct Answer: D**

    Amiodarone and quinidine are antiarrhythmics. Clonidine is an antihypertensive. Adenosine is a naturally occurring substance in the body and has a very short half-life (only a few seconds). Adenosine slows AV nodal conduction or can interrupt it altogether, potentially causing a transient AV block (seen as asystole). The patient may experience mild to moderate chest discomfort, slight hypotension, bradycardia, and possibly flushing.

52. **Correct Answer: C**

    Answers A, B, and D are causes of non-oliguria (> 400 mL/d of urine output). Hepatorenal syndrome is another cause of oliguria.

53. **Correct Answer: D**

    Mesothelioma is a cancer of the mesothelium. Most cases begin in the pleura or peritoneum. Mesothelioma is relatively rare, with only 2,000 new cases of mesothelioma being diagnosed in the United States each year. It occurs more often in men than in women, and the risk of developing this disease increases with age. Symptoms of mesothelioma may not appear until 30–50 years after exposure to asbestos. An increased risk of developing mesothelioma later in life has been found among shipyard workers, people who work in asbestos mines and mills, producers of asbestos products, workers in the heating and construction industries, and other trades people. Symptoms include dyspnea, pleural effusions, weight loss, and abdominal pain and swelling due to an excess of fluid in the abdomen. Other symptoms of peritoneal mesothelioma may include bowel obstruction, clotting disorders, anemia, and fever. Symptoms with metastases may include pain, dysphagia, or swelling of the neck or face.

    Asbestos has been widely used in many industrial products, including cement, duct linings, sound insulation, brake linings, roof shingles, flooring products, textiles, and thermal insulation. If tiny asbestos particles float in the air, especially during the manufacturing process, they may be inhaled or swallowed, and can cause serious health problems. In addition to mesothelioma, exposure to asbestos increases the risk of lung cancer, asbestosis, and cancers of the trachea, larynx, and kidney. Smoking does not appear to increase the risk of mesothelioma, but the combination of smoking and exposure increases a person's risk of developing bronchial cancer.

While we were researching this topic, we discovered a sobering piece of information: More than 110,000 schools in the U.S. still contain some form of asbestos.

54. **Correct Answer: A**

Rapid and pressured speech is a sign of tension and indicates that the patient still needs support and assistance in coping with his diagnosis. Humor and social activities can be positive coping techniques as long as they are not used to avoid the stressful situation. The patient will need assistance and education regarding his diagnosis to effectively identify positive lifestyle changes.

55. **Correct Answer: B**

A heart murmur is a sound produced from turbulent blood flow. By definition, a systolic murmur is heard during systole when the ventricles are contracting. The mitral and tricuspid valves should be closed. If these valves are incompetent (insufficiency), blood will flow back through the valve (regurgitation). Thus, pulmonic and aortic stenosis, as well as mitral and tricuspid insufficiency, are all systolic murmurs.

56. **Correct Answer: A**

Early surgery (within 7 days of signs and symptoms of onset) is usually associated with a shorter hospital stay. It is more appropriate for the nurse to refer treatment options to the physician. Delay in surgery may lead to increased severity of symptoms, although it does not change the mortality or complication rate. Only 25% of delayed surgeries become urgent. Laparoscopic surgeries are associated with shorter hospital stays compared to open surgeries, but there is an increased risk of bile duct injuries and 25% of surgeries may require open surgical interventions due to complications. The nurse should not mention bile duct injury in this case, because the patient has yet to be diagnosed.

57. **Correct Answer: C**

Hepatitis B vaccine is given in three doses. The initial dose is given, followed by the second dose at 1–2 months, and finally the third dose at 4–6 months. Blood titers can be drawn to determine an individual's level of protection and need for a booster shot.

58. **Correct Answer: B**

Pericarditis results in inflamed layers of the pericardial sac. Deep respirations, trunk rotation, and flat positioning allow the parietal and visceral layers of the pericardial sac to rub against each other. Upright and forward positioning pulls the heart away from the diaphragmatic pleura of the lungs and eases the cardiac pain.

59. **Correct Answer: C**

Cerebrospinal fluid (CSF) should be clear, colorless, with a protein count of 16–45 mg/dL. The WBC count should be 0–5 cells/mm^2, with the glucose level in CSF being approximately 80% of serum glucose.

60. **Correct Answer: C**

Because of a defect in chromosome 7, patients with cystic fibrosis lose sodium through their skin and mucous membranes. This results in a thickening of the mucous layers, leading to infection and hyponatremia.

61. **Correct Answer: C**

Systemic lupus erythematosus (SLE) is a chronic inflammatory autoimmune disease that affects the vascular and connective tissues within any body system and organ. As a result of the disease, inflammation may be increased, and the stress of injury further exacerbates the SLE. Symptoms and conditions to monitor closely for include pericarditis, hypertension, diarrhea, thrombocytopenia, anemia, leucopenia, joint and muscle pain, vasculitis, proteinurea, seizures, depression, pneumonia, pleural effusions, nausea, and ulcers.

62. **Correct Answer: C**

Restraints should be used only if alternative methods for behavioral correction are ineffective. There is no indication that this patient is violent or has threatened either staff or self. Restraints should be used only as a last resort to prevent injury to self and staff. Reorientation, medication, and controlling external stimulation are all effective methods for controlling behavior.

63. **Correct Answer: C**

Normal hematocrit levels for adult females are in the range of 37–47%.

64. **Correct Answer: B**

Answers A, C, and D decrease the INR only moderately. Other drugs that significantly decrease the INR include rifampin, phenobarbital, and glutethimide. Vitamin K is widely used as an antidote for warfarin, but it can actually decrease the INR too far and increase warfarin resistance, so careful monitoring is required if INR is critical. Warfarin breakdown is also accelerated by barbiturates.

65. **Correct Answer: D**

These findings describe uncompensated respiratory alkalosis. The pH is greater than 7.45, so the patient has uncompensated alkalosis. To determine whether the alkalosis is respiratory or metabolic, find the value that represents alkalosis:$CO_2 < 35$ mm Hg.

66. **Correct Answer: C**

The goal when working with bulimic and anorexic patients is to support positive nutritional changes while acknowledging and supporting the psychological changes in body and food perception. By acknowledging the difficulties the patient has with food perception and being willing to provide support and counseling with a nutritionist, dietician, and psychologist, the nurse encourages the patient to find foods that are both appealing and provide needed nutrition. The remaining answers are abrasive or do not address the patient's physiological or psychological struggle with eating.

67. **Correct Answer: D**

The MI has impaired the heart's ability to pump effectively. The cardiac output falls and the body reacts by vasoconstricting peripheral circulation and increasing the heart rate. Tachycardia is another result of catecholamine release. The myocardial oxygen consumption is also increased. The left ventricle works harder, but has been compromised by the MI. Preload increases because fluid cannot be pumped out of the heart chambers effectively. The S_3 heart sound is a signal of increased preload. Pulmonary congestion occurs due to increased left heart pressures.

68. **Correct Answer: A**

    Approximately 2% of potassium is extracellular, while the remaining 98% is intracellular. Intracellular electrolytes cannot be directly measured, but extracellular levels can be measured. The normal value for extracellular potassium is in the range of 3.5–5.0 mEq/L.

69. **Correct Answer: A**

    Physical needs must come before psychological needs in a disaster or crisis. According to Maslow's hierarchy of needs, the physical needs must be met first before lower-level needs can be considered. Once the physical needs have been met, then one can focus on locating family, providing social services, and disseminating information to the media.

70. **Correct Answer: C**

    New evidence indicates that an ejection fraction of 35% or less may predispose an individual to sudden cardiac death. A low ejection fraction and existing CAD mean the likelihood of a cardiac event is increased. Generally, if an individual has disease in the left main artery, any three vessels, or the proximal LAD with one additional vessel, he or she is a candidate for a CABG. Emergent conditions necessitating a CABG include MI with shock or refractory pain or unstable angina. Patients who dissect during a stent placement require immediate surgery.

71. **Correct Answer: A**

    Hepatitis A is often misdiagnosed initially as gastroenteritis because its symptoms are usually self-limiting. Infection spread by the fecal–oral route may also be mistaken as food poisoning.

72. **Correct Answer: D**

    The patient may feel as if he has failed the nurse by not remaining sober and that assistance may be withdrawn. The statement in answer D does not judge the patient, but rather shows him the help is still available by initiating communication and encouraging the patient to talk about his struggles with maintaining sobriety. Answer A is judgmental and demeaning. Answer B limits support and indicates to the patient that he is unable to succeed. Answer C focuses on the nurse's feelings, and not those of the patient.

73. **Correct Answer: A**

    TIAs typically last a very short time, sometimes less than an hour, but no longer than 24 hours and there are no neurologic deficits. With a RIND, the symptoms last more than 24 hours but the patient still has a complete recovery. Both types of events are possible precursors of a major stroke within a year.

74. **Correct Answer: D**

    Nitroglycerin is a vasodilator for both arterial and venous systems. Sometimes the diseased coronary vessels are stiff and calcified. If the patient has good collateral circulation, oxygen and blood can reach the ischemic areas. Nitroglycerin is now available in a metered-dose oral spray, as well as in pressed tablets, paste, and intravenous (nitroprusside) formulations.

75. **Correct Answer: C**
Potassium and hydrogen move in opposition to each other. With hypokalemia, hydrogen moves into the extracellular fluid, leading to both respiratory and metabolic alkalosis.

76. **Correct Answer: B**
Prevention of aspiration should be the nurse's priority. The other answers are also a part of caring for a patient who has experienced a cerebrovascular accident—but the ABCs (airway, breathing, circulation) are always the first priority.

77. **Correct Answer: D**
Sometimes, families do not have enough education to make proper decisions. In this case, the family needs to know that the patient is still quite capable of making decisions and that his wishes will be honored.

78. **Correct Answer: B**
An infarct in the left main coronary artery is ominous. Sudden death may occur, as may heart blocks and atrial and ventricular dysrhythmias.

79. **Correct Answer: C**
These findings describe compensated respiratory alkalosis. The pH is between 7.35 and 7.45, so the value is compensated; because it is closer to 7.45, the value is considered alkalotic. To determine whether the alkalosis is respiratory or metabolic, find the value that represents alkalosis: $CO_2 < 35$ mm Hg.

80. **Correct Answer: C**
Pulsus paradoxus may be present in people with asthma, emphysema, cardiac tamponade, restrictive pericarditis, or hemorrhagic shock. Pulse pressure is the difference between systolic and diastolic blood pressure. Pulsus parvus means a small or weak pulse. Pulsus alternans means the upstroke is more powerful than the downstroke— that is, the stroke alternates in strength.

81. **Correct Answer: A**
The Whipple procedure removes the tip or head of the pancreas, the gallbladder, the duodenum, and part of the bile duct. Occasionally, part of the stomach may also be removed. The extent of the cancerous pancreatic tumor will dictate the extent of removal.

82. **Correct Answer: A**
Patients with Guillain-Barré syndrome experience motor weakness, impaired respiratory function, and acute pain; these are the most important nursing diagnoses. The pain is due to accentuated sympathetic response secondary to loss of parasympathetic counterbalance.

83. **Correct Answer: D**
The religious preference of the patient must be respected. The only acceptable form of transfusion in this case is auto-transfusion.

84. **Correct Answer: C**
This response acknowledges the patient's situation without allowing him to manipulate the nurse and indicates that the nurse takes his warning of suicidal talk seriously. This patient should be placed on suicide precautions and moved to a room where he is under direct supervision at all times. The doctor and psychological services should also

be notified immediately. The patient will need continued physical and psychological support during his recovery. Careful monitoring for depression and suicidal thoughts and attempts should be initiated. At this point, the patient is unable to see options or acknowledge positive facts of being alive. Visitors may be seen as pitying and not supportive by the patient. Medication may be necessary, but not until the situation has been fully assessed.

85. **Correct Answer: C**
Some people may take in 800–11,000 mg of potassium per day through their diet.

86. **Correct Answer: D**
Reglan increases gastric emptying by increasing peristalsis, thereby exacerbating the effects of dumping syndrome. Reglan may be used post gastrectomy when gastroparesis is present, but once peristalsis has resumed it should be stopped.

87. **Correct Answer: B**
Even if this patient signed a consent form, she is not certain about the procedure or is not fully informed. The nurse must act as her advocate and notify the physician.

88. **Correct Answer: C**
The antagonist for morphine or other opioids is Narcan (naloxone). Generally, the naloxone dose is 0.4 mg IV. This dose can be repeated about every three to four minutes for a total of three times. When you give Narcan, you must always be alert for the patient to relapse once the dose wears off. Administering multiple follow-up doses is not uncommon.

89. **Correct Answer: B**
Respiratory status and neurologic signs are the most important nursing management issues, especially during the early onset of the demyelinating process.

90. **Correct Answer: D**
If the patient is bleeding, the blood may settle into the lumbar area. Blood is heavy and will flow into the retroperitoneal area because of gravity. More than an hour may pass and the patient may lose several hundred milliliters of blood before his vital signs are affected.

91. **Correct Answer: C**
The laryngeal mask airway (LMA) is intended for use as a temporary airway. It requires minimal training to insert, but it cannot be placed by RNs as a matter of course. The patient must be unconscious and/or lack a gag reflex. The mask is secured by a low-pressure seal, so it cannot be used on patients with high peak ventilator pressures. The LMA carries a significant risk of aspiration; it is also associated with laryngospasm. Advantages when using this airway are that it is blindly inserted into the hypopharynx, does not require visualization of the vocal cords, and does not traumatize the trachea. Patients will not have hoarseness or lose their voice altogether. At best, patients will complain of a mild sore throat.

92. **Correct Answer: B**
The abdominal area is most commonly affected by aortic aneurysms and usually offers good surgical access. Aneurysms in the aortic arch are sometimes not accessible surgically and may pose a high risk during procedures.

93. **Correct Answer: A**

Safety is your highest priority. By removing the daughter from the unit, her behavior and anger can be managed more safely. It is important to address the daughter directly, acknowledge her anger, and avoid trapping her physically in any corner. Use quiet and even tones that will not escalate her emotions. Ignoring the behavior and making jokes will further anger the daughter and may lead to physical acts of violence. Calling the police may elevate the situation if she has not directly made or acted on threats. If security is unable to assist in diffusing the situation, then hospital personnel may need to call the police.

94. **Correct Answer: A**

Due to the patient's pregnancy and resulting HELLP syndrome, she is at increased risk for fluid accumulation in the abdominal cavity and for tissue edema. Signs and symptoms of IAH and ACS include increased ICP, hypercarbia, decreased platelet values, decreased cardiac output, poor or absent urinary output, and abdominal wall rigidity. We deliberately made this mother quite young. This information serves as a distracter of sorts. You probably found yourself thinking, "How can this mother be so young and already have all these kids and be pregnant again?" This line of thought keeps you from focusing on the point of the question, which is HELLP syndrome.

95. **Correct Answer: C**

Sometimes, the bed is emergently needed. In the best possible world, the military could arrange for compassionate leave for the military service member. Nurses certainly should not go ahead and try to procure organs as soon as the family leaves.

96. **Correct Answer: C**

The best option for pheochromocytoma is surgical removal of the tumor. Alpha-adrenergic blockers or beta-adrenergic blockers may be used to treat hypertension until surgery—the definitive treatment—can be performed.

97. **Correct Answer: C**

The P wave represents depolarization of the atrium and the QRS wave represents depolarization of the ventricles; the size difference is related to the muscle mass involved in the polarization. The P wave amplitude indicates the amount or size of the muscle mass involved in the depolarization of the atrium. The QRS wave indicates the amount or size of the muscle mass involved in the depolarization of the ventricles. The greater the muscle mass, the greater the change in amplitude. Nonpatient factors that affect amplitude may be related to gain setting, lead placement, and interference. Patient-related factors that affect readings include electrolyte imbalances, hypertrophy, and cardiac injury.

98. **Correct Answer: C**

Flail chest is a very painful condition that limits respiratory effort because of the pain or analgesia and sedation required to mitigate the pain. CO_2 will increase, PaO_2 will decrease, and the pH will fall below 7.35. The patient will develop respiratory acidosis.

99. **Correct Answer: A**

Addison's disease results in a decrease in aldosterone secretion. This change in hormonal production leads to hyperkalemia and hyponatremia because sodium cannot be retained and potassium cannot be removed.

100. **Correct Answer: B**

Patients with heart transplants do not feel cardiac pain because the heart has been denervated.

101. **Correct Answer: C**

The goal at this point is to regulate the patient's breathing and stabilize her vital signs. Using a firm and quiet voice with simple sentences can help the severely anxious patient focus and diffuse the anxiety. Severely anxious individuals are less able to see options and cope at this stage. Goals should include decreasing any unnecessary stress and remaining available to the patient for communication. The other answers speak to facts not in the nurse's knowledge and may increase the patient's fear or lead to false hope.

102. **Correct Answer: A**

Pain is a cardinal sign of an arterial obstruction. The nurse should check for pallor, another sign of an arterial blockage, sensation, and quality of pulses. If the obstruction is venous, the limb may exhibit cyanosis.

103. **Correct Answer: D**

Dairy products may actually increase both bronchospasm and phlegm. Fluid intake should be increased to approximately 3 L per day. Serevent is a long-lasting inhaler and can take up to an hour to work.

104. **Correct Answer: C**

Family members are probably quite used to providing care for this patient. Do not ignore the patient, and there is no point in speaking slowly unless the caregiver or the patient has difficulty understanding instructions. Teaching quickly is counterproductive and may be considered both rude and unprofessional. Allow time for a return demonstration of skills and encourage questions to ensure full understanding.

105. **Correct Answer: A**

The timing of the patient's symptoms is consistent with alcohol withdrawal or delirium tremens (DTs). DTs are usually seen 12–24 hours after the individual's last ingestion of alcohol, appearing as blood alcohol levels drop. Effects may peak as long as 15 days after DTs begin. Fluids, vitamins, nutrition, and short-term pharmacological treatments are appropriate therapies. The severity of the patient's symptoms will be affected by the amount and duration of alcohol ingestion as well as his underlying physical health, combination of other drugs used, and existing psychological status. There are no indications at this time that the patient is septic or has schizophrenia. He may have underlying drug withdrawal symptoms, but patient history does not provide any indication of this possibility.

106. **Correct Answer: D**

Albuterol administration would decrease lung resistance; resistance means how easy it is to move gases through airways. Albuterol is a bronchodilator that increases the size of the lumen making it easier for ventilation through the bronchi. Conditions that decrease the size of the bronchi lumens increase resistance.

107. **Correct Answer: B**

Monitoring neurologic signs, urinary output, and moustache dressing changes are the most important postoperative care for a patient who has undergone a transsphenoidal resection of a pituitary tumor. Daily weights are important, as are vital signs. Patients undergoing this surgery are also at risk for diabetes insipidus due to a lack of ADH.

108. **Correct Answer: B**

These waves actually heat the tissue around the active sites and prevent the reentry loop from occurring. Once the temperature reaches 50°C, cell damage and death occur. The continuing heat creates a lesion approximately 2–5 mm in diameter. This "burned" area causes necrosis and will not conduct electricity.

109. **Correct Answer: C**

Answer C is the best nursing response, as it allows all members of the healthcare team to join in the decision-making process. Visiting policies vary, but are primarily designed to protect children from disease and from being overwhelmed by equipment and the PCU milieu. Under the circumstances, you would probably want to sneak the kid in on night shift, but many factors should be weighed here. This visit could produce the child's last memory of his mother. The conference will weigh the child's maturity and coping ability. He and the father will probably lose the mother and the sibling. There is no simple answer.

110. **Correct Answer: A**

The correct order for these interventions when assisting with a paracentesis is (1) have the patient void or insert a Foley catheter, (2) order an upright X-ray of the abdomen, (3) position the patient with the affected side up, and (4) examine the abdomen for dullness.

111. **Correct Answer: D**

Headaches may be caused by multiple factors, but are not a cardinal sign of respiratory failure. Patients will exhibit tachypnea, diaphoresis, and restlessness as the body attempts to compensate for the respiratory distress and then exhibit signs of oxygen deprivation and starvation.

112. **Correct Answer: C**

Renal failure and sepsis may lead to pericarditis, so A.M. labs should show an increased WBC, increased ESR, cardiac tissue involvement, and elevated CK-MB. An additional lab would possibly indicate uremia. Assessment findings would also include elevated ST segments, arrhythmias, and pleural effusions on echocardiography.

113. **Correct Answer: A**

Magnesium usually acts synergistically with calcium to control neuromuscular function within all muscle groups.

114. **Correct Answer: A**

The circumflex artery feeds the left atrium and left ventricle. Infarctions as a result of occlusion of this artery result in lateral or left-sided heart damage. The left anterior descending artery and the circumflex artery both branch off from the left coronary artery.

115. **Correct Answer: D**

CBC, CMP, sedimentation rate, CRP, RPR, and toxicology screen are the tests that need to be performed to establish the cause of John Doe's seizures. Seizures can be caused by illness, infection, overdose on drugs or alcohol, tertiary syphilis, dehydration, electrolyte imbalances, and cardiac arrhythmia.

116. **Correct Answer: D**
Surveys can be used to anonymously identify staff perceptions and determine educational opportunities. Mental health issues will likely affect every person at some point in his or her life. Whether due to a catastrophic event or ongoing psychological issues, it is important that nurses understand their own biases regarding mental health and be able to identify resources when caring for this population. If nurses believe the survey will be used punitively, then data may be skewed to what the staff believe the surveyor is looking for, not the truth. Instead of changing assignments immediately, it is best to use the opportunity for education and professional growth.

117. **Correct Answer: D**
Stress-related erosive syndrome (SRES) was once cited as an explanation for gastric complications related to critical care illnesses. The stress response within the patient may lead to rapid erosion of the mucosal lining, resulting in ulcerations. Patients suffering from severe physiological illnesses are at high risk of SRES; if it is left untreated, they may experience gastric bleeding.

118. **Correct Answer: B**
Double effect is a commonly encountered ethical dilemma. Here an action is justified as long as there is no intent to do further harm. Neither the physician nor the wife wants to hasten the patient's death, but they do want to make him more comfortable. It is the intent underlying the use of the narcotic, rather than the use itself, that defines the double effect. At least some good is done through the outcome of the discussion and resolution of the dilemma.

119. **Correct Answer: A**
Gina has endocarditis. Janeway lesions are flat and painless erythematous areas on the palms and soles of the feet predominately. Osler's nodes are small painful nodules that are also associated with endocarditis; they are found on the fingers and toes. Roth spots are seen when examining the retina. These rounded, white lesions are associated with endocarditis as well. Pella's sign is not a medical term. With endocarditis, it is thought that microvascular clots form in the heart, pass through the microcirculation, and impede peripheral circulation, sometimes causing necrosis.

120. **Correct Answer: C**
During ventricular diastole, both the aortic and pulmonic valves close. If a valve is incompetent, the blood will flow backward through the valve, causing turbulent blood flow. The result is a murmur.

121. **Correct Answer: A**
Honey contains the smallest amount of magnesium. It is better to recommend foods such as leafy vegetables with a deep green color, whole grains, nuts, legumes, seafood, cocoa, and chocolate.

122. **Correct Answer: B**
Venturi mask systems allow for high-flow oxygen to be delivered at predetermined concentrations through the use of specific adapters. This method is advantageous for patients who need greater flow or inspiratory pressure without the high oxygen concentration.

123. **Correct Answer: B**

     A psychological crisis may precede an emergency, but not always. Although there is no specific definition for either term, accepted criteria are as follows: A crisis is a less immediate situation that has developed over time in the presence of a psychological situation. Coping mechanisms may be partially effective in a crisis, but do not address the situation directly so as to lead to a conclusion of the problem. A crisis may develop into an emergency if coping mechanisms fail or additional stressors appear. A psychological emergency has multiple elements. In particular, it incorporates a sense of urgency that if the situation is not resolved, that anxiety may be intolerable and may lead to feelings of being overwhelmed. In this case, coping skills have completely failed and patient recognizes the need for help to alleviate the stressors. Suicide calls, notes, and messages meet these criteria.

124. **Correct Answer: C**

     Any metal within the patient will be attracted to the MRI magnet, causing internal damage as the metal moves within the tissues. Metal heart valves, bullets, shrapnel, pacemakers, surgical clips, ear implants, metal rods and clips, metal plates, and BB shot all pose a risk. Metal dental fillings are not prone to magnetic pull and are safe.

125. **Correct Answer: A**

     Matthew has probably dislodged a lead, or the lead may have been damaged on insertion. Either way, Matthew needs a new AICD or new leads.

PCCN PRACTICE EXAM 2 ANSWER SHEET

Use this sheet to test yourself with the Practice Exam.

1. A B C D	26. A B C D	51. A B C D
2. A B C D	27. A B C D	52. A B C D
3. A B C D	28. A B C D	53. A B C D
4. A B C D	29. A B C D	54. A B C D
5. A B C D	30. A B C D	55. A B C D
6. A B C D	31. A B C D	56. A B C D
7. A B C D	32. A B C D	57. A B C D
8. A B C D	33. A B C D	58. A B C D
9. A B C D	34. A B C D	59. A B C D
10. A B C D	35. A B C D	60. A B C D
11. A B C D	36. A B C D	61. A B C D
12. A B C D	37. A B C D	62. A B C D
13. A B C D	38. A B C D	63. A B C D
14. A B C D	39. A B C D	64. A B C D
15. A B C D	40. A B C D	65. A B C D
16. A B C D	41. A B C D	66. A B C D
17. A B C D	42. A B C D	67. A B C D
18. A B C D	43. A B C D	68. A B C D
19. A B C D	44. A B C D	69. A B C D
20. A B C D	45. A B C D	70. A B C D
21. A B C D	46. A B C D	71. A B C D
22. A B C D	47. A B C D	72. A B C D
23. A B C D	48. A B C D	73. A B C D
24. A B C D	49. A B C D	74. A B C D
25. A B C D	50. A B C D	75. A B C D

(Over for questions 76–150)

76. A B C D	101. A B C D	126. A B C D
77. A B C D	102. A B C D	127. A B C D
78. A B C D	103. A B C D	128. A B C D
79. A B C D	104. A B C D	129. A B C D
80. A B C D	105. A B C D	130. A B C D
81. A B C D	106. A B C D	131. A B C D
82. A B C D	107. A B C D	132. A B C D
83. A B C D	108. A B C D	133. A B C D
84. A B C D	109. A B C D	134. A B C D
85. A B C D	110. A B C D	135. A B C D
86. A B C D	111. A B C D	136. A B C D
87. A B C D	112. A B C D	137. A B C D
88. A B C D	113. A B C D	138. A B C D
89. A B C D	114. A B C D	139. A B C D
90. A B C D	115. A B C D	140. A B C D
91. A B C D	116. A B C D	141. A B C D
92. A B C D	117. A B C D	142. A B C D
93. A B C D	118. A B C D	143. A B C D
94. A B C D	119. A B C D	144. A B C D
95. A B C D	120. A B C D	145. A B C D
96. A B C D	121. A B C D	146. A B C D
97. A B C D	122. A B C D	147. A B C D
98. A B C D	123. A B C D	148. A B C D
99. A B C D	124. A B C D	149. A B C D
100. A B C D	125. A B C D	150. A B C D

PCCN PRACTICE EXAM 2 ANSWER SHEET

Use this sheet to test yourself with the Practice Exam.

1. A B C D	26. A B C D	51. A B C D
2. A B C D	27. A B C D	52. A B C D
3. A B C D	28. A B C D	53. A B C D
4. A B C D	29. A B C D	54. A B C D
5. A B C D	30. A B C D	55. A B C D
6. A B C D	31. A B C D	56. A B C D
7. A B C D	32. A B C D	57. A B C D
8. A B C D	33. A B C D	58. A B C D
9. A B C D	34. A B C D	59. A B C D
10. A B C D	35. A B C D	60. A B C D
11. A B C D	36. A B C D	61. A B C D
12. A B C D	37. A B C D	62. A B C D
13. A B C D	38. A B C D	63. A B C D
14. A B C D	39. A B C D	64. A B C D
15. A B C D	40. A B C D	65. A B C D
16. A B C D	41. A B C D	66. A B C D
17. A B C D	42. A B C D	67. A B C D
18. A B C D	43. A B C D	68. A B C D
19. A B C D	44. A B C D	69. A B C D
20. A B C D	45. A B C D	70. A B C D
21. A B C D	46. A B C D	71. A B C D
22. A B C D	47. A B C D	72. A B C D
23. A B C D	48. A B C D	73. A B C D
24. A B C D	49. A B C D	74. A B C D
25. A B C D	50. A B C D	75. A B C D

(Over for questions 76–150)

76.	A B C D	101.	A B C D	126.	A B C D
77.	A B C D	102.	A B C D	127.	A B C D
78.	A B C D	103.	A B C D	128.	A B C D
79.	A B C D	104.	A B C D	129.	A B C D
80.	A B C D	105.	A B C D	130.	A B C D
81.	A B C D	106.	A B C D	131.	A B C D
82.	A B C D	107.	A B C D	132.	A B C D
83.	A B C D	108.	A B C D	133.	A B C D
84.	A B C D	109.	A B C D	134.	A B C D
85.	A B C D	110.	A B C D	135.	A B C D
86.	A B C D	111.	A B C D	136.	A B C D
87.	A B C D	112.	A B C D	137.	A B C D
88.	A B C D	113.	A B C D	138.	A B C D
89.	A B C D	114.	A B C D	139.	A B C D
90.	A B C D	115.	A B C D	140.	A B C D
91.	A B C D	116.	A B C D	141.	A B C D
92.	A B C D	117.	A B C D	142.	A B C D
93.	A B C D	118.	A B C D	143.	A B C D
94.	A B C D	119.	A B C D	144.	A B C D
95.	A B C D	120.	A B C D	145.	A B C D
96.	A B C D	121.	A B C D	146.	A B C D
97.	A B C D	122.	A B C D	147.	A B C D
98.	A B C D	123.	A B C D	148.	A B C D
99.	A B C D	124.	A B C D	149.	A B C D
100.	A B C D	125.	A B C D	150.	A B C D